Plasticity and Recovery of Function in the Central Nervous System

ACADEMIC PRESS RAPID MANUSCRIPT REPRODUCTION

Proceedings of a Conference
held at Clark University, Worcester, Massachusetts
September 24–September 26, 1973

Plasticity and Recovery of Function in the Central Nervous System

Edited by

Donald G. Stein

Department of Psychology
Clark University
Worcester, Massachusetts

Jeffrey J. Rosen

Department of Psychology
Boston University
Boston, Massachusetts

Nelson Butters

Veterans Administration Hospital
Boston, Massachusetts

Academic Press, Inc.   New York   San Francisco   London   1974

A Subsidiary of Harcourt Brace Jovanovich, Publishers

ACADEMIC PRESS, INC.
111 Fifth Avenue, New York, New York 10003

United Kingdom Edition published by
ACADEMIC PRESS, INC. (LONDON) LTD.
24/28 Oval Road, London NW1

Library of Congress Cataloging in Publication Data
Main entry under title:

Plasticity and recovery of function in the central
    nervous system.

    Bibliography: p.
    1.   Central nervous system–Diseases–Congresses.
2.   Neurophysiology–Congresses.   I.   Stein, Donald G.,
ed.   II.   Rosen, Jeffrey J., ed.   III.   Butters, Nelson,
ed.   [DNLM: 1.   Behavior–Congresses.   2.   Brain
diseases–Physiopathology–Congresses.   3.   Central
nervous system diseases–Physiopathology–Congresses.
WL300 P698 1973]
RC361.P56   616.8   74-18449
ISBN 0–12–664350–4

CONTENTS

Participants   vii
Preface   ix
Acknowledgments   xi

Recovery of Function and Localization of Function in Historical
    Perspective
    Burton S. Rosner   1

Neuronal Plasticity: Concepts in Pursuit of Cellular Mechanisms
    Marcus Jacobson   31

Explanatory Models for Neuroplasticity in Retinotectal Connections
    R. L. Meyer and R. W. Sperry   45

Neuroanatomical Correlates of Spared or Altered Function After Brain
    Lesions in the Newborn Hamster
    Gerald E. Schneider and Sonal R. Jhaveri   65

Central Regeneration and Recovery of Function: The Problem of
    Collateral Reinnervation
    Robert Y. Moore   111

The Effects of Interference with the Maturation of the Cerebellum and
    Hippocampus on the Development of Adult Behavior
    Robert L. Brunner and Joseph Altman   129

An Alternative to Developmental Plasticity: Heterology of CNS
    Structures in Infants and Adults
    Patricia S. Goldman   149

Differential Changes in the Acquisition of Developmental Skills in
    Children Who Later Become Dyslexic. A Three Year Follow Up
    Paul Satz, Janette Friel, and Fran Rudegeair   175

Determinants of Cerebral Recovery
    M. S. Gazzaniga   203

Recovery of Function Following Lesions of the Subcortex and
    Neocortex
    Patricia Morgan Meyer   217

CONTENTS

Recovery after Somatosensory Forebrain Damage
Stanley Finger   237

Recovery of Movement after CNS Lesions in Monkeys
Michael E. Goldberger   265

Changes in Drug Sensitivity and Mechanisms of Functional Recovery
following Brain Damage
Stanley D. Glick   339

Some Variables Influencing Recovery of Function after Central Nervous
System Lesions in the Rat
Donald G. Stein   373

Recovery of Behavioral Functions after Sequential Ablation of the
Frontal Lobes of Monkeys
Nelson Butters, Jeffrey Rosen, and Donald Stein   429

Late Changes in the Nervous System: An Overview
Norman Geschwind   467

Subject Index   509

PARTICIPANTS

Dr. Joseph Altman, Department of Biological Sciences, Purdue University, Lafayette, Indiana 47907

Dr. Nelson Butters, Boston V. A. Hospital, 150 South Huntington Avenue, Boston, Massachusetts

Dr. Stanley Finger, Department of Psychology, Washington University, St. Louis, Missouri 63130

Dr. Michael S. Gazzaniga, Department of Psychology, State University of New York at Stony Brook, Stony Brook, New York 11790

Dr. Norman Geschwind, Neurological Unit, Boston City Hospital, Boston, Massachusetts

Dr. Stanley D. Glick, Herbert M. Singer Laboratory of Neurosciences, Beth Israel Medical Center, 307 Second Ave. New York, New York 10003

Dr. Michael Goldberger, Medical College of Pennsylvania, Philadelphia, Pennsylvania

Dr. Patricia S. Goldman, Section on Neuropsychology, Laboratory of Psychology, NIMH, 9000 Rockville Pike, Bethesda, Maryland 20014

Dr. Marcus Jacobson, Department of Physiology and Biophysics, School of Medicine, University of Miami, P. O. Box 875, Biscayne Annex. Miami, Florida 33152

Dr. Patricia M. Meyer, Laboratory Area 6, Ohio State University, 1314 Kinnear Rd., Colombus, Ohio 43212

Dr. Ronald Meyer, Division of Biology, California Institute of Technology, Pasadena, California 91109

Dr. Robert Y. Moore, Box 228, The University of Chicago Clinic, 950 E. 59th Street, Chicago, Illinois 60637

LIST OF PARTICIPANTS

Dr. Jeffrey J. Rosen, Department of Psychology, Boston University, Boston, Massachusetts

Dr. Burton S. Rosner, Department of Psychology, University of Pennsylvania, 3813-15 Walnut Street, Philadelphia, Pennsylvania 19104

Dr. Paul Satz, Director, Neuropsychology Laboratory, University of Florida Gainesville, Florida 32601

Dr. Gerald E. Schneider, Department of Psychology, Massachusetts Institute of Technology, Cambridge, Massachusetts

Dr. Donald G. Stein, Department of Psychology, Clark University, 950 Main Street, Worcester, Massachusetts 01610

PREFACE

One of the most exciting problems in the neurosciences is the question of morphological plasticity in the Central Nervous System and its relationship to functional recovery after brain damage. For the most part however, neurophysiologists and neuroanatomists have preferred to concentrate their efforts on histological or cellular studies of reorganization and they have not been particularly concerned with the functional, or behavioral aspects of neural sprouting or regeneration. Likewise, their colleagues in the behavioral sciences have not been particularly concerned with the physiological substrates that play a role in mediating recovery of function after CNS damage, although there are encouraging signs that this gap between the two domains is beginning to narrow.

This book is an attempt to narrow the gap even further by bringing together the ideas and original research of a group of neuroscientists representing a variety of interests within this broad field. All of the investigators shared a common interest in the problem of CNS and behavioral plasticity but their ideas and approaches to research on this question varied considerably.

To facilitate communication and to provide the opportunity to learn from one another, a conference on CNS Plasticity and Recovery of Function was held at Clark University, September 24–26, 1973. The atmosphere was relaxed and informal and the group was purposely kept small to achieve this effect.

When my colleagues and I organized this conference, with the help of funds from the National Science Foundation (Departmental Development Award to Clark University # GU-3173), we wanted to bring together not only those workers that were committed to the ideas of CNS plasticity, but also those who felt that reorganization of the CNS after damage was of a questionable nature at best. However, we also wanted to demonstrate that plasticity, when it is observed, is not limited only to neonatal or phylogenetically simple organisms, but can be found in adult, higher mammals as well. In addition we thought that a conference and book on the subject of CNS recovery should also be relevant to those with clinical interests so there are also chapters concerned with aspects of recovery in children and adults with damaged brains.

As with most areas of the neurosciences, the pace of change in ideas, theories and techniques is very rapid and this particular aspect of psychobiology is no exception. What is considered as exciting and appropriate today may be thought of as naive and unsophisticated tomorrow. The purpose of this volume, then, is to stimulate further the search for new ideas and better understanding of the nature of CNS organization in normal and damaged organisms. If we have accomplished this goal then the fruits of our labors will have been worthwhile.

ACKNOWLEDGMENTS

The planning of this conference was easy but organizing the details and getting everything to work smoothly was quite another matter. For the former, my colleagues and friends, Drs. Nelson Butters and Jeffry Rosen and I take responsibility. Fortunately, the number of workers interested in behavioral recovery and neural plasticity are small and they are already distinguished, so it was not hard to seek them out. The credit for all of the hard work goes first to Mrs. Alfhild Bassett without whom there would have been chaos. She was there, as always, whenever she was needed. Thanks must also go to Evelyn Piano who has with patience and skill typed the entire manuscript. Each of the participants also deserves sincere thanks. Almost to a person, there was hardly any cajoling needed to get them to send their manuscripts in on time. It's been a pleasure and an honor to work with them.

Finally, a word of appreciation for our host, Clark University. The staff of the university did what it could to make the meetings as comfortable and as pleasant as possible.

RECOVERY OF FUNCTION AND LOCALIZATION OF FUNCTION

IN HISTORICAL PERSPECTIVE

Burton S. Rosner
University of Pennsylvania
Philadelphia, Pennsylvania

On the afternoon of June 16, 1783, Dr. Samuel Johnson, the famed English lexicographer, sat for his portrait in the studio of Miss Frances Reynolds, the sadly untalented sister of Sir Joshua Reynolds. Despite his 73 years and his marked obesity, Johnson afterwards walked the considerable distance from the studio to his home. He went to sleep at his usual hour in the evening and awoke according to his account around 3 A.M. on June 17. To his surprise and horror, he found that he could not speak. He immediately tested his mental faculties by successfully composing a prayer in Latin verse. Next he tried to loosen his powers of speech by drinking some wine, violating his recently acquired habits of temperance. The wine only put him back to sleep. Upon reawakening after sunrise, Johnson still could not speak. He found, however, that he could understand others and that he could write. His penmanship and composition were somewhat defective (Critchley 1962). Johnson proceeded to summon his physicians, Drs. Brocklesby and Heberden, who came and examined him. They prescribed blisters on each side of the throat up to the ear, one on the head, and one on the back, along with salts of hartshorn (ammonium carbonate). Heberden, who was one of London's leading doctors, predicted a speedy recovery. His confidence proved quite justified: the therapeutic regimen was so efficacious that Johnson's speech began returning within a day or two. Recovery proceeded smoothly over the next month, and even the mild disorders in writing lessened. Johnson finally was left with a slight but stable dysarthria until he succumbed to other causes late in the next year.

Heberden's optimism over Johnson's recovery suggests that British physicians of that time had accumulated experience with such cases. Practitioners apparently knew that recovery was possible but had no clear theory of the etiology and course

1

of these disorders. Indeed, they seemed to attribute what we know as aphasia to disturbances of the
vocal apparatus. Thus, Johnson's doctors applied a
wrong treatment, blisters, to a wrong place, the
throat. Happily, these two wrongs only added up to
discomfort for the patient. Heberden ultimately
expressed doubts about a peripheral origin for all
speech disorders but could not advance his thinking
beyond this. Further progress required a theory of
brain function and organization, which finally
matured in the nineteenth century. Only then did
phenomena of recovery of function acquire clear
scientific significance by sharply challenging the
doctrine of localization of function (Riese 1959).
Accordingly, to understand fully the relatively
short history of explanations of recovery of
function, we must trace the much longer history of
ideas about localization of function which finally
forced the birth of these explanations. The complete story begins with ancient Greek thought.

CLASSICAL THOUGHT: GREECE AND ROME

The first obvious question about localization
of function is whether mental processes reside
anywhere in particular in the body. By the middle
of the fifth century B.C., the Greeks had produced
two positive but opposing answers. Alcmaeon of
Croton (ca. 500 B.C.) located mental functions in
the substance of the brain (Castiglione 1947;
Woollam 1958). Soon thereafter Empedocles (ca. 490-
430 B.C.) reasserted an apparently older notion
that the soul dwelt in the heart and blood (Gordon
1949; Phillips 1957). These two theories, the
encephalic and the cardiovascular, were destined to
compete with each other for the next two thousand
years.

Many physicians, especially those of the
Hippocratic school, adopted the encephalic theory
of mind. Hippocrates himself lived sometime
between 460 and 360 B.C., but his reputed writings
were never assembled until about two centuries
after his death. The overseers of the great
library at Alexandria finally ordered this project
(Castiglione 1947). The resulting collection
included treatises by more or less faithful students of Hippocrates and quite possibly contained

nothing by the master himself (Phillips 1957). This
corpus was the source of copies through which
future generations came to know "Hippocrates." Now
the Hippocratic text which deals most extensively
with the brain concerns epilepsy and bears the
famous title On the Sacred Disease (adams 1939). It
makes the brain the "interpreter of consciousness"
(Penfield 1958) and the mediator of feelings,
intellect, and sensations. The treatise argues that
epilepsy is not really a sacred disease but instead
has perfectly natural and understandable causes.
The clinical descriptions of seizures are remarkably clear and direct. Although Adams concurred
with previous attributions of this work to
Hippocrates, later scholarship (Castiglione 1947)
suggests that it was composed well after the
master's death. Two other treatises in the
Hippocratic corpus, Breaths and Heart, maintain the
Empedoclean tradition which placed the mind in the
heart and blood (Phillips 1957). These works do not
seem part of genuine Hippocratic thought, but they
demonstrate that the cardiovascular theory maintained a foothold in Greek medical theory.

Plato and Aristotle in the fourth century B.C.
continued the conflict between encephalic and
cardiovascular theories. Plato's position is somewhat complicated. The Timaeus (Jowett 1953)
locates the immortal and rational soul in the
"marrow" of the head, clearly the brain, but puts
the passions between neck and midriff and the
appetites between midriff and navel. In the Phaedo,
however, Socrates recalls just before his death
that he had wondered as a youth whether man thinks
with his blood or with air or fire or whether the
brain is the organ of perception. He finally concluded, Socrates says that he is incapable of such
inquiries. Thus, Plato's loyalties to the encephalic theory were not very certain. In contrast,
Aristotle, as everybody knows, unambivalently
localized the soul in the heart (Ross 1931; Smith
and Ross 1910; Thompson 1913). One reason was his
accurate observation of the beating heart in a
chick embryo of three days age. The heart is the
first organ formed, and Aristotle therefore
thought that it must carry the soul. He also noted
that wasps and centipedes survive decapitation and
that the tortoise heart still beats after excision

from the body. Being a good biologist, moreover, he recognized that the brain must serve some function. He noticed that it was moist and cool to the touch and concluded that it refrigerated the blood (Clarke 1963).

The Stoic philosophers of Rome accepted the Aristotelian views and transmitted them to Tertullian (160-230 A.D.), an early Church Father (Castiglione 1947). The encephalic theory continued on through the work of Rome's greatest physician, Galen (130-200). Like his model Hippocrates, on whose treatises he wrote long commentaries, Galen was a keen observer. Both men described hemiplegia contralateral to the side of a head injury and Galen provided a magnificent account of Jacksonian seizures (Major 1961). Dissections of fresh ox brains supplied Galen with new anatomical data, especially concerning the ventricles (Woollam 1958) which Herophilos had first described some five centuries previously (McHenry 1969). The new anatomy turned up in Galen's physiological theory (Singer and Rabin 1946). The theory starts with the intestines converting food into chyle which the mesenteric veins bear to the liver. The liver turns this substance into venous blood and adds "natural spirits" to it. The blood then travels to the right ventricle of the heart; some of it passes through invisible pores into the left ventricle where it interacts with *pneuma* (spirit) inspired into the lungs and carried by the pulmonary vein to the heart. This interaction changes the natural spirits into "vital spirits" of which some reach the brain through blood flow in the carotid arteries. At the base of the brain Galen had observed a fine network of vessels, the *rete mirabile*. He proposed that this network distilled vital spirits into "animal spirits." The latter were stored in the ventricles of the brain (Magoun 1958) before distribution to the body via the brain substance and finally the nerves during execution of mental functions. Galen's encephalic theory of mind thus related the brain to the rest of the body.

FROM THE DECLINE OF ROME TO THE FIFTEENTH CENTURY

Shortly after the time of Galen's death, the Germanic invasions occurred which undermined the

western part of the Roman Empire. These incursions
finally forced the transfer of the imperial capitol
to Constantinople in the fourth century. The Eastern Empire was essentially Greek in orientation,
preserving that language and its literature. Western Europe lost its knowledge of Greek classics,
which the Romans had never greatly admired in any
case. Snatches of Aristotle and the first parts of
Timaeus were all that were available in Latin
translation (Haskins 1927). The translation of
Plato did not include the passages which mention
the tripartite division of the soul (Gilson 1955).
Greek influences and culture remained fitfully
alive in southern Italy and Sicily, which were old
Hellenic areas of colonization. The Byzantine
Empire thus became the chief repository of Plato
and Aristotle (Castiglione 1947). It also preserved
the works of Galen, who had been born and trained
in the eastern provinces. Although Galen composed
his treatises while residing in Rome, he still
wrote in Greek rather than Latin. If he had used
Latin, the intellectual history of western Europe
might have been somewhat different, because Latin
and the Latin classics remained alive in the west
after the fall of Rome.

Byzantium became something more for our history,
however, than a mere repository. In the fourth
century A.D., Nemesius, bishop of Emesa in Syria,
produced a new theory of the physical basis of mind
(Telfer 1955). Although he claimed that he was
following Galen, with whom he was perfectly
familiar, Nemesius in fact went further. He first
distinguished three sets of mental faculties:
sensation and imagination; thought and judgment;
and memory. He localized the first set in the
anterior ventricles of the brain, the second set in
the "middle of the brain," and the third in the
"cerebellum and hinderbrain." The sequence followed
a sensible rostrocaudal order. Man derived information about the world from his senses and gets ideas
through imagination. He reflects upon this material
and forms judgments about it. The results are
stored away in memory for future reference.
Nemesius was the first to distribute psychological
functions differentially within the encephalon. He
also was the first to localize functions in the
ventricles, although he seems to have involved only

the anterior cavities.

The intellectual treasures of the Byzantine Empire spread into the medical schools of Syria and Persia, where Aristotle and Galen became objects of careful study and commentary (Castiglione 1947). When the Islamic religion swept the Arab world and sparked the conquest of the Near East and Middle East in the seventh century, Arabian physicians found the medical schools awaiting them. They explored the Syrian and Persian teachings and thereby moved into absorbing and reworking the old Greek store of scientific, medical, and philoso- phical materials. Among the Arabian writers and commentators of the ninth century was one Costa ben Luca or Qusta ibn Luqa (Thorndike 1923). He offered a theory of mind in which sensation seems to have dwelt in the anterior ventricles while the posterior chambers mediated imagination, reason, and memory. A valve or "vermis" between the two sets of cavities controlled interaction among the faculties. Although it is not clear whether Costa ben Luca knew the writings of Nemesius, he might well have since he read Greek.

The Arabian conquests had staggering effects on the Christian world of the seventh through tenth centuries. Saracen naval fleets abruptly halted trade between eastern and western Mediterranean lands. Western Europe suffered a frightful social and economic decline (Pirenne 1925) and conse- quently underwent further intellectual isolation. The energies of Byzantium were devoted to resisting the Moslems (Guerdan 1957), with little remaining for new modes of creativity. In the eleventh century, however, came the reopening of commerce between different Mediterranean regions. Cities such as Venice developed sufficient maritime power to break Islamic domination of the Mediterranean and to reestablish contact with Byzantium. The Crusades began to push back the Moslems in the Near East, in Spain, and in Sicily. Growing parity of political and economic power brought in its wake growing intellectual parity. A lively inter- change of ideas occurred in Spain, Sicily, and North Africa which funneled Arabian medical, scientific, and philosophical knowledge into western Europe. The Greek traditions as sustained by the Arabs flowed along in this development and were reinforced by direct contact of Christian translators with Greek sources preserved in Sicily. One of these translators was Alfanus, archbishop of Salerno from 1058 to 1087, who rendered Nemesius into Latin. The ideas of Nemesius may have influenced an adventurous eleventh century figure, Constantinus Africanus, who lived in North Africa and then Sicily before finally becoming a monk at Monte Cassino (Haskins 1927; Thorndike 1923). Constantinus apparently decided that all mental functions were localized in the ventricles, as had Costa ben Luca. From the traditions of Nemesius, Costa ben Luca, and Constantinus Africanus sprang the mediaeval theory of the basis of mind. It held that sensation and fantasy occur in the anterior ventricles, judgment and reason in the middle (IIIrd) ventricles, and memory in the posterior (IVth) ventricle. An eleventh century manuscript at Caius College, Cambridge, represents at least part of this theory (Singer 1957). It depicts the brain divided into portions for "fantasy," "intellect," and "memory."

Intellectual exchange primarily in Spain reintroduced Aristotle and Galen into western European thought. Arabs, Jews, and Christians participated in this development (Castiglione 1947) which also gave to the West texts of Arabian medical encyclopedias such as that of Avicenna (980-1037). Thus, encephalic and cardiovascular theories of the basis of mind joined the ventricular theory in spreading throughout Europe. Three groups of partisans soon formed. For example, William of Saliceto (1210-1270) was a sophisticated Bolognese physician who contended that the cerebellum mediated involuntary and the cerebrum voluntary motion (McHenry 1969) and so took an encephalic stance. Alfred of Sarashel, a leading English scholar of the thirteenth century, argued for the Aristotelian cardiovascular position (Pagel 1958). Many clerics and some physicians upheld the ventricular theory; somebody even concocted a book containing this view and attributed the work to St. Augustine (Thorndike 1923; Gilson 1955). Several hundred years had to elapse after the end of the Middle Ages before one of the three rival theories could emerge triumphant.

FROM THE FIFTEENTH TO THE NINETEENTH CENTURIES

Andreas Vesalius (1514-1564) struck the first major blow against the ventricular theory through his dissections of the human body, previously forbidden on theological grounds. He observed the ventricles of the human brain as well as those in animals and reached the following devastating argument (Singer 1952):

> "All our contemporaries, so far as I can understand them, deny to apes, dogs, horses, sheep, cattle, and other animals, the main powers of the Reigning Soul - not to speak of other (powers) - and attribute to man alone the faculty of reasoning; and ascribe this faculty in equal degree to all men. And yet we clearly see in dissecting that men do not excel those animals by (possessing) any special cavity (in the brain). Not only is the number (of ventricles) the same, but also all other things (in the brain) are similar, except only in size and in the complete consonance (of the parts) for virtue."

This shrewd combination of comparative psychology and comparative anatomy began the downfall of the ventricular theory. Further evidence against it came from vivisection experiments by Volcher Coitier (1534-1600) who opened the brains of animals down to the ventricles without very striking effects (McHenry 1969). Coitier also found that removal of considerable chunks of the brain had few obvious effects on behavior or vital functions. The growing body of anatomical and physiological knowledge also offered no support to the cardiovascular view. Harvey's analysis of the circulation of the blood further discredited it, although Aristotle's ideas had influenced Harvey (Clarke 1963). Nevertheless, theories of the material basis of mind were still in confused competition at the close of the sixteenth century, as three quotations from Shakespeare attest. The first one is from The Merchant of Venice (Act III Scene ii) where Bassanio chooses between the three caskets while Portia sings:

> "Tell me where is fancy bred,

Or in the heart or in the Head?"
Portia like a true barrister neatly sidesteps this
difficult scientific question and opts for the
eyes. She is neither encephalic nor cardiovascular
in the end.

The next passage comes from Henry IV, Part II
(Act IV Scene ii). Sir John Falstaff has just
informed the Chief Justice that King Henry has
returned in poor health from Wales:

"Chief Justice: I talk not of his majesty.
You would not come when I sent for you.
Falstaff: And I hear, moreover, that his
highness is fallen into this same whoreson
apoplexy.
Chief Justice: Well, God mend him. I pray
you, let me speak with you.
Falstaff: This apoplexy is, as I take it,
a kind of lethargy, an't please your
lordship; a kind of sleeping in the blood,
a whoreson tingling.
Chief Justice: What tell me of it? Be it
as it is.
Falstaff: It hath it original from much
grief, from study and perturbation of
the brain. I have read the causes of its
effects in Galen: it is a kind of deafness."

Sir John takes a mixed cardiovascular and encephalic view. Finally, consider what the school-
master Holofernes says in Act IV Scene ii of Loves
Labour's Lost:

"This is a gift that I have, simple, simple;
a foolish extravagant spirit, full of forms,
figures, shapes, objects, ideas, apprehen-
sions, motions, revolutions. These are
begot in the ventricle of memory, nourished
in the womb of the *pia mater*, and delivered
upon the mellowing of the occasion. But the
gift is good in those in whom it is acute,
and I am thankful for it."

Holofernes is a self-satisfied Nemesian. It is
worth noting that all three plays were written in
the 1590's, possibly within a period of five
years. Shakespeare could select his theory of mind
to fit his dramatic purposes. Few of his contemp-
oraries had a better basis of choice.

During the two centuries after Shakespeare,
however, the ventricular and cardiovascular

theories finally vanished. Their abandoment was
not due to sudden, dramatic disproofs but instead
reflected slowly developing knowledge and concepts
about brain function. Furthermore, these developments occurred within the framework of the old
Galenic notion of animal spirits. Descartes (1596-
1650) stated clearly in The Passions of the Soul
(Haldane and Ross 1931) that the substance of the
brain provides channels through which animal
spirits move in order to control psychological
functioning. Sensations, thoughts, movements, and
memories reflect the particular paths which the
spirits take. This was the first time that repeti-
tion of a specific experience had been related to
recurrent activation of a special small subsystem
within the brain. The problem of the "locus of the
engram" grew from this beginning. Thomas Willis
(1621-1675), who coined the term "neurology," also
retained the idea of animal spirits, despite
Vesalius' earlier demonstration that man unlike the
ox has no *rete mirabile* and despite his own
description of the vascular circle at the base of
the brain (Feindel 1962; Meyer and Hierons 1965).
Willis proposed, however, that they were not stored
in the ventricles but rather reside in the
substance of the brain. He also distributed
different functions to various parts of the brain.
The cerebellum was said to control involuntary
movement, while perception and voluntary motion
were located in the corpus striatum, imagination in
the corpus callosum, memory in the cortex, and
instinctual behavior in the middle of the brain.
This was not a bad start.

Along with the growing acceptance of some form
of encephalic theory came new observations on brain
function in the seventeenth and eighteenth
centuries. Robert Boyle (1627-1691) described a
patient who had contralateral paralysis following a
depressed fracture of the skull. When the surgeon
raised the fracture and removed a piece of bone
from the cerebral surface, voluntary movement soon
returned (Gibson 1962). The phenomenon of contralateral paralysis became more understandable when
Pourfour du Petit (1664-1741) clearly observed the
decussation of the pyramids around 1710 (Thomas
1910). He also proposed that contralateral
paralysis and contralateral weakness signalled two

different disorders (McHenry 1969). A.C. Lorry
(1725-1783) distinguished the motor functions of
the cerebellum from the vital functions of the
medulla (Walker 1957). The notion of a functional
organization of the brain seemed to be in the air.
        The most astonishing figure of this era,
however, must be Emanuel Swedenborg (1688-1772).
To begin with, he arrived at a crude neuron theory
in which "cerebellula" or "glands" in the cortex
gave rise to nerve fibers. We know the "cerebellula" today as cell bodies. Swedenborg thought that
the cerebellula were the termini of sensation
(Akert and Hammond 1962) and that different sensory
systems ended in different cortical areas. This
spatial organization was necessary in his view for
keeping different experiences separate and distinct. Thus, Swedenborg anticipated the modern form
of the law of specific nerve energies. He even had
some notions about differential cerebral localization of more complex mental functions (Schwedenberg
1960). Perhaps his greatest triumph was to infer
the correct order in which the body is represented
in the motor strip of the cortex. All of these
enormously important ideas had absolutely no
influence whatsoever. Shortly after finishing his
neurological writings, Swedenborg had a mystical
experience which turned him to religious
preoccupations. The eventual outcome was the
Swedenborgian Church. The manuscripts on brain
function lay unpublished until their discovery
around 1885. By then, of course, they had nothing
startling to announce.
        Here was the situation at the end of the
eighteenth century, around the time of
Dr. Johnson's aphasic episode described at the
beginning of this paper. The encephalic theory of
the basis of mind had long ago ousted its two
rivals. The winning theory had undergone some
elaboration, consisting of tentative and usually
unsystematic assignments of different functions
to different parts of the brain. In this form the
theory had relatively little scientific or clinical
force. Conditions obviously were ripe for the
appearance of an organized approach to localization
of function. Just precisely such an approach grew
up in the early nineteenth century, and we know it
today under the name "phrenology."

THE NINETEENTH CENTURY STRUGGLE OVER LOCALIZATION

The first organized scientific formulation of localization of function was the work of an anatomist, Franz Joseph Gall (1758-1828), and his pupil, Johann Caspar Spurzheim (1776-1832). Their *magnum opus* is a publication in four volumes which emerged between 1810 and 1819 entitled, Anatomie et Physiologie du Systeme Nerveux en General, et du Cerbeau en Particular. Spurzheim worked with Gall on the first volume and on part of the second, thereafter leaving his teacher (Ackerknecht 1958). Their achievements constitute quite an impressive record (Critchley 1965; Temkin 1953). They recognized that white matter consisted of nerve fibers and held that grey matter constituted the organs of mental life. Nerve fibers in their view began in and ended in grey matter. Gall and Spurzheim also clearly demonstrated the decussation of the pyramids. Their major advance, however, was to divide psychological functioning into 27 "faculties" or classes of abilities and to assign each faculty a particular cortical area as its seat. All cerebral cortical regions were used up in this parcellation. Eight of the faculties were unique to humans, while man and animals shared the other 19 (Ackerknecht 1958). Gall and Spurzheim thus integrated comparative psychology with comparative anatomy. Young (1970) has beautifully analyzed how Gall inferred different faculties from striking variations in human behavior and how he confirmed the inferences by examining animals. The division of functions among different cortical areas raised the question of how mental functioning was coordinated into a phenomenologically unified whole. Gall and Spurzheim neatly gave this job to intracortical fibers running between the cortical "organs" for the different faculties.

Along with this brilliance went a fatal piece of foolishness. Gall and Spurzheim argued, perhaps acceptably, that the relative prominence of a faculty in an individual depended on the relative size of the corresponding cortical organ. But then they insisted that the size of this organ in turn determined the shape and relative elevation of the overlying skull. Through "cranioscopy," as Gall termed it, one could evaluate character by superficial examination of the skull. The procedure traces back to Gall's much earlier interest in physiognomy, which purported to tell how to read character from an individual's face and body. This adolescent fixation apparently blinded Gall to the fact that the inner and outer surfaces of the skull are not topographic images of each other.

Gall and Spurzheim had great influence on investigations in France and England. In France, Pierre Flourens (1824) launched a major assault against the idea of localization in the cerebrum. Ablation experiments on pigeons showed him that cerebellar lesions disturbed coordination while removal of the cerebral hemispheres impaired intelligence, memory, and voluntary action. Removal of small parts of the cerebrum led to recovery of the higher functions, after transient disturbances (Krech 1962). Thus, Flourens seems to have been the first to recognize clearly the phenomenon of recovery of function after brain injury. Progressive enlargement of cerebral lesions finally reached a point where all higher faculties vanished permanently at once. This observation clearly contradicted Gall and Spurzheim. Despite bitter opposition from the prestigous Flourens (Young 1970), localizationist ideas still influenced French neurology. Bouillaud (1825) published a paper arguing that his collection of pathological human cases showed that speech was located in the anterior frontal lobes, just as Gall had said. This is a careful paper, discussing cases with frontal lesions and deficits and those with non-frontal lesions without deficits. In 1836 Marc Dax reportedly read a paper in Montpelier in which he claimed that lesions of the left hemisphere produce loss of speech and of other signs of thought (Stookey 1954). His son finally published the manuscript in 1865. By then, of course, Paul Broca (1861) had demonstrated two cases of aphasia with lesions in the left frontal lobe. Wernicke's work some ten years later further developed the basic concept of a restricted cortical representation for speech (Gibson 1962).

Localizationist doctrine reached nineteenth century England when Spurzheim settled there after leaving Gall (Ackerknecht 1958). In fact, Spurzheim was the one who coined the term "phrenology"

(Temkin 1947) and gave it a moralizing aura. The movement soon gained adherents among British intellectuals and physicians, just as it did among the French. One of its earliest English partisans was Herbert Spencer who published three phrenological papers while in his twenties. Although Spencer later abandoned phrenology (Jefferson 1955), he kept the idea of localization of function and wove it into an evolutionary view of the nervous system. Adopting the associationistic psychology formulated by Alexander Bain (Young 1970), Spencer argued that the nervous system evolved into an increasingly complex and differentiated structure which improves the efficiency of adaptation by adjusting inner subjective relationships to outer objective ones. Evolution of the nervous system might become so complex, however, as to produce dissolution of its functioning. Spencer's writings exerted enormous influence on Hughlings Jackson who liberally credits his inspiration (Taylor 1958). Jackson took over the evolutionary view of the nervous system, altered the idea of dissolution to describe the effects of brain injury, and contributed to the development of the doctrine of localization. Thus phrenology exercises an important if indirect influence on perhaps the greatest neurologist of the last century. As an organized movement phrenology began to decay at about the same time.

The closing decades of the nineteenth century were a period of major achievements for the doctrine of localization of function. The outstanding discovery probably was Fritsch and Hitzig's (1870) demonstration of the cortical motor strip. Besides directly establishing localization of motor control, their work demolished the views of Flourens who insisted that cortex as the seat of unified mind was inexcitable (Young 1970). This brought the cerebral cortex out of any unique status relative to other parts of the brain and showed that regions above the brainstem and spinal cord also guided movement (Jefferson 1953). Bartholow (1874) and Sciamanni (1883) confirmed that man also has a cortical motor strip. Besides enlarging on the work of Fritsch and Hitzig, Ferrier (1876) joined Munk (1881) in providing evidence for differential perceptual modalities. Although Goltz vigorously attacked the validity of

14

Munk's findings (Riese and Hoff 1951), the localizationist view soon prevailed. A further advance
in the study of localization came when Franz (1902)
introduced the use of animal training procedures
which had recently developed in experimental
psychology. He showed that lesions in different
cortical areas could have different effects on
retention of a learned response. Other results,
however, led Franz to doubts about localization.
This skeptical view was taken up by Lashley, who
made the last major attack against localization in
his monograph, <u>Brain</u> <u>mechanisms</u> <u>and</u> <u>intelligence</u>
(Lashley 1929). The doctrine of localization
weathered that storm and today stands as a
fundamental tenet of the neural sciences.

RECOVERY OF FUNCTION IN THE LOCALIZATIONIST CONTEXT

        Those like Flourens who believed that the
cerebrum acts in a unitary, undifferentiated
fashion had no problem with recovery of function
after brain injury. The intact parts of the
injured structure simply would continue to work in
their accustomed ways, after some initial period of
non-specific shock. At worst, mild loss of efficiency might occur. The phenomena of recovery,
however, do challenge the doctrine of localization:
If functions are differentially distributed in the
cerebrum, how can those disrupted by a given lesion
regain effectiveness? Neuropathology showed that
nerve cell bodies in the mammalian nervous system
cannot regenerate. Thus, solutions to the problem
of recovery had to come from other directions.
Within a relatively short time, three different
explanations of recovery were offered.
        Hughlings Jackson proposed that a given
function is represented several times at different
levels of the nervous system. The function therefore does not dwell exclusively in a given region,
as Gall and Spurzheim had assumed. According to
Jackson, higher levels of the nervous system
evolved later, mediate a given function in a more
finely tuned fashion, are more easily excited, and
inhibit lower levels. Damage at a higher level
releases the lower ones from inhibition, and they
carry out the function as best they can. Since
higher levels are more excitable, partial injury

of a higher representation of a function permits more complete recovery. Jackson thus held that hierarchical representation underlay what he called "Principle of Compensation" in neural functioning. This view of recovery is somewhat related to explanations based on Flourens' idea of uniform representation of a function throughout many neural regions which work by mass action. After injury, the surviving representations again do their best. Mass action, of course, does not include any hierarchical arrangement and thus does not recognize the descending inhibition which Jackson emphasized.

A second explanation of the phenomena of recovery came from Munk. He argued that regions of the brain which were not otherwise occupied could assume functions mediated previously by an injured area. This is a substitutionist view, and it differs sharply from explanations of recovery based on hierarchical or nonhierarchical representation. According to Munk, the area substituting for the damaged one would never have become involved otherwise in mediating the function in question. Furthermore, the substituent area must be available due to current lack of other duties. Of course, it must also have the capacity to perform its adopted role. A variant of Munk's view would assume that any cortical area, for example, could take on functions lost by injury to some particular region. This is the theory of recovery due to equipotentiality (Lashley 1929).

The theories of Jackson and Munk appeared in the latter part of the nineteenth century. A third explanation of recovery was offered by von Monakow (1914) in the early years of the present century. He argued that damage to the brain deprives other intact regions of normal afferent inflows from the injured area. The sudden loss of input to the otherwise normal areas produces in them a particular type of shock, which he called diaschisis. The intact areas thereby would function poorly, producing symptoms. As the diaschisis dissipated, the intact regions would regain their old modes of operation and the corresponding symptoms would vanish. This would leave the symptoms for which loss of the damaged area was directly responsible.

Besides rerepresentation, substitution, and

diaschisis, a fourth theory of recovery has developed in the past fifty years. On this theory, parts of the brain remaining after injury reorganize dynamically in order to carry out lost functions in new ways. Subroutines which previously had entered into the lost functions may be dropped or even new ones may be substituted. Luria, Naydin, Tsvetkova, and Vinarskaya (1969) have offered the clearest formulation of this theory, which we may label as "retraining." Indeed, in their view, specific rehabilitative therapy is necessary for recovery in higher organisms such as man after brain damage. Retraining theory raises in very clear form an issue which has been latent in our presentation so far. The issue is, just what is localized and just how do we define a function for purposes of localization? The facts of development raise the same issue. During maturation, external stimulation is necessary for elaboration of various behaviors. As these behaviors develop, however, they become independent of external stimuli for their organization. The execution of a "function" and thus its definition shifts with development.

Further consideration of this problem brings us to a general realization. Neurological observations on symptoms of brain injury and on the course of recovery are always interpreted and perhaps are even made within the framework of prevailing psychological concepts (Riese and Hoff 1950; Tizard 1959). It would seem rash to try to define "function" for once and for ever. In fact, the history of ideas about localization of function inextricably involves the history of psychological concepts. The transition from the faculty psychology of Gall to the associationism of Spencer and Hughlings Jackson exemplifies the point. It follows that progress in understanding recovery of function depends partly on improvements in psychological theory, methods, and modes of analysis. In turn, phenomena of deficits after brain injury and of recovery can sharpen or even transform psychological conceptions.

RECENT DEVELOPMENTS IN UNDERSTANDING RECOVERY OF FUNCTION

This history which we have traced across a span of twenty-five centuries shows that the doctrine of localization of function synthesizes two venerable traditions: The encephalic theory of mind and the spatial parcellation of psychological functions first propounded by Nemesius. Credit for the first systematic elaboration of the doctrine must go to Gall and Spurzheim. Once the localizationist view took hold, it confronted the problem of recovery. Four plausible answers to this problem appeared: hierarchical rerepresentation, substitution, diaschisis, and retraining. Each is compatible with various interpretations of the doctrine of localization. Furthermore, the four explanations are not logical rivals, since each could apply in various degrees to particular situations. Given this historical background, we now may ask whether any significant new developments have occurred in the study of recovery of function after brain injury. At least four advances come to mind.

The first new development actually is a rediscovery. By 1876, Soltmann (1876) had observed that lesions of motor cortex in young subjects had less severe effects than in adult animals. Fifty years later, Kennard attacked this problem again (Kennard 1936, 1938, 1940, 1942; Kennard and McCulloch 1943). Her findings show that unilateral lesions in precentral areas in infant animals have minimal effects compared to the same lesions in adults; the contralateral motor areas as well as ipsilateral frontal and postcentral regions seem to take over for the damaged tissue. The relationship between age of injury and severity of deficit is fairly general (Rosner 1970) but it is somewhat task-dependent also (Nonneman and Isaacson 1973). The greater plasticity in younger animals is reminiscent of a general situation in embryology to which the terms "prospective significance" and "prospective potency" apply (Balinsky 1970). The prospective significance of a given embryonic zone is the particular tissue into which it normally differentiates. The prospective potency of that zone is the set of different tissues into which it could develop if circumstances such as injury

elsewhere so demanded. As normal ontogenesis proceeds, "determination" occurs, and the embryonic
region loses prospective potency as it achieves
prospective significance. The same concepts seem
applicable to functional development of the brain.
The prospective significance of a particular
infantile cortical zone, for example, is the set of
functions which it comes to mediate through normal
development. The prospective potency of the region
is the set of functions which it can mediate when
challenged by damage to other parts of the brain.
As normal development proceeds, determination
occurs and prospective potency diminishes as
prospective significance is realized. This argument
suggests that determination of regional function,
like determination of tissue structure, may involve
repression of genes. Perhaps depression would give
new capacities for recovery of function in brain-
damaged adults. If so, there would undoubtedly be
a price, since we cannot assume that plasticity
demands no payment.

    Ades and Raab (1946) discovered that a two-
stage seriatim bilateral removal of precentral
area 4 in adult monkeys is far less deleterious
than a single-stage one. This finding has appeared
in many other contexts (Rosner 1970). Ades and
Raab found that postcentral cortex played a role in
cushioning the effects of a two-stage removal.
Kennard (1940) had observed the differences between
one-stage and two-stage lesions of areas 4 and 6 in
infants and had found evidence that postcentral
cortex plays a role in this phenomenon and also in
compensating for infantile lesions (Kennard and
McCulloch 1943). These various findings suggest
that seriatim removals in adult animals may unmask
the prospective potency of other areas.

    A second new development in studies of
recovery of function is evidence for denervation
supersensitivity in the central nervous system.
Denervated central neurons, like denervated peripheral structures (Trendelenburg 1963), may
acquire supersensitivity to the transmitters which
normally impinge upon them (Schoenfeld and Uretsky
1967, 1972; Ungerstedt 1971; Uretsky and Schoenfeld
1971). Any remaining fibers which released the same
transmitters would have a much larger effect than
usual. Such fibers could include some from the

damaged system which were somehow spared. A
fraction of the injured system thus could produce
recovery.

Central supersensitivity has a peripheral
analogue. A third new set of findings on recovery
of function, however, seem to lack a similar
parallel. Various drugs, such as cholinergic
agents (Ward and Kennard 1942), anticholinesterases
(Luria, Naydin, Tsvetkova and Vinarskaya 1969), or
amphetamine (Braun, Meyer and Meyer 1966), can
accelerate recovery from brain injury. Other
agents, such as barbiturates (Watson and Kennard
1945), slow recovery. Although these effects may
be useful clinically, their basis is unknown.

The final new advance in work on recovery is
the finding of axonal growth in the damaged central
nervous system. This growth takes two forms, direct
and collateral. Björklund and his colleagues
(Björklund and Stenevi 1971, 1972; Katzman,
Björklund, Owman, Stenevi and West 1971) found
that ascending catecholaminergic fibers begin
growing after interruption by electrolytic or
mechanical lesions. The fibers invade the area of
damage, advance along nearby blood vessels, and can
enter transplanted adrenergically innervated tissue
such as iris. Nerve growth factor facilitates fiber
growth. After about seven weeks, however, the new
stretches of axons seem to decrease in prominence.
This may reflect establishment of synapses with
lessening of the histofluorescence by which
regrowth is demonstrated; alternatively, it could
signal degeneration. Experiments on spinal cord by
Nygren, Olson and Seiger (1971) indicate that
regrowing transected fibers may not be able to
break the region of a lesion. These investigators
suggest that mechanical factors associated with
the lesion rather than limitations on fiber
regeneration may block invasion of the damaged
area. Elimination of such mechanical barriers could
promote recovery of function.

The phenomenon of collateral sprouting in the
central nervous system is a different form of
axonal growth. Uninjured fibers can form new
collaterals which invade regions deprived of their
normal afferent inflow by damage elsewhere (Lynch,
Deadwyler and Cotman 1973; Moore, Björklund and
Stenevi 1971; Raisman 1969). The new collaterals

make synaptic contacts with denervated postsnyaptic membrane. Collateral sprouting might explain the recent findings of Berger, Wise and Stein (1973) that nerve growth factor facilitates recovery from lateral hypothalamic lesions. They interpret their results as reflecting faster regeneration in damaged fibers or as due to enhanced supersensitivity.

Collateral sprouting poses a curious problem when considered as a possible mechanism for recovery of function. It is not self-evident that sprouts from a system different than the damaged one must always improve functioning. Conceivably, such new sprouts could disrupt the activity of cells which receive them. The literature on sprouting contains an undercurrent of thought to the effect that all contacts must be good. Currently, there is no compelling reason to accept that proposition.

THEORIES OF RECOVERY IN LIGHT OF NEW DEVELOPMENTS

We may finally ask about the implications of recent developments in the study of recovery of function for the future form of theories of recovery. Of the four traditional theories, hierarchical rerepresentation, substitution, diaschisis, and retraining, the first and last seem least affected by specific contemporary advances. This is quite understandable. Recovery due to rerepresentation fundamentally reflects the evolution of neuronal connections within the nervous system. As the neural control of particular functions becomes better known, the particular bases for recovery through rerepresentation will become clearer. Similarly, retraining utilizes a general property of the nervous system. The more we come to understand the neurology of learning, the better will we comprehend retraining. Finally, all four theories are quite compatible with observations on facilitation of recovery by drugs; these findings have no differential implications for the theories at present.

Studies of lesions in young animals have an obvious implication for recovery by substitution. This mechanism seems more available to a younger subject and becomes progressively inaccessible as determination proceeds. Munk's insistence that a substituent area must be "unoccupied" now seems a remarkably shrewd idea. Furthermore, if a neural region substitutes for an injured one, the functions normally mediated by the former may be blocked from full expression. The cost of prospective potency as a device for recovery remains to be investigated.

Lastly, von Monakow's theory of diaschisis may be reinterpreted in terms of development of denervation supersensitivity. This would be one way in which nerve cells subjected to deafferentation could resume normal function. Recovery from diaschisis through axonal growth, direct or collateral, would afford another possible version of von Monakow's views. This reinterpretation seems remote from the spirit of his thinking, however, since he viewed disappearance of diaschisis as a process within the affected nerve cells themselves. Instead, central axonal growth following brain damage provides an entirely new explanation of recovery of function beyond the sphere of the four older theories. Thus, we should add this new conception to the set of major theories of recovery of function after brain injury. The newcomer will undoubtedly be the object of fascinated attention in the future.

Acknowledgments. I wish to thank my colleagues, Drs. Oscar S.M. Marin and C.R. Gallistel, for their incisive comments on an earlier version of this paper. A valuable conversation with Dr. John Marshall in an early stage of preparing this essay helped organize my views on several points.

Postscript. Since completing this manuscript, I have seen Edwin Clarke's and Kenneth Dewhurst's new book, An Illustrated History of Brain Function, published in 1972 by the University of California Press. This beautiful collection of drawings and diagrams illustrating concepts of brain function contains an extensive section on the different versions of ventricular theory in medieval times. Anybody interested in localization of function will spend a delightful evening with this book.

REFERENCES

Ackerknecht, E.H. (1958). Contributions of Gall and the phrenologists to knowledge of brain function. *In* F.N.L. Poynter (Ed.) "The History and Philosophy of Knowledge of the Brain and its Functions," pp. 149-153. Oxford: Blackwell.

Adams, F. (1939). "The Genuine Works of Hippocrates," Baltimore: Williams and Wilkins.

Ades, H.W. and Raab, D.H. (1946). Recovery of motor function after two-stage extirpation of area 4 in monkeys. *J. Neurophysiol.* 9, 55-60.

Akert, K. and Hammond, M.P. (1962). Emanuel Swedenborg (1688-1772) and his contribution to neurology. *Med. Hist.* 6, 255-266.

Bartholow, R. (1874). Experimental investigations into the functions of the human brain. *Amer. J. Med. Sci. (New Series)* 67, 305-313.

Balinsky, B.I. (1970). "An Introduction to Embryology," 3rd ed. Philadelphia: W.B. Saunders

Berger, B.D., Wise, C.D. and Stein, L. (1973). Nerve growth factor: enhanced recovery of feeding after lateral hypothalamic damage. *Science* 180, 506-508.

Björklund, A. and Stenevi, U. (1971). Growth of central catecholamine neurones into smooth muscle grafts in the rat mesencephalon. *Brain Res.* 31, 1-20.

Björklund, A. and Stenevi, U. (1972). Nerve growth factor: stimulation of regenerative growth in central noradrenergic neurons. *Science* 125, 1251-1253.

Bouillaud, J. (1825). Recherches cliniques propre à demontrer que le perte de la parole correspond à la lésion de lobules anterieurs du cerveau et à confirmer l'opinïon de M. Gall sur le siège de l'organe du language articulé. *Arch. Gen. Med.* 8, 25-45.

Braun, J.J., Meyer, P.M. and Meyer, D.R. (1966). Sparing of a brightness habit in rats following visual decortication. *J. Comp. Physiol. Psychol.* 61, 79-82.

Brocco, P. (1861). Remarques sur le siège de la faculté du language articulé, suivies d'une observation d'aphémie (perte de la parole). *Bull. Soc. Anat. Paris* 36, 330-357.

Castiglione, A. (1947). "A History of Medicine,"
2nd ed. New York: Alfred Knopf.

Clarke, E. (1963). Aristotelian concepts of the
form and function of the brain. *Bull. Hist. Med.*
37, 1-14.

Critchley, M. (1962). Dr. Samuel Johnson's aphasia.
Med. Hist. 6, 27-44.

Critchley, M. (1965). Neurology's debt to F.J. Gall
(1758-1828). *Brit. Med. J.* 2, 775-781.

Feindel, W. (1962). Thomas Willis (1621-1675): The
founder of neurology. *Canad. Med. Assn. J.* 87,
289-296.

Ferrier, D. (1876). "The Functions of the Brain,"
London: Smith Elder and Co.

Flourens, P. (1824). "Recherches experimentales sur
les propriétés et les fonctions du système
nerveux dans les animaux vertébrés," Paris:
Crevot.

Franz, S.I. (1902). On the functions of the cerebrum: I. The frontal lobes in relation to the
production and retention of simple sensory-
motor habits. *Amer. J. Physiol.* 8, 1-22.

Fritsch, G. and Hitzig, E. (1870). Ueber die
elektrische Erregbarkeit des Grosshirns. *Arch.
Anat. Physiol. Wiss. Med.* 37, 300-332.

Gibson, W.C. (1962). Pioneers in localization of
function in the brain. *J. Amer. Med. Assn.* 180,
944-951.

Gilson, E. (1955). "History of Christian Philosophy
in the Middle Ages," New York: Random House.

Gordon, B.L. (1949). "Medicine throughout Antiquity," Philadelphia: F.A. Davis.

Guerdan, R. (1957). "Byzantium: Its Triumphs and
Tragedy," New York: Capricorn Books.

Haldane, E.S. and Ross, G.R.T. (Transl.) (1968).
"The Philosophical Works of Rene Descartes,"
2 Vols. Cambridge, England: Cambridge University
Press.

Haskins, G.H. (1927). "The Renaissance of the
Twelfth Century," Cambridge, Mass.: Harvard
University Press.

Jefferson, G. (1953). The prodromes to cortical
localization. *J. Neurol. Neurosurg. Psychiat.*
16, 59-72.

Jefferson, G. (1955). Variations on a neurological
theme - cortical localization. (Herbert Spencer
and phrenology) *Brit. Med. J.* 2, 1405-1408.

Jowett, B. (Transl.) (1953). "The Dialogues of Plato," 4 vols. 4th ed. London: Oxford University Press.

Katzman, R., Björklund, A., Owman, C., Stenevi, U. and West, K.A. (1971). Evidence for regenerative axon sprouting of central catecholamine neurons in the rat mesencephalon following electrolytic lesions. *Brain Res*. 25, 579-596.

Kennard, M.A. (1936). Age and other factors in motor recovery from precentral lesions in monkeys. *Amer. J. Physiol*. 115, 138-146.

Kennard, M.A. (1938). Reorganization of motor function in the cerebral cortex of monkeys deprived of motor and premotor areas in infancy. *J. Neurophysiol*. 1, 477-496.

Kennard, M.A. (1940). Relation of age to motor impairment in man and subhuman primates. *A.M.A. Arch. Neurol. Psychiat*. 44, 377-397.

Kennard, M.A. (1942). Cortical reorganization of motor function. Studies on series of monkeys of various ages from infancy to maturity. *A.M.A. Arch. Neurol. Psychiat*. 48, 227-240.

Kennard, M.A. and McCulloch, W.S. (1943). Motor response to stimulation of cerebral cortex in absence of areas 4 and 6 (*Macaca mulatta*). *J. Neurophysiol*. 6, 181-190.

Krech, D. (1962). Cortical localization of function *In* L. Postman (Ed.) "Psychology in the making. Histories of Selected Research Problems," pp. 31-72. New York: Alfred Knopf.

Lashley, K.S. (1929). "Brain Mechanisms and Intelligence," Chicago: University of Chicago Press.

Luria, A.R., Naydin, V.L., Tsvetkova, L.S. and Vinarskaya, E.N. (1969). Restoration of higher cortical function following local brain damage. *In* R.J. Vinken and G,W, Bruyn (Eds.) "Handbook of Clinical Neurology," Vol. 3. pp. 368-433. Amsterdam: North-Holland.

Lynch, G., Deadwyler, S. and Cotman, C. (1973). Postlesion axonal growth produces permanent functional corrections. *Science* 180, 1364-1366.

Magoun, H.W. (1959). Development of ideas relating the mind to the brain. *In* C. McC. Brooks and P.F. Cranefield (Eds.) "The Historical Development of Physiological Thought," pp. 81-107. New York: Hafner.

Major, R.H. (1961). Galen as a neurologist. *World Neurol.* 2, 372-380.

McHenry, L.C. (1969). "Garrison's History of Neurology," Springfield, Illinois: Thomas.

Meyer, A. and Hierons, R. (1965). On Thomas Willis' concepts of neurophysiology. *Med. Hist.* 9, 1-15.

Monakow, C.V. (1914). "Die Lokalisation im Grosshirnrinde und der Abbau der Funktion durch korticale Herde," Wiesbaden: J.F. Bergmann.

Moore, R.Y., Bjorklund, A. and Stenevi, U. (1971). Plastic changes in the adrenergic innervation of the rat septal area in response to denervation. *Brain Res.* 33, 13-35.

Munk, H. (1881). "Ueber die funktionen der Grosshirnrinde. Gesammelte Mitteilungen aus den Jahren 1877-1880," Berlin: August Hirshwald.

Nonneman, A.J. and Isaacson, R.L. (1973). Task dependent recovery after early brain damage. *Behav. Biol.* 8, 143-172.

Nygren, L.G., Olson, L. and Seiger, A. (1971). Regeneration of monoamine-containing axons in the developing and adult spinal cord of the rat following intraspinal 6-OH-dopamine injections or transections. *Histochemie* 28, 1-15.

Pagel, W. (1958). Medieval and renaissance contributions to knowledge of the brain and its functions. *In* F.N.L. Poynter (Ed.) "The History and Philosophy of Knowledge of the Brain and its Functions," pp. 95-114. Oxford: Blackwell.

Penfield, W.D. (1958). Hippocratic preamble: the brain and intelligence. *In* F.N.L. Poynter (Ed.) "The History and Philosophy of Knowledge of the Brain and its Functions," pp. 1-4. Oxford: Blackwell.

Phillips, E.D. (1957). The brain and nervous phenomena in the hippocratic writings. *Irish J. Med. Sci.* 381, 377-390.

Pirenne, H. (1925). "Medieval Cities: Their Origins and the Revival of Trade," Princeton: Princeton University Press.

Raisman, G. (1969). Neuronal plasticity in the septal nuclei of the adult rat. *Brain Res.* 14, 25-48.

Riese, W. (1959). "A History of Neurology," New York: M.D. Publications.

Riese, W. and Hoff, E.C. (1950). A History of the doctrine of cerebral localization. I. Sources, anticipations, and basic reasoning. *J. Hist. Med.* 5, 50-71.

Riese, W. and Hoff, E.C. (1951). A history of the doctrine of cerebral localization. II. Methods and main results. *J. Hist. Med.* 6, 439-470.

Rosner, B.S. (1970). Brain Functions. *Ann. Rev. Psychol.* 21, 555-594.

Ross, W.D. (Ed.) (1931). "The Works of Aristotle Translated into English," Vol. 3. Oxford: Clarendon.

Schoenfeld, R.I. and Uretsky, N.J. (1967). Operant behavior and catecholamine-containing neurons: prolonged increase in lever-pressing after 6-hydroxydopamine. *Eur. J. Pharmacol.* 20, 357-362.

Schoenfeld, R.I. and Uretsky, N.J. (1972). Altered response to apomorphine in 6-hydroxydopamine-treated rats. *Eur. J. Pharmacol.* 19, 115-118.

Schwedenberg, T.H. (1960). The Swedenborg manuscripts: a forgotten introduction to cerebral physiology. *A.M.A. Arch. Neurol.* 2, 407-409.

Sciamanni, E. (1883). Fenomeni produtti dall'applicazione della corrente elettrica sulla e dura madre e modificazione del polso cerebrale. *Atti d. r. Acad. d. Lincei., Roma* 13, 25-42.

Singer, C. (1952). "Vesalius on the Human Brain," London: Oxford University Press.

Singer, C. (1957). "A Short History of Anatomy and Physiology from the Greeks to Harvey," New York: Dover.

Singer, C. and Rabin, C. (1946). "A Prelude to Modern Science," Cambridge, England: Cambridge University Press.

Smith, J.A. and Ross, W.D. (Eds.) (1910). "The Works of Aristotle Translated into English," Vol. 4, Oxford: Clarendon.

Soltmann, O. (1876). Experimentelle Studien uber die Functionen des Grosshirns der Neugeborenen. *Jb. F. Kinderheilk. (n.F.)* 9, 106-148.

Stookey, B. (1954). A note on the early history of cerebral localization. *Bull. N.Y. Acad. Med.* 30, 559-578.

Taylor, J. (Ed.) (1958). "Selected Writings of John Hughlings Jackson," 2 vols. London: Staples

Telfer, W. (Transl.) (1955). "Cyril of Jerusalem and Nemesius of Emesa. Library of Christian Classics," vol. 4. Philadelphia: Westminster Press.

Temkin, O. (1947). Gall and the phrenological movement. *Bull. Hist. Med.* 21, 275-321.

Temkin, O. (1953). The neurology of Gall and Spurzheim. *In* E.A. Underwood (Ed.) "Science, Medicine, and History," vol. 2. pp. 282-289. London: Oxford University Press.

Thomas, H.M. (1910). Decussation of the pyramids - an historical inquiry. *Johns Hopk. Hosp. Bull.* 21, 304-311.

Thompson, D.W. (1913). "On Aristotle as a Biologist," Oxford: Clarendon.

Thorndike, L. (1923). "A History of Magic and Experimental Science," vol. 1. New York: Macmillan.

Tizard, B. (1959). Theories of brain localization from Flourens to Lashley. *Med. Hist.* 3, 132-145.

Trendelenburg, U. (1963). Supersensitivity and subsensitivity to sympathomimetic amines. *Pharmacol. Rev.* 15, 225-276.

Ungerstedt, U. (1971). Postsynaptic supersensitivity after 6-hydroxydopamine-induced degeneration of the nigro-striatal dopamine system. *Acta Physiol. Scand. Suppl.* 367, 69-93.

Uretsky, N.J. and Schoenfeld, R.I. (1971). Effects of l-Dopa on the locomotor activity of rats pretreated with 6-hydroxydopamine. *Nature: New Biol.* 234, 157-159.

Walker, A.E. (1957). Stimulation and ablation, their role in the history of cerebral physiology. *J. Neurophysiol.* 20, 435-449.

Ward, A.A., Jr. and Kennard, M.A. (1942). Effect of cholinergic drugs on recovery of function following lesions of the central nervous system. *Yale J. Biol. Med.* 15, 189-229.

Watson, C.W. and Kennard, M.A. (1945). The effect of anticonvulsant drugs on recovery of function following cerebral cortical lesions. *J. Neurophysiol.* 8, 221-231.

Woollam, D.H.M. (1958). Concepts of the brain and its functions in classical antiquity. *In* F.N.L. Poynter (Ed.) "The History and Philosophy of Knowledge of the Brain and its Functions," pp. 5-18. Oxford: Blackwell.

Young, R.M. (1970). "Mind, Brain, and Adaptation in the Nineteenth Century," Oxford: Clarendon.

NEURONAL PLASTICITY:
CONCEPTS IN PURSUIT OF CELLULAR MECHANISMS

Marcus Jacobson
University of Miami School of Medicine
Miami, Florida

In our efforts to wrest some understanding of
neuronal plasticity from our inadequate experimental results we show that we share the conviction,
derived from Classical Greece, that mere knowledge
of facts for their own sake is pointless (and sometimes harmful) and that anyone serious enough to
inquire into such matters wants to know not merely
what happens but why, and by what fixed principles
or laws of nature. Sadly, our dream of arriving at
such an understanding by the unassisted efforts of
reason has long been shattered by our adoption of
the experimental method. Having embarked on the
Baconian program of investigation by experiment we
are compelled to consider not merely the possible
fallacies of logic (which may be a pretty exercise
in logic itself) but perforce have to deal with
such nasty matters as the limitations of our
materials and experimental methods. It turns out
that a failure to acknowledge and respect the
limitations of our techniques results at best in
overinterpretation and at worst in misinterpreta-
tion of our data. Particularly, in respect to the
topic of this symposium we tend to find plasticity
in the brain when it really belongs only to our
methodology or to our interpetation of the experimental results. The dangers of being too generous
to our experimental data have come out very clearly
in the history of studies of the retino-tectal
system. For that reason, I am making an effort to
arrive at an objective view of our achievements in
that field of research.

Let us consider the ways of using (and abusing)
a familiar experimental strategy, namely mapping
the distribution of nerve terminals originating in
a set of nerve cells in one part of the brain (set
A) and projecting to another part of the nervous
system to connect with neuron set B. In normal
animals a regular spatial deployment of terminals
is mapped, and we want to find out how the map is
altered by experimental surgery to neuron set A

and/or set B. The retino-tectal system serves to
illustrate my point. Normally, a ganglion cell at
a particular retinal position always projects its
axon to a particular position in the tectum. Thus
the axon terminals originating in the retina are
deployed in the tectum in a spatial pattern or map
which reduplicates the pattern of deployment of the
ganglion cells in the retina. To demonstrate this,
we lower a microelectrode into the tectum at a suc-
cession of positions further and further back on
the tectum, and we find that we can record nerve
action potentials at each of these successive positions only by providing the frog or fish with a
visual stimulus at an appropriate and successively
temporal position in the visual field. In this
manner we can map the retino-tectal projection of
the optic nerve terminals to the tectum. Such a map
gives an indication of the position-dependent
properties of the retinal ganglion cells, which we
term locus specificities (Jacobson and Hunt 1973),
that predispose each axon to terminate at a unique
locus in the tectum. Because the map is obtained
from pre-synaptic terminals, it does not show
whether those terminals have formed functional
synaptic connections in the tectum. The retino-
tectal projection does provide a convenient assay
of the position-dependent specificities of the
retinal ganglion cells (set A), but does not provide an assay of functional connectivity between
neuron set A and neuron set B in the tectum. Such
an assay can only be obtained by recording beyond
the synapse, that is, by assaying the post-synaptic
potentials arising in neuron set B when neuron set
A is stimulated appropriately. The map is also
limited in respect to the information that can be
obtained from it. It provides no more than relative information about the disposition of the
position-dependent properties across the retinal
cell population. The map does not show which
locus specificities are present, it only shows that
the order of their spatial deployment in a retinal
population occurs in a particular direction and
across a particular population of cells. Thus, it
is extremely risky to try to correlate discontinuities or continuities in the retinal fiber
projection to the tectum with a history of surgical
manipulation of the retino-tectal system. At best,

the map permits a correlation between the direction
in which these locus specificities are finally
deployed in the eye and the previous developmental
history of the eye's position with respect to the
body. The main limitation of the mapping technique
is that after experimental surgery to either the
eye or the tectum, it cannot assay the range of the
position-dependent properties in the retinal cell
population, or tell whether the set of properties
that is finally expressed is complete, reduced, or
augmented. But the map can provide information
about the relative order with which the set of
position-dependent properties has been spatially
deployed in the retina.
     When we consider the experimental strategies
that have been used to study plasticity in the
nervous system we are struck by the lack of critical appreciation of the limitations of the methodology. For example, a classical strategy is to
make size disparities between neuron set A and set
B, by removing parts, for example, of retina or
tectum during embryonic development and ultimately
mapping the final configuration of connections or
projections between the two sets. "Plasticity" in
the system is assayed by determining whether the
final map is normal or compressed, expanded or
distorted in any other way. Unfortunately, this
strategy is intrinsically limited because the
result can never be interpreted unambigously,
either when "plasticity" is manifested or when it
appears to be absent. One cannot tell, without
other controls, whether the set of elements present
in the altered map is the same as the set that
would have developed without surgical interference.
Thus the cells in set A (retina) and/or set B
(tectum) might have been replaced by new cells. Or
the cells might have changed their properties; or
if their properties were retained, their expression
might have been altered in the novel context produced by the experimental situation. Attempts to
force such maps to yield or reveal the rules
governing connectivity between two sets of nerve
cells leads inevitably to circular arguments: the
map is an operational indication of the relatively
orderly expression of position-dependent properties
in a set of elements, but after experimental
surgery neither the identity of the set or the

expression of its properties can be determined from the map. It is not known whether the same elements are present or the same properties persist nor whether the expression of the properties has been altered under the experimental conditions. Realization of these limitations of our experimental methods reduces our confidence in many conclusions that have been reached about neuroplasticity in the retino-tectal system or in other systems in which uncontrolled changes may result from ablation of part of the brain. Absence of plasticity under one set of conditions does not mean that the same system might not show plasticity under other conditions, and conversely, we should not be ready to assert that plasticity occurs unless experimental controls have been done to deal with changes in cell production and deployment.

In the light of these considerations of the limitations of the methodology let us recount the main experimental results of producing size disparities in the retino-tectal system. In the initial study of the effects of making size disparities in the retino-tectal system, Attardi and Sperry (1963) removed part of the retina and cut the optic nerve in goldfish. They showed histologically that after 3 to 67 days the optic nerve fibers had grown back only to the appropriate parts of the tectum. They concluded that the regenerating optic nerve fibers were "destination bound" and that the optic nerve fibers grew by the most direct pathway to their proper synaptic slots in the tectum, bypassing inappropriate slots on the way. Each fish was studied at only one postoperative stage, and whether the system had arrived at a steady state or was at an intermediate state could not be known. A similar criticism can be levelled at the study of retino-tectal size disparities in the goldfish by Jacobson and Gaze (1965). We did two kinds of experiments; in the first the entire population of optic nerve fibers was allowed to regenerate into a residual lateral or medial part of the tectum; in the second we studied the regeneration of about half the normal number of optic nerve fibers to the intact tectum. In both experiments, it seemed as if, by 139 days, the optic fibers had returned only to the appropriate positions in the tectum, and the assumption was made that the system had reached its final state.

The first evidence of plasticity in the retino-tectal system of the goldfish appeared after regeneration of the optic nerve into a residual rostral half tectum (Gaze and Sharma 1970). In those studies the entire retina was found to send its fibers into the rostral part of the tectum: the optic fibers were deployed in the correct order, but were compressed by a factor of about two into the rostro-caudal axis of the tectum. Yoon (1971; 1972 a, b, c) showed that such compression of the optic nerve fibers into the residual part of the tectum could occur into either medio-lateral or rostro-caudal axis of the tectum, and was reversible. We had thus reached a position in which the nervous system, or at least the visual system, seemed to behave as a rigidly determined system in some experiments and as a plastic system in others. The physicist would not be upset by this, for he knows that the electron, in DeBroglie's approximate words "behaves like a wave on Mondays, Wednesdays and Fridays, and like a particle on the other days of the week," depending on the point of view of the observer and on the terms of his description. But the biologist is disconcerted when a system exhibits what seems to be contradictory behavior under different sets of conditions. However, I am not in the least dis-comforted by this, and such apparent contradictions appeal to me. If it is indeed correct that the system does behave in a paradoxical manner (and we have first to exclude any experimental errors or fallacies in interpretation of the experimental results) the paradox may be resolved in several different ways.

First, different results may be obtained when observations are made at different times of a system in the process of change: at early stages, the kinetics of the change may be seen, while the dynamics are observed after the system has reached a steady state. This is what appears to be hap-pening in the case of the projection of the retina to the optic tectum in the goldfish, after removal of parts of the tectum. Secondly, the system may behave invariantly, in fact, but appear to have two different modes of behavior according to the level of description that is used: macroscopically it may not show the changes that appear on examination at a higher resolution. Thirdly, the system may behave according to an invariant rule, but the outcome may vary according to the context. Such a system is said to be context sensitive. Another reason for apparently paradoxical behavior may be that the system is not homogeneous but is actually composed of more than one subset with different behaviors, and the outcome of an experimental manipulation will depend on which set is observed or upon which set responds to the manipulation.

There is some evidence that the result of removing part of the tectum may depend on the time after the operation. Thus Sharma (1972b) found that a few weeks after removing the central part of the goldfish tectum and crushing the optic nerve, the regenerated optic nerve fibers had returned to their correct places in the tectum, leaving a large central scotoma in the visual field. In other fish, examined months after removal of the central part of the tectum, the scotoma was not present and the fibers from the entire retina seemed to be compressed into the residual tectum. These results suggest that the optic nerve fibers had initially returned to their proper places in the tectum (as shown by Attardi and Sperry in 1963 and by Jacobson and Gaze in 1965) but later the optic nerve terminals were repositioned in order to accommodate all the regenerating optic fibers into the residual part of the tectum, as found by Yoon (1971; 1972a, b).

The experiments on adult goldfish have given quite different results from similar experiments done on adult frogs (Straznicky 1973; Meyer and Sperry 1973). Removal of part of the tectum and section of the optic nerve in frogs is followed by regeneration of the optic nerve fibers only to the correct positions in the tectum. We lack enough information to enable us to understand why frogs have failed to show retino-tectal plasticity. After removing part of the tectum in the adult frog we do not know what becomes of the retinal fibers that were destined for the ablated tectum; do the retinal ganglion cells perish if deprived of synaptic targets; do the fibers project to anomalous regions of the brain; are synaptic connections formed by optic fibers that terminate

at the correct tectal loci, by fibers that terminate anomalously, or by neither; are there changes
in the residual population of tectal neurons?

Another limitation of these experiments is that
they did not show whether the regenerated optic
nerve fibers had formed functional synaptic connections in the tectum. This essential information
was precluded by the experimental methods employed
in all studies so far cited: because the electrical
potentials that are recorded in the tectum arise
from presynaptic terminals of optic nerve fibers,
there was no way of knowing whether such fibers had
formed functional synaptic connections with tectal
cells. The presynaptic potentials that are used to
indicate the positions of optic nerve fibers in the
tectum may originate from a sessile nerve terminal
or from one that is moving about; from a fiber that
ends in a non-functional synapse, or as we usually
assume, from a fiber that terminates in a functional synapse at the position at which we record the
presynaptic potentials. If the fibers ultimately
form connections, do they connect initially at the
correct synaptic loci and later move to new loci
during compression of the projection; or do they
connect only once at the final, compressed position? In addition, we want to know whether the
connections are reformed with the appropriate type
of tectal neurons at the correct depth in the
tectum as is found in normal goldfish (Jacobson and
Gaze 1964). Whatever the final configuration of
connections, we want to know whether it was
produced *ab initio* or only after a period of trial
and error -- and if so whether malconnections were
eliminated by error-elimination, error-correction,
or error-neutralization. To study the kinetics of
regrowth of the optic nerve fibers in the tectum
will require repeated mapping of the retino-tectal
projection in the same animal at close intervals
during the process of regeneration of the optic
nerve. To determine whether the regenerated optic
nerve fibers have formed functional connections in
the tectum will require postsynaptic recording
(Skarf 1972; Skarf and Jacobson 1974).

We are attended by similar doubts and uncer-
tainties when we come to consider the effects of
creating retino-tectal size disparities in
embryonic frogs. Thus, by removal of the nasal or

the temporal half of an eye rudiment in the tailbud
frog embryo, and replacements with a temporal or
nasal half eye respectively, we constructed double
nasal (NN) or double temporal (TT) eyes (Gaze,
Jacobson, Székely 1963; 1965). When the projection
of the compound eye to the tectum was mapped in the
adult frog, we found that each half eye projected
to the entire tectum. In our interpretation of this
result we made the assumption that each half eye
had expressed the properties of half the set of
elements normally present in an entire eye, but no
control experiments were done to justify such an
assumption. We cannot know from those experiments
whether the elements in each half eye might have
been replaced by a full set of elements; or whether
the properties of the elements might have altered
to those of a full set of properties; or whether
the properties of the half set of elements in the
retina might have been expressed as a full set of
elements in the development of the retino-tectal
map. More recently we have performed additional
controls (Jacobson and Hunt 1973; Hunt and
Jacobson 1973 b) in which we made compound eyes by
combining different retinal halves, a nasal half
retina and a ventral half retina were fused
together, or a right nasal half retina was combined
with an inverted left temporal half retina, for
example. In all cases, the half eye, regardless of
its site of origin in the retina, projected to the
entire tectum. The most likely explanation of these
results is that regulation had occurred, meaning
either that the half eye had acquired a full set of
properties or that the half set of properties was
expressed as a full set in the formation of a
retino-tectal map.

Without knowing the mechanism of expression of
the ganglion cell locus specificities during formation of the retino-tectal map, we cannot deduce
from the map which specificities are present in the
retina as a whole or at any particular retinal
position. Thus, the main limitation of the technique is that, in an experimentally manipulated
retino-tectal system, it cannot assay the range of
the properties of cells in retina or tectum or tell
whether the set of properties is complete, reduced
or augmented, but it can determine whether the
relative order of the set of properties in the

retina has been altered (inverted, for example)
within the limits of the spatial resolution of the
mapping method. With such limitations, is it at all
surprising, therefore, that when the question is
asked about the behavior of the system in terms of
its metrics (the total range and intervals between
the elements) the answer is that it behaves with
considerable plasticity, for the metrics (the number and range of elements) cannot be determined
from the assay. Alternatively, if the question is
asked about the topological invariance (for
example, the relative order of the elements) we
should not be surprised if the answer is that it
behaves with considerable rigidity. If in addition
we consider that it is unusual for the experiment-
alist to indicate whether his map was obtained at
an intermediate stage of development or in the
final state of the system, we suspect that the
interpretation of retino-tectal maps may sometimes
move out of the realm of scientific inference into
that of prophecy.

Because there is no absolute measure of the
specific properties of the elements that compose
a neuronal set, the set of ganglion cells in the
retina for example, we are compelled to use some
form of comparative or relative measure. The
retino-tectal map, for example, gives us only a
relative measure of some parameters within a set,
and permits us to map the relative order of elements within the set, but provides no information
about the identity of individual elements.
Inversions or translocations may be detected
directly, but deletions or additions that did not
alter the relative order of the elements in the map
could only be detected by comparing the unknown set
directly with a neuron set of known composition.
Thus we lose information about the completeness of
the set of nerve fibers projecting from the retina
to the tectum because there is nothing in the
tectum to compare with an unknown set of optic
nerve fibers. A possible means of avoiding this
theoretical impasse was suggested to me by an
article on holography (Gabor, Kock and Stroke
1971). In holography, two sets of coherent waves
are projected onto a screen, and the hologram is
produced by interference between the object waves
and the reference or background waves. Why not

project two sets of optic nerve fibers into the
same tectum, one from a test eye and another from
a normal or reference eye grafted into the same
socket? The way in which the two sets of optic
nerve fibers mingle in the tectum provides a
measure of their shared locus specificities, while
the regions of the tectum in which the two sets of
optic fibers do not mingle shows which specificities are not common to both sets (Jacobson and
Hunt 1973). This strategy must be used with adequate controls to deal with the effects of experimental surgery on cell proliferation, cell
migration and cell death in the retina and tectum,
and is potentially able to give information about
the completeness and range of a neuron set that
has been surgically reduced in numbers or deranged
in any other way.

Enough has been stated to indicate that the
"plastic" changes that appear to occur in the
retino-tectal maps cannot be interpreted solely in
terms of nerve growth and synapse formation without
also considering the changes in histogenesis,
differentiation and morphogenesis of the retinal
and tectal cell population. By so doing we bring
the problems of neuronal plasticity into the domain
of embryonic cell regulation. It seems obvious
that the regulative capacities that exist in the
embryo, for example the capacity of a surgically
reduced embryonic rudiment to develop into a whole
structure of diminished size, is in some respects
analogous to neuronal plasticity. There is
undeniable heuristic value in considering neuronal
plasticity in relation to the phenomena of regulation in morphogenetic fields. However, the phenomena of embryonic regulation are largely
inexplicable and are hardly ready to serve as
useful models of neuronal plasticity. Thus, to
call neuronal plasticity a mode of regulation in
morphogenetic fields is merely to beg the question
of the mechanism of both embryonic regulation and
neuronal plasticity. There is probably at least one
cellular mechanism that embryonic regulation and
neuronal plasticity have in common, namely a
mechanism of cell communication whereby any
reduction in the cell population is signalled to
the residual cells, which are then capable of
regulating their programs of cellular differenti-

ation. In the embryo the channels for cell communication that are necessary for regulation are probably provided by gap junctions (Dixon and Cronly-Dillon 1972; Jacobson and Hunt 1973). Gap junctions are found quite ubiquitously in the central nervous system in adult animals (Waxman and Pappas 1971; Sloper 1972), and they may serve as channels for the intercellular signals mediating the plastic responses of nerve cell populations to injury. The gap junctions may serve not merely to couple neurons electrically, but also as an essential part of the mechanisms that regulate the growth and differentiation of nerve cells.

In conclusion, when we consider all the uncontrolled variables that operate in neural systems that have been experimentally deranged and injured, the variability of the results is hardly surprising. Even when control experiments are performed to determine whether new elements arise to replace old ones, or to determine whether the old elements adopt new properties that are expressed as new kinds of interneuronal associations, each experiment permits us no more than a partial characterization of the system, and none has yet provided us with a means of explaining neuronal plasticity in terms of cellular properties and operations. Yet, to return once again to my opening remarks, there exists a strong propensity to invent explanations even when the facts are few and their provenance is uncertain. Our yearning for explanations should not serve as a license for the uninhibited indulgence in our craving for conjectures. Even if the conjecture ultimately proved to be correct, it would be only a triumph of hope over reason.

REFERENCES

Attardi, D.G. and Sperry, R.W. (1963). Preferential selection of central pathways by regenerating optic fibers. *Exp. Neurol.* 7, 46-64.

Dixon, J.S. and Cronly-Dillon, J.R. (1972). The fine structure of the developing retina in *Xenopus laevis. J. Embryol. Exp. Morphol.* 28, 659-666.

Gabor, D., Kock, W.E. and Stroke, G.W. (1971). Holography. *Science* 173, 11-15.

Gaze, R.M. and Sharma, S.C. (1970). Axial difference in the reinnervation of the goldfish optic tectum by regenerating optic nerve fibres. *Exp. Brain Res.* 10, 171-181.

Gaze, R.M., Jacobson, M. and Székely, G. (1963). The retino-tectal projection in *Xenopus* with compound eyes. *J. Physiol. (Lond.)* 165, 484-499.

Gaze, R.M., Jacobson, M. and Székely, G. (1965). On the formation of connections by compound eyes in *Xenopus. J. Physiol. (Lond.)* 176, 409-417.

Hunt, R.K. and Jacobson, M. (1973 a). Neuronal locus specificity: altered pattern of spatial deployment in fused fragments of embryonic *Xenopus* eyes. *Science* 180, 509-511.

Hunt, R.K. and Jacobson, M. (1973 b). Neuronal specificity revisited. *In* A.A. Moscona and A. Monroy (Eds.), "Current Topics in Developmental Biology," New York: Academic Press.

Meyer, R.L. and Sperry, R.W. (1973). Tests for neuroplasticity in the anuran retino-tectal system. *Exp. Neurol.* 40, 525-539.

Jacobson, M. (1974). Through the jungle of the brain: Neuronal specificity and typology re-explored. *Ann. N.Y. Acad. Sci. (In Press).*

Jacobson, M. and Gaze, R.M. (1964). Types of visual response from single units in the optic nerve of the goldfish. *Quart. J. Exp. Physiol.* 49, 199-209.

Jacobson, M. and Gaze, R.M. (1965). Selection of appropriate tectal connections by regenerating optic nerve fibers in adult goldfish. *Exp. Neurol.* 13, 418-430.

Jacobson, M. and Hunt, R.K. (1973). The origins of nerve-cell specificity. *Sci. Amer.* 228, 26-35.

Sharma, S.C. (1972 a). Redistribution of visual projections in altered optic tecta of adult goldfish. *Proc. Nat. Acad. Sci. U.S.A.* 69, 2637-2639.

Sharma, S.C. (1972 b). Reformation of retino-tectal projections after various tectal ablations in adult goldfish. *Exp. Neurol.* 34, 171-182.

Sharma, S.C. and Gaze, R.M. (1971). The retino-topic organization of visual responses from tectal reimplants in adult goldfish. *Arch. Ital. Biol.* 109, 357-366.

Skarf, B. (1973). Development of binocular single units in the optic tectum of frogs raised with disparate stimulation to the eyes. *Brain Res.* 51, 352-357.

Skarf, B. and Jacobson, M. (1974). Development of binocularly driven single units in frogs raised with asymmetrical visual stimulation. *Brain Res. (In Press)*.

Sloper, J.J. (1972). Gap junctions between dendrites in the primate neocortex. *Brain Res.* 44, 641-646.

Straznicky, K. (1973). The formation of the optic fibre projection after partial tectal removal in *Xenopus. J. Embryol. Exp. Morphol.* 29, 397-409.

Waxman, S.G. and Pappas, G.D. (1971). An electron microscopic study of synaptic morphology in the oculomotor nuclei of three inframammalian species. *J. Comp. Neurol.* 143, 41-72.

Yoon, M. (1971). Reorganization of retino-tectal projection following surgical operations on the optic tectum in goldfish. *Exp. Neurol.* 33, 395-411.

Yoon, M. (1972 a). Reversibility of the reorganization of retino-tectal projection in goldfish. *Exp. Neurol.* 35, 565-577.

Yoon, M. (1972 b). Transposition of the visual projection from the nasal hemiretina onto the foreign rostral zone of the optic tectum in goldfish. *Exp. Neurol.* 37, 451-462.

Yoon, M. (1972 c). Synaptic plasticities of the retina and of the optic tectum in goldfish. *Amer. Zool.* 12, 106.

EXPLANATORY MODELS FOR NEUROPLASTICITY IN RETINOTECTAL CONNECTIONS

R. L. Meyer and R. W. Sperry
California Institute of Technology
Pasadena, California

There has been a certain amount of controversy and confusion of late in the literature that deals with the growth and maintenance of retinotectal connections. In brief, the original explanatory model advanced back in the early 1940's is now being questioned by a number of people in the light of some new and apparently conflicting findings, creating a situation that now prompts us to undertake some further experiments.

First by way of background, the eye and the brain of the goldfish on which much of the work has been done, shown in Figure 1, is a relatively

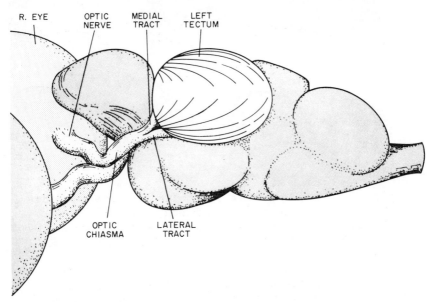

Figure 1. A drawing of the brain of the common goldfish, Carassius auratus, with the retinotectal system shown in white. Each optic nerve completely crosses at the chiasm and divides into two brachia which run along the medial and lateral tectal margins sending off fascicles of fibers in the directions indicated by the black lines.

simple system in which nerve fibers arising from
cell bodies in the retinal layer of the eye grow
centrally to connect directly in topographical
fashion with the optic lobe or tectum of the midbrain on the opposite side.

The earlier work of Attardi and Sperry (1963)
summarized in Figure 2 shows the types of growth

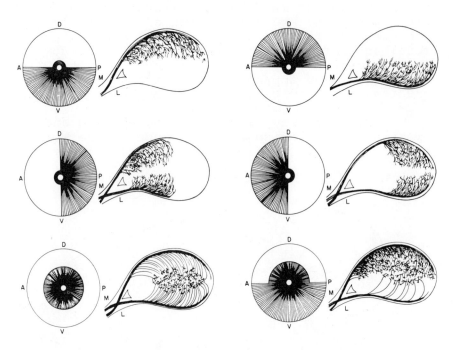

*Figure 2. Diagrammatic reconstructions of regen-
eration patterns formed in optic tracts and tectum
by fibers originating in different retinal halves,
as indicated (After Attardi and Sperry 1963).*

patterns, seen with a modified Bodian stain
selective for regenerating fibers, that were
obtained from different sectors of retinal field
when the rest of the retina was removed. This
illustrates the main point at issue: namely the
conclusion that fibers of the optic nerve grow
selectively along specific routes to reach specific
target points in the tectum, to establish thereby
an orderly topographic map of the retinal field on
this brain center.

This same kind of orderly mapping is found in the initial development in the embryo and also in regeneration in the adult amphibian or fish when the nerves are divided and the hundreds of thousands of fibers scrambled (Sperry 1943; 1944; 1948). The scrambled fibers somehow unsort themselves and regrow the appropriate topographic connections required for optokinetic, orienting and visual discrimination behavior. The more recent techniques of microelectrode mapping of the visual field (Cronly-Dillon 1968; Gaze 1959; Jacobson and Gaze 1965; Maturana *et al*. 1959) and Nauta degeneration stains suitable for fish (Roth 1972) confirm in general these earlier observations of selective optic nerve growth. The same holds even when the eye is rotated or inverted so that the animals are obliged to view everything upside down and backward after regeneration (Sperry 1943; 1944) and also when the nerves are crossed to the wrong side of the brain, producing a left-right reversal in visual perception (Sperry 1945). These maladaptations in visual orientation remain uncorrected by experience.

It was concluded from these and related findings that each retinal point is pre-programmed to connect with a corresponding complimentary point in the tectum. It was inferred that the nerve cells of the retina and tectum must acquire cell-unique cytochemical tags that serve as markers to identify each cell and its fiber according to the precise location of the cell body within the retina or tectum. Each locus in the retina was inferred further to have a corresponding complimentary or matching locus in the tectum for which it possesses a selective preferential chemical affinity or selective adhesivity (Sperry 1943; 1944; 1945; 1951; 1965).

This kind of refined chemical labeling of hundreds of thousands of individual cells in an adult tissue seemingly homogeneous in appearance was a bit hard to accept back in early days, and apparently still is in some places. It was suggested (Sperry 1945; 1951; 1963) that such chemical labeling could easily be brought about by a polarized field-like or gradient type of differentiation on at least two, perhaps three axes in the developing retinal and tectal fields. The

latitude and longitude of each cell, so to speak,
becomes stamped on the cell in some chemical form.
        The same scheme will work and is assumed to
apply also to the visual system of higher forms
(Sperry 1963) and also to other systems like the
vestibular system and the cutaneous system where
we have the same kinds of gradients and topographic
mapping on the brain centers (Sperry 1951). In
other words, this retino-tectal model and the
points that are at issue here involve general
principles that have wide applicability to the
formation of nerve connections throughout the
nervous system.
        We can now consider some of the subsequent
seemingly discrepant findings that have been
obtained largely by Gaze and his associates, by
Sharma, by Yoon, and others. Compound eyes (Figure
3) formed experimentally in the early amphibian

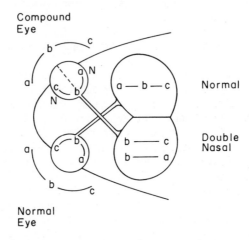

*Figure 3. Diagram of the visual field to retina
to tectum projection in Xenopus with a double
nasal compound eye.*

embryo by uniting two nasal half retinas or two
temporal halves come to project not to just the
corresponding half of the tectum but to the whole
tectum, each half spreading across the entire
tectum in a mirror image pattern (Gaze *et al.* 1965;
Straznicky *et al.* 1971). In goldfish (Figure 4),
when the posterior half of the tectum is removed,
it is reported that the whole retina in time will

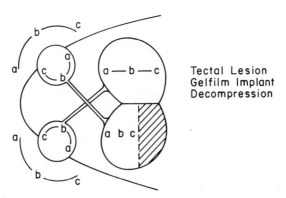

Tectal Lesion
Gelfilm Implant
Decompression

Figure 4. Diagram of the visual field to retina to tectum projection in a goldfish with either a caudal tectal ablation or a mechanical barrier inserted along the dotted line.

come to project in an apparently orderly but compressed pattern upon the remaining half tectum (Gaze and Sharma 1970) and this can occur under conditions where regeneration of tectal cells appears unlikely (Yoon 1971). A gelfilm implant separating rostral and caudal tecta induces a similar compression followed by expansion over the entire tectum after absorption of the gelfilm (Yoon 1972a). This must involve a considerable rearrangement of retino-tectal connections throughout the whole remaining tectal half field. Similarly, as illustrated in Figure 5, it is reported that when half of the retina is removed and sufficient time is allowed, that the remaining half retina will expand its projection to effect an orderly coverage of the whole extent of the tectal field (Horder 1971; Yoon 1972b). Again this would involve a considerable reorganization of the original pattern of retino-tectal connections.

These and similar findings have been taken to mean by a number of investigators (Gaze 1970; Gaze and Keating 1972; Gaze and Sharma 1970; Sharma 1972a; Straznicky *et al.* 1971) that the old explanatory model is not quite adequate and Gaze (Gaze 1970; Gaze and Keating 1972) proposes a modified hypothesis. This would retain the concept of gradients and of chemical ordering, but the

49

Retinal Lesion

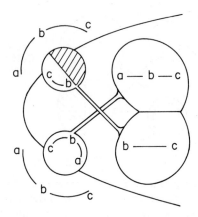

Figure 5. Diagram of the visual field to retina to tectum projection in a goldfish sustaining a temporal retinectomy.

optic fibers instead of finding predetermined targets are hypothesized to arrange themselves in the course of growth in an orderly way and on a competitive basis to fill up whatever gradient is available, establishing their connections on a kind of sliding scale, instead of one that is pre-fixed.

Assuming these findings hold up, our own interpretation has been that these apparent discrepancies are not necessarily in conflict at all, but are readily and better accounted for in terms of the original model than in terms of the sliding scale concept (Sperry 1965; Meyer and Sperry 1973). The polarized field-like retinal or tectal differentiation system on which the original explanation was based is almost by definition as a morphogenetic field (Weiss 1939), something which if cut in half will automatically regulate itself into a whole.

Thus the compound eyes, formed in the early stages of growth and development may be assumed, by the time testing occurs, to no longer contain two half retinas as supposed, but rather two whole twin retinal fields. This would explain why the two nasal or temporal halves overlap across the whole tectum in mirror image alignment. Similar surgical manipulations on the developing limb bud are known to produce the growth of duplicate limbs (Weiss 1939; Saunders and Gasseling 1968). Similarly after removal of the half tectum or retina in the goldfish, it is possible that there is still sufficient developmental plasticity so that the remaining half field of the tectum or retina regulates into a whole field and changes accordingly the chemical labels for cell localization. Recent experiments (Sharma and Gaze 1971; Yoon 1973) suggest that this regulative plasticity with respect to compression and expansion may persist after the capacity for reversal of polarity is lost. Goldfish of the size used are still growing rapidly and the retinotectal system appears to be still growing by cell division (Kirsche and Kirsche 1961).

In other words, the observed plasticity in these experiments is not, in our view, a plasticity in the process by which nerves grow and form their connections. Instead the plasticity is in the precursor process by which the nerve cells differentiate and acquire their local chemical tags. The plasticity that is, is in the organizational dynamics of the developing morphogenetic fields.

We have recently attempted a critical test between these alternatives in a system in which tectal growth is complete and regulation therefore improbable (Meyer and Sperry 1973). In the tree frog *Hyla regilla* tectal growth by cell addition appears to end by metamorphosis (Larsell 1929; Straznicky and Gaze 1972), and if our view is correct, one would not predict these same kinds of plasticity or "sliding scale" effects to obtain in this adult animal. Repeating the procedures used in some of the previous experiments, the posterior half of the tectum was ablated and in many cases the optic nerve was divided and allowed to regenerate. As indicated in Figure 6, if the model of Gaze is correct, one would expect to eventually get a compression of the whole retina onto the remaining front half of the tectum. According to the original model, on the other hand, one would expect to find no such compression and that the scotoma or blind area would remain unchanged.

The results both electrophysiological and

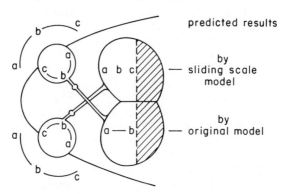

Figure 6. Predicted retinotectal projection
patterns of the adult frog following caudal tectal
ablation and optic nerve crush.

behavioral were clearly in favor of the original
hypothesis. The behavioral data were based on a
perimetry technique for which these animals are
well suited. Like most anurans *Hyla* are typically
quiescent but readily orient to potential food
objects moving in their visual field. By aligning
a calibrated glass hemisphere over a frog resting
on a table top, visual stimuli could be presented
near the glass surface to precise locations in the
visual field. In practice this was done by blinding
the right visual field by an optic nerve crush.
From the blind area a 1-4° black disc mounted on a
glass rod was slowly advanced into the left
posterior field. At some point this typically
produced a sudden turning of head and body toward
the stimulus. By this procedure the temporal
contour of the left visual field from the horizon
to 50° upwards could be mapped with an accuracy of
about 10°.

Figure 7A shows such a contour indicated by the
front edge of the stippling obtained from a normal
animal. The superior field is, as expected, quite
large extending in parts to 180° behind the frog.
After a caudal right half tectum ablation this
field contour regresses to near the 60° meridian.
Considering the 55-60° optic axis divergence from
the midline, this represents an approximate half
field scotoma. This is illustrated in Figure 7B,
in the map of an animal which sustained this

surgery 7 to 10 days prior. Figure 7C shows this same animal remapped 124 days after surgery, a time more than sufficient for the elimination of the scotoma in goldfish. The extent of the field is found not significantly altered.

Three other animals with both complete maps also showed an essentially unchanged scotoma. In addition, there was a small region at the temporal extreme, shown on the figure by the circled numbers, from which false counterreversal responses to the mirror image position could be obtained. Previous work has shown that optic fibers terminating on the wrong tectum mediate these responses (Sperry 1945). Thus fibers corresponding to the ablated tectum appear to grow out of their usual course all the way to the appropriate region of the contralateral tectum rather than terminate in the inappropriate rostral tectum. This presence of alternative correct sites, however, is not the reason for the absence of field expansion since, as will be described, this also fails to occur after bilateral ablations.

The electrophysiological unit recording results obtained with a method similar to Gaze's (1959) also demonstrate the apparent permanency of these scotomas. In Figure 8A is seen a map of the left superior visual field onto the dorsal right tectum of a normal animal. The numbers and letters indicate corresponding electrode placements and receptive field positions, a measure of the respective optic axon terminal and ganglion cell locations (Gaze 1958; Lettvin *et al.* 1960). The retinotectal projection pattern obtained is similar to that reported for other frogs (Gaze 1958; Jacobson 1962). After an optic nerve crush this same organization could again be recorded as early as 60 days postoperatively. Electrophysiological maps were obtained from 9 animals with right caudal tectal ablations and from 4 with bilateral ablations combined in most cases with optic nerve section. In contrast to goldfish where the scotoma vanishes only 90 days after this surgery (Yoon 1971), the blind area remained essentially unaltered up to 339 days after tectal ablation. The longest surviving animal, shown in Figure 8B, demonstrates a typical scotoma of the appropriate size and location. Other scotomas produced by

mid tectal ablations were preserved, contrary to
the case in goldfish (Sharma 1972a), up to 171
days in the four animals measured. A map illustrated in Figure 8C from one of these frogs 106
days after the ablation and left optic nerve
section shows the missing retinal representation.
Similarly in 3 other animals medio-laterally
oriented pieces of gelatin film implanted into
the tectum failed to induce the fiber compression
reported in goldfish despite survival periods of
up to 291 days. Thus both the electrophysiological
results and the behavioral data appear to rule out
the "sliding scale" model.

Very recently Straznicky (1973) has demonstrated a similar lack of plasticity in the adult
Xenopus using electrophysiological measurements
subsequent to various unilateral tectal ablations,
and Gaze (1970) has previously reported these
kinds of results after similar lesions in the late
tadpole stages. We might also add that in the
chick embryo DeLong and Coulombre (1965) and later
Kelly (1970) have shown that optic axons from
surgically reduced retinas grow only to the
appropriate tectal regions leaving the inappropriate regions uninnervated. The apparent
plasticity shown in the *Xenopus* compound eye
experiments almost certainly involves regulative
type changes in the locus specificity properties
of retinal neurons and in reality these experiments
also conform to the idea of selective innervation.
The recent compound eye results of Hunt and

---

*Figure 7. Behaviorally obtained maps showing the
posterior contour of left visual space. The
stimulus was advanced in a temporal nasal direction along each tested 10° parallel until an
orienting response was obtained. The number of
responses at each position is shown and the
stippling indicates the visual field giving no
responses. The right eye was blinded by nerve
interruption in all cases. A. Normal. B. Frog
with right caudal half tectum ablation sustained
7-10 days prior. C. Same animal as in B but tested
124 days after tectal surgery. Circled numbers
represent contralateral orientation movements to
the mirror image position.*

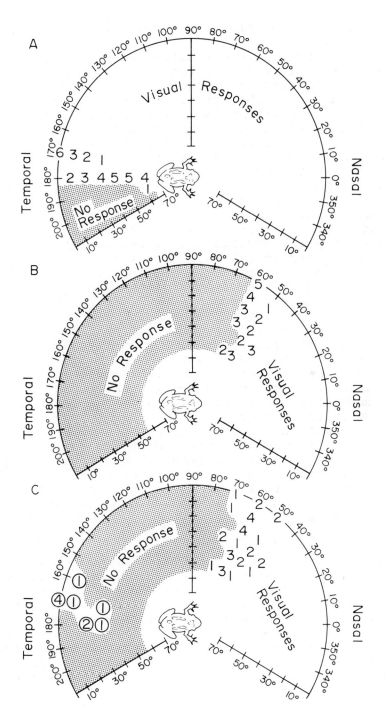

Jacobson (1973) directly supported the same interpretation.

Firm inferences about neuroplasticity and
regulation in the goldfish, however, are hindered
by some apparent inconsistencies in the goldfish
work and by an absence of critical experiments.
There is disturbing lack of agreement between the
electrophysiological data on which all of the
evidence for plasticity rests and the correlated
anatomical data. Yoon (1972b) and Horder (1971)
both report electrical evidence for uniform
spreading of a surgically formed half retina over
an entire normal tectum. In contradiction to this,
the original study of Attardi and Sperry (1963)
using Bodian staining, Roth's (1972) recent
similar work, and our own autoradiography experiments (Meyer 1973a) show that these same half
retinas preferentially terminate in the appropriate
tectal region even after long survival periods.
Yoon (1972d) and Horder (1971) have further
electrophysiological data apparently showing that
if noncomplimentary retinal and tectal halves are
removed, the remaining retina spreads over the
entire inappropriate half tectum. Under these same
conditions the anatomical evidence of Roth (1972)
indicates that innervation is restricted to the
region near the lesion leaving much of the tectum
without optic fibers.

Worse yet, the electrophysiological evidence
seems self-contradictory. While Yoon (1972b)
claims both nasal and temporal hemiretinas show
plasticity, Horder (1971) has evidence that only a
nasal half retina expands in this manner and
Jacobson and Gaze (1965) have data suggesting
neither half does this. Although only a rough

---

*Figure 8. Electrophysiological map of left visual
space onto right tectum with numbers and letters
indicating corresponding electrode placements and
receptive field location. A. Normal. B. Right
caudal half tectum ablation and left optic nerve
crush 339 days prior. C. Ablation of a rectangular
piece of dorsal right tectum and left optic crush
106 days prior. Crosshatching indicates pia
covered ablation area with o indicating electrode
positions giving no responses.*

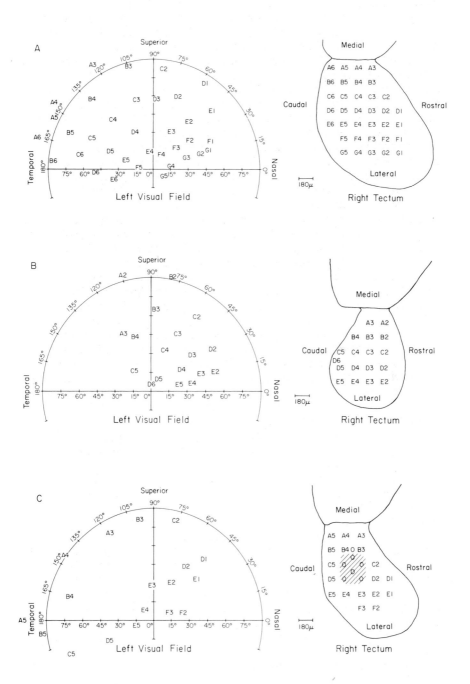

mediolateral incision is sufficient to induce
complete field compression onto the rostral tectum
in Yoon's hands (1971), a similarly placed even
larger lesion does not produce this result in
Sharma's (1972b) experiment. Medial or lateral
tectal ablations have been reported not to cause
plasticity (Gaze and Jacobson 1965) and the thought
that this may be a consequence of interference with
the medial optic tract is supported by Yoon (1971).
Yet after removal of rostral tectum causing
comparable tract damage, a compressed visual field
representation onto caudal tectum is nevertheless
found, according to Sharma (1972b). In the original
Gaze and Sharma (1970) study simple removal of
caudal tectum invariably resulted in tectal
positions from which two widely separated receptive
fields could be recorded. Not one instance of this
field reduplication was found by Yoon (1971).

Many of these apparently conflicting electrophysiological results may very possibly be
accounted for by differences in postoperative
survival periods or subtle surgical variables.
However, there is as yet no direct evidence or
convincing arguments that would resolve these
discrepancies. In the additional light of the
chick, adult frog, and goldfish anatomical investigations all showing selective innervation, one may
perhaps question whether some of these goldfish
electrophysiological experiments accurately
describe the distribution of optic axon terminals
on the tectum. The recordings from goldfish with
retinal lesions, at variance with anatomical
results, would seem particularly suspect because
of possible optic aberrations, changes in retinal
topography, and regeneration of new retina
consequent to surgery. While the electrical
measurements following tectal lesions would seem
to indicate some genuine change in fiber distribution, better techniques may be called for. We
have recently employed a more refined electrophysiological method recording with the eye under
water instead of in air, as previously done, and
with more precise electrode placement and eye
alignment techniques (Meyer 1973b). Initial results
raise in our minds the possibility that some
measurement errors may exist in previous work.
Whatever is the case, it seems to us that the

goldfish electrophysiology work showing plasticity
needs further analysis and some validation of the
inferred fiber distribution and connectivity
pattern by anatomical behavioral or postsynaptic
recording methods.

REFERENCES

Attardi, D.G. and Sperry, R.W. (1963). Preferential selection of central pathways by regenerating optic fibers. *Exp. Neurol.* 7, 46–64.

Cronly-Dillon, J. (1968). Pattern of retinotectal connections after retinal regeneration. *J. Neurophysiol.* 31, 410–418.

DeLong, R.C. and Coulombre, A.J. (1965). Development of the retinotectal topographic projection in the chick embryo. *Exp. Neurol.* 13, 351–363.

Gaze, R.M. (1958). The representation of the retina on the optic lobe of the frog. *Q.J. Exp. Physiol.* 43, 209–214.

Gaze, R.M. (1959). Regeneration of the optic nerve in *Xenopus laevis*. *Q.J. Exp. Physiol.* 44, 290–308.

Gaze, R.M. (1970). "The Formation of Nerve Connections." New York: Academic Press.

Gaze, R.M., Jacobson, M. and Székely, G. (1963). The retinotectal projection in *Xenopus* with compound eyes. *J. Physiol.* 165, 484–499.

Gaze, R.M., Jacobson, M. and Székely, G. (1965). On the formation of connexions by compound eyes in *Xenopus*. *J. Physiol.* 176, 409–417.

Gaze, R.M. and Keating, M.J. (1972). The visual system and "neuronal specificity." *Nature (Lond.)* 237, 375–378.

Gaze, R.M. and Sharma, S.C. (1970). Axial differences in the reinnervation of the goldfish optic tectum by regenerating optic nerve fibres. *Exp. Brain Res.* 10, 171–181.

Horder, T.J. (1971). Retention by fish optic nerve fibers regenerating to new terminal sites in the tectum, of "chemospecific" affinity for their original sites. *J. Physiol. (Lond.)* 216, 53P–55P.

Hunt, R.K. and Jacobson, M. (1973). Neuronal locus specificity: altered pattern of spatial deployment in fused fragments of embryonic *Xenopus* eyes. *Science* 180, 509–511.

Jacobson, M. (1962). The representation of the retina on the optic tectum of the frog. Correlation between retinotectal magnification factor and retinal ganglion cell count. *Q.J. Exp. Physiol.* 47, 170–178.

Jacobson, M. and Gaze, R.M. (1965). Selection of appropriate tectal connections by regenerating optic nerve fibers in adult goldfish. *Exp. Neurol.* 13, 418-430.

Kelly, J.P. (1970). The specification of retino-tectal connections in the avian embryo. *Anat. Rec.* 166, 329.

Kirsche, W. and Kirsche, K. (1961). Experimentelle Untersuchungen zur Frage Regeneration und Funktion des Tectum opticum von *Carassius carassius. L.Z. Mikroskop Anat. Forsch.* 67, 140-182.

Larsell, O. (1929). The effects of experimental excision of one eye on the development of the optic lobe and optic layer in larvae of the tree frog. *J. Comp. Neurol.* 48, 331-353.

Lettvin, J.Y., Maturana, H.R., McCulloch, W.S. and Pitts, W.H. (1960). Anatomy and physiology of vision in the frog *(Rana pipiens). J. Neurophysiol.* 43, 129-175.

Maturana, H.R., Lettvin, J.Y., McCulloch, W.S. and Pitts, W.H. (1959). Physiological evidence that cut optic nerve fibers in the frog regenerate to their proper places in the tectum. *Science* 130, 1709.

Meyer, R.L. (1973a). Growth of half eyes onto the optic tectum of goldfish. *Calif. Inst. Technol. Div. of Biol. Ann. Rep.* N. 36, p. 45.

Meyer, R.L. (1973b). Underwater mapping of the visual field of fish. *Calif. Inst. Technol. Div. of Biol. Ann. Rep.* No. 35, pp. 44-45.

Meyer, R.L. and Sperry, R.W. (1973). Tests for neuroplasticity in the anuran retinotectal system. *Exp. Neurol.* 40, 525-539.

Roth, R. (1972). Normal and regenerated retino-tectal projections in the goldfish. Ph.D. Thesis. Case Western Reserve University.

Saunders, J.W. and Gasseling, M.T. (1968). Ectodermal-mesenchymal interactions in the origin of limb symmetry. *In* R. Fleischmajer and R.E. Billingham (Eds.), "Epithelian-Mesenchymal Interactions," Baltimore: Williams and Wilkins pp. 78-97.

Sharma, S.C. (1972a). Redistribution of visual projections in altered optic tecta of adult goldfish. *Proc. Nat. Acad. Sci. USA* 69, 2637-2639.

Sharma, S.C. (1972b). Reformation of retinotectal projections after various tectal ablations in adult goldfish. *Exp. Neurol.* 34, 171-182.

Sharma, S.C. and Gaze, R.M. (1971). The retinotopic organization of visual responses from tectal reimplants in adult goldfish. *Arch. Ital. Biol.* 109, 357-366.

Sperry, R.W. (1943). Visuomotor coordination in the newt *(Triturus viridescens)* after regeneration of the optic nerve. *J. Comp. Neurol.* 79, 33-55.

Sperry, R.W. (1944). Optic nerve regeneration with return of vision in anurans. *J. Neurophysiol.* 7, 57-69.

Sperry, R.W. (1945). Restoration of vision after crossing of optic nerves and after contralateral transposition of the eye. *J. Neurophysiol.* 8, 15-28.

Sperry, R.W. (1948). Patterning of central synapses in regeneration of the optic nerve in teleosts. *Physiol. Zool.* 28, 351-361.

Sperry, R.W. (1951). Mechanisms of neural maturation. *In* S.S. Stevens (Ed.), "Handbook of Experimental Psychology," New York: Wiley. pp. 236-280.

Sperry, R.W. (1963). Chemoaffinity in the orderly growth of nerve fiber patterns and connections. *Proc. Nat. Acad. Sci. USA.* 50, 703-710.

Sperry, R.W. (1965). Embryogenesis of behavioral nerve nets. *In* R.L. Dehan and H. Ursprung (Eds.) "Organogenesis," New York: Holt. pp. 161-186.

Straznicky, K. (1973). The formation of the optic fibre projection after partial tectal removal in *Xenopus*. *J. Embryol. Exp. Morph.* 29, 397-409.

Straznicky, K. and Gaze, R.M. (1972). The development of the tectum in *Xenopus laevis:* An autoradiographic study. *J. Embryol. Exp. Morph.* 28, 87-115.

Straznicky, K., Gaze, R.M. and Keating, M.J. (1971). The retinotectal projections after uncrossing the optic chiasma in *Xenopus* with one compound eye. *J. Embryol. Exp. Morph.* 26, 523-542.

Weiss, P. (1939). "Principles of Development." New York: Holt.

Yoon, M. (1971). Reorganization of retinotectal projection following surgical operations on the optic tectum in goldfish. *Exp. Neurol.* 33, 395-411.

Yoon, M. (1972a). Reversibility of the reorganization of retinotectal projection in goldfish. *Exp. Neurol.* 35, 565-577.

Yoon, M. (1972b). Synaptic plasticities of the retina and of the optic tectum in goldfish. *Amer. Zool.* 12, 106.

Yoon, M. (1972c). Transposition of the visual projection from the nasal hemiretina onto the foreign rostral zone of the optic tectum in goldfish. *Exp. Neurol.* 37, 451-462.

Yoon, M. (1973). Retention of the original topographic polarity by the 180° rotated tectal reimplant in young adult goldfish. *J. Physiol.* 233, 575-588.

Supported by the F.P. Hixon Fund of the California Institute of Technology, U.S. Public Health Service grant No. MH-03372, and training grant Nos. GM-00086 and GM-02031 from the National Institutes of Health.

NEUROANATOMICAL CORRELATES OF
SPARED OR ALTERED FUNCTION
AFTER BRAIN LESIONS IN THE NEWBORN HAMSTER

Gerald E. Schneider and Sonal R. Jhaveri
Massachusetts Institute of Technology
Cambridge, Massachusetts

Comparisons of the effects of surgical lesions
in the visual system of adult and neonatal
hamsters provide examples of sparing of function,
loss of function, and maladaptive alterations of
function after damage inflicted early in life. In
this paper, we will review these examples, adding
to them some previously unpublished findings.
Experimental neuroanatomical evidence will be
cited for each example to argue that sparing or
alteration of function can be due to a post-
traumatic growth of anomalous axonal connections.
The formation of such connections is influenced
by several factors governing the growth or
regeneration of axons; these factors have been
specified in a further series of experiments on
the neuroanatomical bases of plasticity.

Effects of lesions on visually guided behavior in the hamster: the role of age at time of injury

The Syrian golden hamster (*Mesocricetus
auratus*) is particularly useful for studies of
neuroanatomical plasticity and recovery of
function. The gestation period of only 16 days
is among the shortest for eutherian mammals, and
the central nervous system at birth is corres-
pondingly immature; yet the animal grows rapidly,
and the brain reaches full size in only 3 months.
In both the neonate and the adult, two major
visual structures, the superior colliculus and
the striate cortex, can each be readily manipulated surgically. Behavioral studies following
surgical ablation of these structures in the adult
hamster have revealed exceptionally clear and
long-lasting symptoms. Thus, this species seemed
ideally suited to a comparison of effects of
lesions inflicted early or late in life.
The development of the brain at birth differs
widely among various mammals. The short gestation

65

period of the Syrian hamster makes it possible to
study effects of injury to the immature brain
without using *in utero* surgery, a procedure which
would be required for similar investigation of
other species. The immature state of the hamster
brain appears comparable in development to that
of a 2 1/2 - 3 month human fetus, judging from
photographs of whole fetuses in Hamilton, Boyd,
and Mossman (1962) and in Ferm (1967), and by
comparing notes on myelination of central-nervous-
system pathways (Clark and Telford 1964;
Kretschman 1967; Yakovlev and Lecours 1967).
According to the light-microscopy data of Clark
(1966), myelination in the central nervous system
of the hamster does not begin until the end of
the first postnatal week. The major cell migra-
tions in the developing neocortex are still taking
place at the time of birth (Shimada and Langman
1970). The cerebral hemispheres have not yet grown
posteriorly to cover the midbrain, and the surface
of the superior colliculus is completely exposed
beneath a thin cartilagenous interparietal bone
(see fig. 1 in Schneider 1973). Hence, the
colliculus at birth is more readily accessible to
surgical manipulation than in other commonly used
laboratory animals.

Three comparisons of the behavioral effects
of lesions made in neonates and adults are
summarized in figure 1:

Visual-cortex ablation. In the first example,
surgical ablations of neocortical area 17 and some
bordering cortex were made by aspiration in 8-day-
old pups ("early" cortex lesions) or in fully
grown hamsters ("late" lesions). A well-restricted
bilateral lesion in the adult, even if it spared a
small portion of caudal area 17, was sufficient in
many cases to cause a failure to learn a simple
pattern discrimination, involving a choice between
simultaneously presented horizontal and vertical
stripes (Schneider 1969, 1970). Animals with early
lesions, when allowed to grow to 3 or more months
of age and tested on the same problem, showed
some ability to learn this pattern discrimination
task (5 out of 7 hamsters with complete removal of
area 17 reached criterion), even when the early
lesion was considerably larger than in the adult-
operated animals (Schneider 1970). However, the

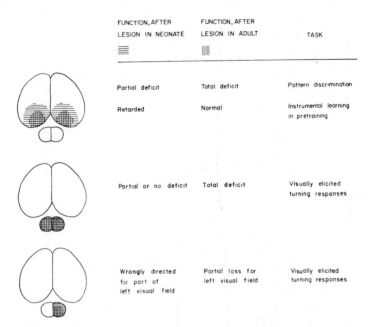

	FUNCTION, AFTER LESION IN NEONATE ≣	FUNCTION, AFTER LESION IN ADULT ⦀	TASK
	Partial deficit	Total deficit	Pattern discrimination
	Retarded	Normal	Instrumental learning in pretraining
	Partial or no deficit	Total deficit	Visually elicited turning responses
	Wrongly directed for part of left visual field	Partial loss for left visual field	Visually elicited turning responses

Figure 1. Summary of behavioral effects of brain lesions in the Syrian hamster. The left-hand column depicts the lesions on dorsal-view diagrams of the cerebral hemispheres and the superior colliculi. Early lesions of cortex were made in 8-day-old animals; early lesions of the colliculi were made, in most cases, on the day of birth (16 days after conception); lesions in adulthood were made in animals at least 12 weeks old. All animals were tested in adulthood. (From Schneider, in Stein and Eidelberg, in press.)

animals operated as neonates did reveal deficiencies in their performance in that they were slower in learning the task when compared to normal controls.

The relative sparing of function after early posterior cortex lesions was found to be dependent on the behavior studied, since on a different task, it was found that the animals with early lesions, and not those with late lesions, were deficient. In the pretraining part of the testing, involving an instrumental conditioning procedure in which the animals were required merely to open the doorways and obtain a water reward, the animals with early lesions were severely retarded, while those with lesions acquired in adulthood were normal.

Bilateral lesions of midbrain tectum. In the second example (fig. 1), bilateral lesions of the superior colliculus were made by undercutting this structure in adult hamsters. The procedure resulted in an enduring loss of the turning response which is normally elicited by visual presentation of sunflower seeds. No recovery of head turning, head raising, or rearing in response to presentation of seeds in any part of the visual field was observed in subjects with the most complete lesions, surviving up to 8 months after surgery (Schneider 1966, 1969). Such a complete deficit occurred when the tectal undercut separated the entire extent of the superficial optic layers (site of termination of the visual afferents) from the deeper layers (origin of descending pathways). However, if the superficial tectal layers were completely destroyed at birth by application of heat to the overlying skull, the animals grew up to show a considerable sparing of visually elicited turning (Schneider 1970). We have recently reexamined this finding in a quantitative study of visual orienting movements, using videotape apparatus. With this apparatus, we recorded the behavior of animals with total or partial early tectum lesions and analyzed their turning responses, using slow-motion and single-frame playback. Accurate turning occurred toward stimuli presented in much of the visual field; but, in addition, definite abnormalities in initial head movements (under- or over-shoots) occurred in response to stimuli presented in particular parts of the field (Singer, Schneider, and Jhaveri, unpublished data).

Unilateral lesions of midbrain tectum. In the third example, the midbrain lesions were made on only one side. The surgery in adults, made by unilateral undercutting, resulted in loss of orienting movements toward the visual field contralateral to the lesion. (None of these lesions were complete, and partial return of function was always observed -- Schneider 1966, 1969.) In the cases of unilateral tectum lesions

made in the neonate, the most interesting finding
was a behavioral anomaly scarcely ever seen in
normal control animals: turning in the wrong
direction in response to stimuli presented in
parts of the field of the eye contralateral to the
lesion (Schneider 1973 and unpublished data). Such
misdirected turning was most marked in animals in
which the ipsilateral eye was also removed at
birth. It occurred most often when stimuli were
presented in the upper temporal field (see below).

Mechanisms underlying sparing or alteration of function: the role of anomalous connections

Visual-cortex ablation. Hamsters with early
visual-cortex ablations were able to solve a
pattern discrimination problem which animals with
less extensive lesions sustained in adulthood
failed to solve. Histological analysis revealed a
virtually complete atrophy of the dorsal nucleus
of the lateral geniculate body (LGd) in hamsters
with early lesions which were able to solve the
problem (Schneider 1970). This finding ruled out
the possibility that spared remnants of area 17,
or an anomalous cortical projection of geniculate
body neurons, subserved the functional sparing. By
contrast, the animals with lesions inflicted in
adulthood showed spared remnants of posterior area
17 and a considerable number of surviving neurons
in LGd, including the areas showing retrograde
degenerative changes. Yet, such anatomical sparing,
in many cases, did not suffice for recovery of
pattern vision.
        A search for altered retinal projections in
hamsters with early visual-cortex ablations did
reveal one change (besides the near absence of a
projection to the dorsal thalamus): the projection
to the superficial gray layer of the superior
colliculus showed an altered pattern of lamination.
This change was demonstrated histologically using
the Fink-Heimer method for staining sections from
the brains of adult animals which survived 5-7
days following eye removal. (No degeneration
debris resulting from neonatal lesions could be
observed in the adult animals with the use of the
silver method.) The change is illustrated in
figure 2. It consists of a loss of the contrast,

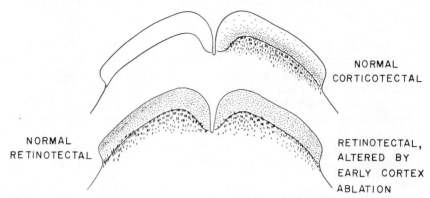

Figure 2. Charts of frontal sections through the superior colliculi of 2 hamster brains, showing the superficial gray layer and the underlying optic fiber layer. (Upper) Axonal and terminal degeneration, depicted by line segments and dots, respectively, in a normal adult hamster which survived 4 days following ablation of the right visual cortex. (Lower) Axonal and terminal degeneration in an adult hamster which had under- gone ablation of posterior cortex on the right side at birth -- so the corticotectal connection illustrated in the upper chart was absent; at age 25 weeks both eyes were removed and the animal was sacrificed after 7 days. The left side shows the normal pattern of retinofugal degeneration for this survival time, with the densest projections in the superficial sublamina; the right side shows an alteration in the laminar pattern. Both brains were stained by the Fink-Heimer modification of a Nauta silver technique. (From Schneider, in Stein and Eidelberg, in press.)

normally conspicuous laterally, between the heavy degeneration in the dorsal part and lighter degeneration in the more ventral part of the superficial gray layer. This could be interpreted as a shifting of some of the more superficial axon endings into the deeper region normally occupied by corticotectal afferents. Alternatively, the deeper endings may have increased in density without a change in the more superficial distri- bution.

This slight anomaly may be relevant to the functional sparing because it could result in some enhancement of function in a pathway whereby visual information can reach the telencephalon. The colliculus has a projection to neocortex by way of a synapse in the nucleus lateralis posterior (LP) of the thalamus (Schneider 1970, 1973). This pathway, unlike the other known routes whereby visual information can reach neocortex (geniculostriate and pretecto-thalamo-cortical), was partially spared by the neonatal cortex lesions. The tectal route to cortex does appear to subserve some pattern discrimination ability in species with a relatively large superior colliculus like the tree shrew (Snyder and Diamond 1968) and the squirrel (Levey, Harris, and Jane 1973). These animals can learn simple pattern discrimination problems after total surgical removal of striate cortex in adulthood. (In the hedgehog, poor but nevertheless above chance performance on such problems can be achieved after total striate cortex ablation -- see Hall and Diamond 1968.) With such evidence at hand, it is not clear why the adult hamster or rat loses pattern discrimination ability after removal of area 17.

It is interesting to contrast the findings on hamsters with those on rats. Rats with early visual-cortex ablations develop several anomalous retinal projections not observed in hamsters, including one directly to LP and a considerably enlarged area of termination in the pretectal region (Cunningham 1972). Yet, such rats have failed to show any evidence of spared pattern vision (Bland and Cooper 1969; Bauer and Hughes 1970; Thompson 1970). Thus, having more anomalous connections does not mean having more sparing of function: some of the altered connections may even be maladaptive.

Bilateral lesions of midbrain tectum. Bilateral ablation of the superficial layers of the superior colliculus at birth results in the development of several anomalous retinal projections (Schneider and Nauta 1969; Schneider 1970, 1973). Figure 3 depicts these alterations which we have seen in dozens of cases. Following eye removal, degenerating axons can be traced to the damaged midbrain

71

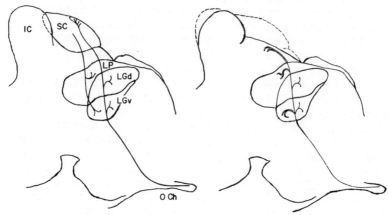

Figure 3. (Left) Lateral-view reconstruction of rostral brainstem of normal adult hamster. Heavy line depicts schematically the course of a group of optic-tract axons and some of their terminations; the tectothalamic pathway is shown in a similar manner. (Right) Similar view of brainstem of adult hamster which had undergone destruction of the superficial layers of the superior colliculus in the neonate. Dotted lines represent the standard outline of a normal case. Anomalous optic-tract connections are depicted by double lines. (From Schneider, 1973.)

region; the majority are found near the surface with some subjacent termination. This represents an abnormal pattern of retinotectal projection for the commonly studied mammals. It is uncertain whether these axons are the fibers which were transected during surgery and have regenerated into the region of damage, or whether they are fibers which had not yet reached the tectum at the time of the neonatal ablation. Both possibilities seem likely. A new projection appears in the LP, revealed by silver staining of a very dense field of terminal degeneration, as dense as that seen in the lateral geniculate body in the same cases. Observations with the electron microscope in one such case confirm the existence of degenerating boutons with axodendritic synapses in LP (Kalil and Schneider, in preparation). There is also an increased amount of optic-tract termination in the ventral nucleus of the lateral geniculate body (LGv). The abnormalities in the diencephalon occur in just those areas normally receiving projections from the superficial layers of the superior colliculus (fig. 3). These normal tectofugal projections are missing after an early lesion of the colliculus (Schneider 1973).

The extent of the retinotectal connection is correlated with the sparing of visually elicited turning behavior. In cases where retinal projections could be traced to the lateral but not to the medial part of the residual tectum, the animals had shown head turning in response to seeds presented in the lower but not the upper visual field (see fig. 1 of Schneider 1970). This defect is similar to one observed in adult-operated hamsters in which only the medial part of the superior colliculus was undercut. In a few cases where the early tectum lesion was very deep and extensive, comparatively few retinofugal axons reached the dorsal midbrain, whereas the abnormal projections to the LP and the LGv were extensive. In these animals, repeated attempts to elicit turning with visually presented sunflower seeds yielded responses only for the lower nasal field -- the area of greatest responsiveness in normal animals. The same animals displayed brisk lateral turning in response to stimulation of the vibrissae. However, hamsters with a larger abnormal projection into the damaged midbrain were found to have visual orienting abilities that were nearly normal during informal testing. Histology in these cases did not reveal heavier abnormal projections in the diencephalon.

The correspondence of the behavioral performance with the retinal projection to the midbrain provides evidence that anomalous axonal connections are responsible for a sparing of function. One must also consider the possible role of visual inputs to the residual tectum other than the direct retinotectal projection. A connection from posterior neocortex (area 17 and bordering areas) to the superior colliculus is apparently not sufficient, since 5 animals with early tectum ablations have been observed to recover their visual orienting ability rapidly following bilateral ablation of this cortex in the adult (unpublished data, including analysis of one case with videotape recording and playback). A possible role of a connection to the tectum which may originate in the LGv cannot be ruled out. Such a connection has been identified recently in the cat and rat by Graybiel (1974) and in the cat by Rosenquist and Edwards (1973).

Unilateral lesions of midbrain tectum. In the third example summarized in figure 1, we have the clearest case of a behavioral effect attributable to an anomalous axonal pathway. Hamsters with unilateral tectum lesions inflicted at birth grow up with the anomalies depicted in figure 3 only on the side of the lesion. In addition, there is a retinal projection to the "wrong" side of the midbrain.

If one eye is removed from a normal adult hamster, and the brain is prepared for silver staining 5 days postoperatively, degenerating axons can be followed in serial sections to the superficial gray layer of the superior colliculus on the contralateral side. Of the degenerating axons that remain uncrossed at the optic chiasm, the small component that reaches the colliculus appears to terminate anteriorly within the layer of optic fibers (stratum opticum) except perhaps for a few scattered axons in the overlying super-ficial gray layer (see Schneider 1970).

If the same experiment is performed with adult hamsters which had suffered unilateral ablation of the superficial layers of the superior colliculus on the day of birth, some striking anomalies are found (Schneider 1973). As in the case of bilateral lesions, axons from the eye contra-lateral to the early lesion can be followed to the damaged area, where evidence of termination appears near the surface. Degenerating axons can also be traced, in most of the cases, into an anomalous decussation across the tectal midline. They terminate in a medial strip of the superficial gray layer on the undamaged side. Axons from the other eye terminate, as expected, in the superfi-cial gray of the undamaged colliculus, except that they do not terminate in a medial strip of tissue which corresponds to the area innervated by the "wrong" eye.

The mutually exclusive distribution of terminating axons from the two eyes might suggest that
normal and anomalous fibers compete for available
terminal space. This suggestion is consistent
with the consequences of removing the axons which
normally project to the undamaged tectum by an eye
removal performed at the same time as the midbrain
lesion. The recrossing axons increase in quantity
and distribute to all or most of the superficial
gray layer on the "wrong" side of the brain. In
the medial third or half of this tectum, the
density of terminal degeneration appears similar
to that seen in normals, but many of the axons are
oriented mediolaterally rather than rostrocaudally.
(If only one eye is removed at birth, leaving the
colliculus undamaged, the normal ipsilateral
projection to the tectum from the remaining eye
does increase, terminating in scattered patches in
the superficial gray, mostly anteriorly. However,
the quantity of this increase is small compared
with the distribution of the abnormal recrossing
bundle.)
These neuroanatomical anomalies lead to a prediction about the behavior of the animals, in
particular those with a lesion of one tectum
combined with a removal of the ipsilateral eye.
Figure 4 (left) shows a diagram of neural pathways
underlying visually elicited head turning in the
Syrian hamster, according to conclusions based on
effects of selective lesions in adult animals.
Visually elicited turns to the left depend on a
pathway from the left eye to the right superior
colliculus, which gives rise to a descending pathway (probably the crossed predorsal bundle) to
the lower motor mechanisms controlling primarily
the axial muscles. Symmetric pathways on the other
side control turning to the right. If the right
tectum is damaged at birth, and the right eye
removed as well, the growth of anomalous retinal
projections to both sides of the midbrain should
lead to turning responses in either direction from
stimulation in the visual field of the remaining
left eye (fig. 4, right). The nature of the
response would be expected to depend on the topography of the projections, at least if other inputs
to the tectum can be ignored.
The results of videotape recording and slow-

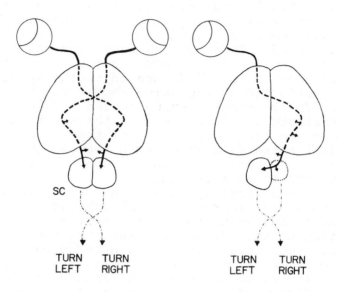

Figure 4. Axonal pathways in the Syrian hamster critical in the control of visually elicited turning of the head. (Left) Top view of eyes, cerebral hemispheres, and superior colliculi (SC); the latter are displaced caudally for the sake of the diagram. The course and termination of axons of the retinal ganglion cells are indicated by the heavy lines and arrows (cf. fig. 3). These axons pass below the forebrain, and most cross at the optic chiasm and rise along the surface of the diencephalon (where some axons terminate), finally reaching the SC. Connections in the right SC mediate turning toward the left via descending pathways to the brainstem and spinal cord; similarly, connections in the left colliculus mediate turning toward the right. (Right) Similar view of brain of hamster in which the right eye and the superficial layers of SC were ablated at birth. Axons from the remaining eye not only form anomalous connections in the diencephalon, but also form an abnormal pattern of termination in the midbrain tectum, some ending in the area of early surgical damage, others recrossing to the left SC. This leads to a prediction of abnormal turning behavior in response to stimuli in at least part of the left visual field (From Schneider, in Stein and Eidelberg, in press.)

motion analysis of visually elicited orienting
movements, using perimetry procedures developed
with the help of David Singer at M.I.T., support
the prediction. The animals were trained to hold
their heads in a relatively constant position with
their noses in a small hole where seeds were
occasionally presented. Turns were elicited by the
appearance of a small black rubber sphere
(diameter 1.2 cm.) from behind a white baffle at a
distance of about 14 cm. from the animal's head.
Responses were rewarded by presentation of sunflower seeds, regardless of the accuracy or
direction of the turns. Figure 5 illustrates
results for two cases (see fig. 17 of Schneider
(1973), for results obtained with an earlier case).
The open circles represent points in the visual
field where the stimulus elicited a turn in the
correct direction. Most of these turns were fairly
accurate in directing the head toward the stimulus.

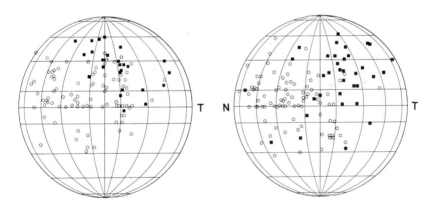

*Figure 5. Results of videotape analyses of the
left visual field in cases 44-8 (left) and 44-10
(right), in which the right eye and the superficial
layers of the right superior colliculus were
ablated at birth. The visual field is represented
as the surface of a sphere with the nasal pole at
the left; grid lines are 20° apart with extra
lines at horizontal eye level and at 90° from the
straight ahead. Open circles represent positions
of the stimulus in the field where turns in the
correct direction were elicited. Black squares
represent turns in the wrong direction.*

Dark squares represent points in the field where stimulus presentations elicited turns in the wrong direction. In these cases the topography of the head movements has not been found to be consistently related to the position of the stimulus in the visual field. A regular finding in such cases is that most of the wrong-direction turns occur in response to stimuli in the upper-temporal field. The relative size of the abnormal region in the field varies from animal to animal.

It is interesting to note what such results imply about the anatomy. For example, if the recrossing fibers terminated on the wrong side in a retinotopic pattern which is mirror symmetric to that observed normally, one would predict that the animals would turn toward points in the visual field symmetrically opposite (with respect to the vertical meridian) to the points of stimulus presentation. Such a result was obtained by Sperry (1945), using frogs in which the optic nerve axons were forced to regenerate at the chiasm into the ipsilateral optic tract, hence growing to the wrong side of the midbrain. The results with hamsters are different in both behavior and morphology. In our cases with neonatal ablation of the right eye and the superficial layers of the right tectum, the population of axons from the remaining eye distribute to both the damaged and undamaged sides of the midbrain surface. The two sides together may form parts of only one continuous tectal space. Thus, a single retinotopic map would be spread over both sides of the midbrain. The details of the actual topography have not been fully studied, but in order to suggest what the pattern might be, we can compare the normal retino-tectal topography (Jhaveri and Schneider 1974) with the overall distribution of retinofugal axons in the residual right tectum, and its continuation through the abnormal decussation into the left side (Schneider 1973; and fig. 4). The representation of the nasal parts of the visual field is closest to the points of entry of optic-tract axons into the colliculus. The axons coursing medially in the colliculus represent the superior visual field. Taking these two facts together with the observation of a medial gathering of axons to form the abnormal decussation, one can

predict that axons representing the more superior
and the more temporal visual field would be the
ones most likely to cross the tectal midline.
This agrees with the behavioral finding that the
head turning directed to the wrong side was most
often in response to stimulation in the upper
temporal field. However, the behavioral findings
also suggest that the recrossing fibers do not
form a mirror image map, or even an orderly one,
on the wrong side. Below we will present anatomical
findings on the topography of recrossing axons
which are consistent with the predictions from
behavior.

Anomalous connections form under the influence of
specific factors governing the growth or regeneration of axons after lesions

The evidence that abnormal axonal connections
are important in accounting for sparing or alteration of function after early brain damage has
encouraged us to investigate the factors
influencing the growth or regeneration of axons
after discrete lesions in the neonatal hamster.
The phenomenon of recrossing retinotectal axons
reviewed above provides the best evidence for the
first factor: a tendency for axons to invade
vacated terminal space, and compete with other
axons for occupancy, in some cases exclusive
occupancy (Schneider 1973). This factor can lead
to dramatic departures from the normal specificity of connections. Optic-tract axons can be
induced to terminate not only in anomalous
locations within the visual system but also
outside the system. For example, if the axons of
the brachium of the inferior colliculus (BIC),
which carry auditory information into the medial
geniculate body (MGB), are transected in hamsters
at birth and simultaneously a lesion of the
superior colliculus is made, then some optic-tract
axons enter the MGB near the caudal pole of the
lateral geniculate and terminate there (Schneider
1973). (The area of entry is the only region where
optic-tract axons normally course over the surface
of the medial geniculate.) This small projection
was found in 13 cases with early midbrain lesions.
In each case the large bundles of fibers of the

BIC were found to be missing on one side along with the superficial layers of the superior colliculus. In 8 additional cases with similar colliculus lesions but with partial sparing of the BIC, no evidence of the abnormal projection to MGB was found. One further case, with a deep unilateral ablation of the superior colliculus combined with a complete transection of the BIC at birth, was studied with the electron microscope. Evidence of degenerating boutons with axodendritic synapses in MGB was obtained on the side of the early lesions, after removal of both eyes in the adult (Kalil and Schneider, in preparation). One cannot help wondering whether these hamsters might be able to hear with their eyes! But we have no information about the functioning of this connection.

Figure 6 illustrates diagrammatically the tendency for axons to invade "open" or vacated terminal space, with competition between axon populations for exclusive occupancy. Concepts

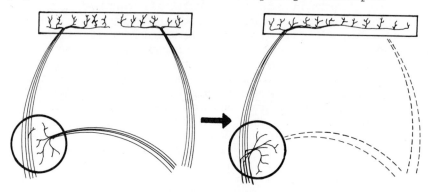

INVASION OF VACATED TERMINAL SPACE

Figure 6. Diagrammatic illustration of the concept of a tendency for axons to invade available or vacated terminal space and compete with other axons for, in some cases, exclusive occupancy. Two hypothetical structures are indicated, each innervated from 2 sources, but the terminal distribution of one is limited by the presence of the other. This is demonstrated by the consequences of removing one of the sources of input to each structure: the other system then expands its terminal field. (Modified from Schneider, 1973.)

similar to this have become popular in reports of neuroplasticity experiments in the literature (e.g., see Bernstein and Goodman 1973), where one can read frequently of the invasion of vacated "synaptic space". We prefer to use the more general term "terminal space" since there may be few, if any, synapses formed at the time the abnormal distribution of axons occurs (e.g., see Lund and Lund (1972) for a study of synaptogenesis in the superior colliculus of the rat). The "space" which different axon populations occupy is not necessarily defined only in terms of available postsynaptic sites

What additional factors can be demonstrated? Consider the anomalous optic-tract termination in the LP (fig. 3): it is always found within the tissue which normally would have received a projection from the superficial layers of the superior colliculus. The amount of abnormal termination can be shown to be influenced by a factor separate from the tendency for innervation of vacated terminal space: a kind of compensatory sprouting, or "pruning effect" (Schneider 1973). Consider the two groups of hamsters with early unilateral tectum lesions described above: the ones in which the ipsilateral eye was also removed developed a much larger projection to the remaining undamaged tectum via the anomalous decussation. The larger projection to the midbrain was found to be correlated with a smaller projection to the LP, although the degree of thalamic denervation was equivalent for the two groups. Apparently, the greater the degree of pruning of the upper branches of the axonal tree (in the colliculus), the greater the compensatory sprouting by lower branches (in LP).

Figure 7 illustrates this second factor which influences the formation of abnormal axonal connections after early lesions. It might be considered to be a tendency for axons to conserve at least a minimum quantity of terminal arborization. An action of this factor independent of the first factor is suggested by the hypertrophy of the dorsal terminal nucleus of the accessory optic tract observed in cases of early tectum lesions (Schneider 1973). This nucleus appears to receive few, if any, connections from the region damaged

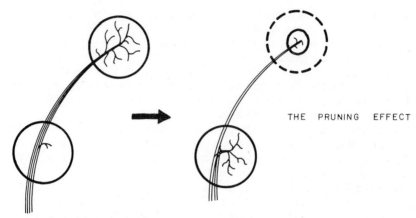

THE PRUNING EFFECT

Figure 7. Diagrammatic illustration of the concept of a tendency for growing axons to conserve at least a minimum quantity of terminal arborization. (Modified from Schneider, 1973.)

by the early lesion, yet it undergoes an enlargement, receiving throughout its increased volume a projection from the upper retina (Jhaveri 1973). We suggest that the hypertrophy is induced by a compensatory sprouting of axons passing near the nucleus on their way to the tectum.

Two additional factors concern the topography of the connections. They were suggested by behavioral analysis of hamsters with tectum lesions made at birth (Schneider 1973; Schneider, Singer, Stevenson, and Jhaveri, unpublished) and were demonstrated by experimental neuroanatomical studies (Jhaveri 1973; Jhaveri and Schneider 1974).

Anatomical methods for study of topography

To study the topography of optic-tract projections in adult Syrian hamsters, we made small retinal lesions by passing radio-frequency current through an electrode which penetrated the schlera at positions measured with respect to the attachments of the rectus muscles. Five days after surgery, each animal was perfused and the brain prepared for the staining of degenerating axons and terminals (Fink and Heimer 1967) in a closely spaced series of sections. The following report is based on

results obtained in 33 normal animals and in 14
animals in which the rostral part of the superficial gray layer of the superior colliculus
had been ablated on the day of birth. In many
cases only one retinal lesion was made but
sometimes one in each eye; as many as three
lesions were made in one eye of a few normal
animals.

After processing the tissue sections, we
used a method of reconstruction which involved
mapping of the observed degeneration argyro-
philia on lateral and dorsal views of the
brainstem surface. Figure 8 shows our standard
dorsal-view reconstruction of a normal adult
hamster, with stereotaxic coordinates indicated.
To use this reconstruction in charting
degeneration in serial, frontal sections from
the brains of experimental cases, we first
placed grid lines on it which corresponded to
each section, matching major landmarks as
closely as possible. Next, a measuring scale
was determined for each section which allowed
the closest match to the standard, and the
outlines of the new brain were redrawn. (Thus,
slight overall differences in size were
corrected for, and minor changes in the scale
from section to section allowed partial
correction for variations in tissue shrinkage.)
Finally, the positions of the observed silver
deposits indicative of either fibers of passage
or fields of terminal degeneration were marked
for each section on the corresponding grid
lines, using the projection onto the horizontal
plane of relevant points on the surface of the
brainstem. (Similarly, projections onto a
vertical plane were used to obtain a lateral-
view reconstruction.) The most useful representation of a subsurface terminal site was
obtained when its position was represented at
the surface by a point along a line drawn
perpendicular to this surface. The usefulness
of such a "surface" reconstruction is
apparently due to the manner in which
terminating fibers branch or bend away from the
main optic tract at the surface of the diencephalon and extend inward along relatively
straight lines ("lines of projection").

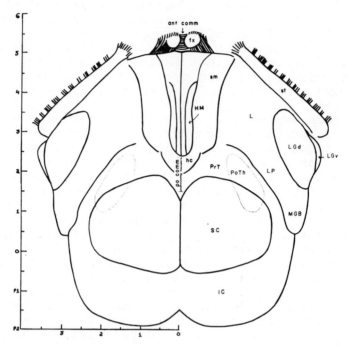

Figure 8. Dorsal view of the rostral brainstem of a 15-week-old Syrian hamster, reconstructed from serial sections cut in the tranverse plane. Surface landmarks and cell-group borders lying just beneath the optic tract are shown in solid line. (These borders were projected to the nearest surface of the tract and then onto a horizontal plane separately for every 5th 30 μm section.) Shown in fine dotted lines are the outlines of the deeplying anterior pretectal nucleus, or nucleus posterior thalami (PoTh), projected directly onto a horizontal plane. The scale units are in mm; the anterior-posterior zero corresponds to the lambda point on the overlying skull. The head is aligned so that the bregma point and the caudal edge of the interparietal bone at the midline are at the same elevation.

One example will serve to illustrate the type of analysis which led to the conclusion, from many cases, that the representation of the whole retina (or most of it) becomes compressed into the remnant of superior colliculus remaining after an early lesion. Figure 9 shows a dorsal-view reconstruction

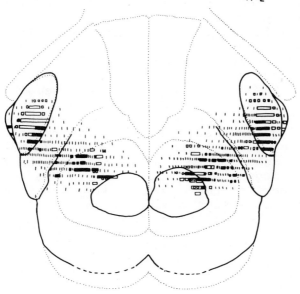

Figure 9. Dorsal-view of brainstem of case 47-2,
reconstructed from serial 30 μm sections spaced
150 μm apart, after matching to the standard reconstruction shown in fig. 8 which is indicated here
in dotted lines. The animal had a bilateral
ablation of the rostral SC at birth and a lesion
restricted to the temporal retina in each eye at
age 7½ months, 5 days before sacrifice. The brain
was prepared for histology using the method of
Fink and Heimer. Solid lines were reconstructed
from the sections and show the differences from the
standard not correctable by overall magnification
changes. Solid bars, terminal degeneration which
extends through the entire depth of the superficial
gray in SC, or which lies immediately subjacent to
the optic tract elsewhere; open bars, terminal
degeneration not contiguous to the optic tract
projected to the nearest point on the surface, or
lying in abnormal position below the optic fibers
in areas where the superficial gray of SC is present; open circles, terminal degeneration which
does not reach the surface in the superficial gray
of SC; short line segments, degenerating axons of
passage in the optic tract. Scale is 1 mm.

of the brainstem of a hamster which on the day of birth had undergone surgical ablation of the rostral superficial layers of the superior colliculus bilaterally. In the adult, a lesion of the temporal retina was made in each eye 5 days before sacrifice. The superficial gray layer of the colliculus was found to be reduced to about a third of its normal area on each side. The remaining caudal part appears to have shifted slightly, moving anteriorly towards the gap produced by the removal of the rostral tectum. Similarly, the inferior colliculi were found slightly anterior to their normal position. Terminal degeneration was found in the rostro-lateral part of the superficial gray of the superior colliculus on the right, as well as in the deeper tectal tissue just anterior to this area -- i.e., in the area of early damage. On the left, where the corresponding retinal lesion had been placed more peripherally, the terminal field of degeneration scarcely reached the spared superficial gray.

To analyze such a result, we had to make careful comparisons with results for control cases which were free of early brain damage. For the right-hand side of the brain illustrated in figure 9, we had a well-matched control case as judged by the areas of terminal degeneration in the dorsal and ventral nuclei of the lateral geniculate body. This is illustrated in figure 10a, which shows a lateral view of the right lateral geniculate body and the areas where the terminal field of degeneration, traced from our reconstruction, was observed immediately subjacent to the optic tract in each of the two cases. Figure 10b shows similar tracings of terminal fields in dorsal views of the superior colliculus, with the results for the experimental and control cases superimposed. Note that the degeneration extends further caudo-medially in the experimental case. The area of degeneration is smaller in the case with the early lesion, if only the superficial gray layer is considered. (The more anterior degeneration, which is seen beneath the optic tract, occupies much less depth and is less homogeneous than that seen in the superficial gray, and it merges with the pretectal area. It originates in the more

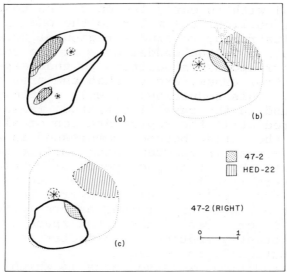

Figure 10. Analysis of the right side of case 47-2 by comparison with control case HED-22, which had a corresponding retinal lesion. (a) Lateral view of lateral geniculate body, showing areas where terminal degeneration reached the optic-tract border in the 2 cases; the star indicates the position of the optic disk area, derived from comparison of many further cases. (b) Superior colliculi of the 2 cases superimposed. (c) Same, but with caudal borders of SC matched to correct for tissue movements consequent to the early lesion. Scale, 1 mm.

peripheral parts of the temporal retina, according to the results for the left side of the experimental case illustrated.) Since the lesion on the day of birth was restricted to the rostral end of the tectum, the caudal edge of the remnant should correspond to the caudal edge of a normal case. This consideration provides justification for superimposing the reconstructions with the caudal edges of the superficial gray layer matched, as shown in figure 10c. Here one can readily see the extreme caudal displacement of the representation of the temporal retina. In the case illustrated, it lies caudal to the position which corresponds to the optic disk in the normal tectum.

If we place a lesion in the nasal retina of

an animal with an early lesion of the rostral
superior colliculus similar to the one in the
case illustrated, we find a region of terminal
degeneration in the caudal pole of the colliculus
which corresponds in position to that expected
from control cases, except that the area is
reduced. This reduction, as well as the displacement found in the case illustrated, is what one
would predict if the representation of all or
most of the retina becomes compressed in an
orderly manner in the remaining small tectum.

We attribute this phenomenon of compression to
an axon-ordering factor of unknown mechanism,
whereby the population of axons from the retina
tends to arrange its terminal arbors in topographic order, even if the total space available
is consistently reduced. This factor is illustrated
diagrammatically in figure 11.

In addition, we have cases in which certain
axons entering the superior colliculus have become
deflected from their normal course, and some of
these terminate in places considerably displaced
from the positions occupied by other fibers from
a similar retinal locus. Thus, discontinuities in
the tectal representation of retinal positions
have been observed. For example, we have four
cases in which we followed a group of fibers which
had their origin in the nasal retina, as
demonstrated by single areas of termination
reaching the ventral borders of each nucleus of
the lateral geniculate body. As they cross the
region of the early tectum lesion, some axons
appear to deviate laterally. A small terminal
field is found along their course at the lateral

Figure 11. (Opposite page) Diagrammatic illustration of the phenomenon of compression of the
retinotectal map. This could happen if the same
groups of axons each terminated in a smaller space
(upper), or if distributed axons degenerated in
numbers proportional to the reduction in terminal
space, leaving the remainder to terminate each
with normal-sized end arbors (lower). In either
case, the axon groups maintain a normal relationship relative to each other.

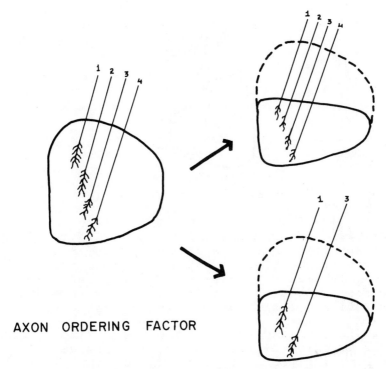

AXON   ORDERING   FACTOR

margins of the superficial gray layer of the
colliculus, while some of the fibers are observed
to curve back medially to join the main population,
terminating in a caudal area of the superficial
gray. The major features of these cases are
illustrated diagrammatically in figure 12.
     This phenomenon provides evidence that
"mechanical" influences can cause a deflection of
growing or regenerating axons, resulting in a
disruption of the orderly topography of their
terminal distribution. Axon-ordering factors
probably still operate on deflected axons, but
they cannot always completely compensate for too
much disarray.
     The importance of this last factor is
supported by our initial experiments in a study
not yet completed. We are investigating the
topography of the retinal projection to the wrong
side of the midbrain in cases with the right
colliculus and right eye ablated at birth. Most of
the axons cross the tectal midline in a large

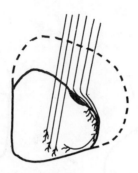

"MECHANICAL" DISTORTION OF AXON DISTRIBUTION

Figure 12. Diagrammatic illustration of results for cases which showed a discontinuity in the retinotectal map, with distorted axonal trajectories. Separated patches of terminal degeneration were found in SC but not in LGd or LGv in 4 cases with lesions of the rostral tectum at birth.

fasciculus, unlike their normal sheet-like spread in the brachium of the superior colliculus. In this bunching together, some "scrambling" seems to occur, according to observations of sections cut in the plane of the decussation and stained for normal fibers. The terminal field of these axons shows topographic discontinuities, as well as other abnormal patterns. For example, consider one such case where in the adult animal we placed a lesion in the lower nasal retina. In the normal hamster, such a lesion would result in terminal degeneration in the caudomedial part of the superior colliculus. In this case, degenerating axons were followed across the midline in the anomalous decussation. Some were traced antero-laterally from the area of crossing to a small terminal region in the anterolateral edge of the superficial gray layer. Other axons were traced caudally in this remaining tectum to several terminal patches which did not completely fill the full depth of the superficial gray layer. Reconstructions of this case and a control case are illustrated in figures 13 and 14.

In another case, we ablated the right tectum

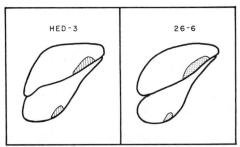

Figure 13. Reconstructed lateral views of dorsal and ventral nuclei of the lateral geniculate body in the 2 cases illustrated in fig. 14. The areas of terminal degeneration which reached the optic-tract border of these cell groups are outlined.

and the right eye at birth, and inadvertently, also ablated the caudomedial part of the left tectum. In the adult, we made a lesion in the lower nasal retina of the remaining left eye. Degenerating axons from the retinal lesion, which normally would have terminated in the caudomedial portion of the right tectum, were followed across the midline into the left superficial gray layer to terminal areas in the medial tectum rostrally, as well as in the medial part of what remained caudally.

Correlations of abnormal retinotectal topography with behavior

Such a scrambling in the retinotectal topography helps to explain why the wrong-direction turning movements observed in many such cases do not show consistent changes in direction of head orientation with changes in visual field positions of the stimulus. Discontinuities in the retinotectal map in cases with rostral tectum lesions could at least partially account for some specific inaccuracies in head-turning responses in such cases, e.g., not turning far enough for a seed in part of the temporal field or not raising the head in a turn towards a stimulus in parts of the upper field. The phenomenon of compression of the retinotectal map probably explains why we find a visual field nearly normal in size, especially in nasotemporal extent, in cases where the area

of retinofugal termination in the tectum is
drastically reduced (to 1/3 of normal, or even
less).

Discussion and conclusions

        Most experiments on effects of early brain
lesions in animals have supported the principle
proposed by Kennard (1942) that early brain
lesions are less disruptive of later performance
than lesions suffered in maturity. However, one
can also find reports of experiments in which
early and late lesions were found to be equally
detrimental to function (e.g., Bland and Cooper
1969; Thompson 1970; Johnson 1972); sparing of
function after neonatal lesions appears to be not
only site dependent, but when it is found, it may
be specific for only certain tasks (Bauer and
Hughes 1970; Hicks and D'Amato 1970; Nonneman and
Isaacson 1973). Some exceptions to the Kennard
principle are also presented in this volume by

Figure 14. (Opposite page) Dorsal view of the
brainstem of control case HED-3 and experimental
case 26-6, which had similar lesions of the nasal
retina in the adult, as indicated by the degeneration patterns found in the lateral geniculate
body, illustrated in fig. 13. Reconstruction
method and conventions as for the case illustrated
in fig. 9. For identification of structures, see
fig. 8. Case 26-6 had an ablation of the right eye
and the superficial layers of the right SC on the
day of birth; the right inferior colliculus has
shifted anteriorly, partly filling the gap left by
the early lesion (cf. fig. 3); the left lateral
geniculate body shows some transneuronal atrophy.
Solid dots, terminal degeneration which reaches
the surface of SC but which does not extend
through the entire depth of the superficial gray
layer; circled dots, small patches of terminal
degeneration not reaching either the surface or
the deep boundary of the superficial gray; oblique
line segments, axonal degeneration of fibers of
passage with anomalous transverse orientation
(precise directions of axon orientation were not
ascertained from the sections).

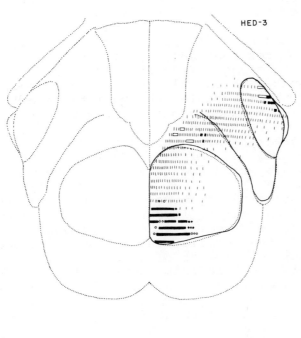

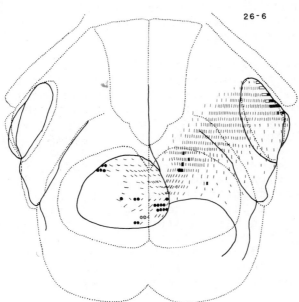

Brunner and Altman, by Goldman, and by ourselves.
Studies of the behavior of Syrian hamsters after
early lesions in the visual system have provided
examples not only of sparing of function, but also
of loss or retardation of function, and of a
maladaptive change of function (see fig. 1). Thus,
experiments with animal subjects have produced
findings which parallel the variety of effects of
early brain damage in man (reviewed by Teuber,
1971).

Some striking alterations in axonal connections
are found in the brains of adult hamsters which
had been subjected soon after birth to specific
lesions (see figs. 2, 3, 4). We are only beginning
to understand the factors which influence the
growth of anomalies. Investigations of these
factors are of special interest because of the
likelihood that similar factors are involved in
the normal development of specific connections.

Causal relationships between the sparing and
alteration of function after early brain lesions
and the accompanying morphological anomalies are
not always clear. In what follows, we would like
to consider these relationships further, then
proceed to discuss the factors underlying the
formation of anomalous connections with respect to
current work on neuronal plasticity and development.

In our example of early lesions of occipital
neocortex, the sparing of pattern vision was
correlated with an alteration in the laminar
pattern of termination of the retinotectal axons
(fig. 2). By itself this correlation provides
little evidence of a causal relationship. However,
since experiments on species other than the
hamster indicate that the retino-tecto-
thalamocortical pathway can mediate some pattern
vision, the suggestion that a morphological
alteration of this system might underlie sparing
of function in the hamster must be considered. In
addition, the possibility of other neuroanatomical
changes should not be ignored. For example, are
the tectal or pretectal projections to the
thalamus altered by an early occipital cortex
lesion?

The hypothesis of an altered role of the
retinotectothalamic connections after early

striate cortex ablation suggests that a pathway to
the neocortex not normally essential for simple
pattern discrimination becomes important for this
function after early ablation of striate cortex.
This may further imply that other functions of
neocortex might be retarded by the change -- i.e.,
a "crowding out" of function may occur, perhaps
related to the competitive crowding of growing
axon populations after early lesions. The idea
that sparing of function may exact a price was
supported by the fact that the hamsters with early
cortex lesions, and not those with lesions in
adulthood, were retarded on a different task,
namely, learning to negotiate the apparatus during
pretraining. For humans with early cerebral
lesions, a sparing of specific sensory, motor, and
language functions linked with a retardation of
other abilities has often been claimed (Hebb 1942;
Teuber and Rudel 1962; Teuber 1971; Woods and
Teuber 1973; Milner 1974; Teuber 1974).

In the examples of early bilateral or unilateral lesions of the superior colliculus, the
arguments that anomalous retinotectal connections
account for the spared and the altered function
are strong ones. However, further neuroanatomical
anomalies in such cases may also be found. Perhaps
the best case for a specific function of an
anomalous connection can be made for the cases of
early unilateral tectum lesions, where abnormal
retinal projections to the wrong side of the midbrain are correlated with visually elicited
turning in the wrong direction. Observations of
the effects of selective transection of the
anomalous pathway and detailed comparisons of
behavioral and electrophysiological mapping
results would be interesting.

The factors which govern the growth and
specificity of axonal connections after brain
lesions can be classified as either intrinsic
(endogenous), presumably determined by intra-
cellular mechanisms, or extrinsic (exogenous),
e.g., involving interactions of axons with each
other or with the substrate (Schneider 1973). The
factor which appears to be an intrinsic one is the
tendency of neurons to conserve some minimal
quantity of their axonal arborization. We have
cited data on populations of axons but propose

that this factor applies to individual cells.   It
manifests itself in the "pruning" effects
observed in cases of early lesions of the superior
colliculus.   One is led to ask about the action of
this factor in the cases of early lesions of
occipital cortex. The LGd atrophies in such cases;
what happens to the axons of retinal origin which
would have terminated in this structure?   Branches
of the same axons may be the ones which sprout to
form altered connections in the superior
colliculus (SC).   There is electrophysiological
evidence for the existence of a population of
retinofugal axons with branches ending in both the
LGd and the SC in the rat (Sefton 1968) and in the
cat (Hoffmann 1973; Hoffmann and Stone 1973). The
axons normally destined for the LGd may show
other changes. Cunningham (1972) has reported
evidence that in cases of early damage to the
visual cortex in the rat, there is a volumetric
hypertrophy of the region of retinal projection
in the pretectal area, accompanied by an increase
in size of the optic tract which extends beyond
the geniculate body.   Our hamster cases provide
only a hint of such an effect, which will require
supplementation and quantification of these
projections before it can be substantiated.   The
kind of hypertrophy described by Cunningham is
reminiscent of the hypertrophy of the dorsal
terminal nucleus of the accessory optic tract in
hamsters after early colliculus lesions.

One extrinsic factor is the tendency for
axons to invade vacated terminal space, competing
with other axons, at least in some cases, for
exclusive occupancy of the "space" (the nature of
which need not be strictly defined at present).
The development of this concept has been discussed
recently (see Bernstein and Goodman 1973).   There
are cases where a structure denervated soon after
birth is not invaded by sprouts from adjacent
axons -- e.g., the optic tract in the hamster
does not invade the hypothalamus or subthalamus
after early hemispherectomy (Schneider 1970). The
reasons for this lack of anomalous growth remain
to be explored (see Schneider 1973).

Chemical factors, usually assumed to be
expressed as chemotropisms within chemical

gradients or as selective chemoaffinities, have often been invoked to account for the specificities in the growth of axonal connections (see Sperry 1963, 1971; Gaze 1970; Jacobson 1970). The alluring, apparent sufficiency of this hypothesis may have led to some neglect of other factors which the results of the experiments with hamsters, reviewed here, have led us to stress. It is not clear that chemoaffinities of retinofugal axons for tectal target cells are crucial in the formation of topographic connections after early partial tectum lesions.

Some "axon-ordering factor" does operate on the optic-tract axons growing into a partially ablated tectum, in such a way that a full map is formed in the reduced space. Mapping of visual receptive fields of retinal axon potentials after regeneration in goldfish with partial tectum ablations has led to similar conclusions (Gaze and Sharma 1970; Yoon 1971, 1972; Sharma 1972a, b). Similar experiments on toads and frogs have not yet given clear evidence of the compressed map phenomenon (Straznicky 1973; Meyer and Sperry 1973; but cf. Straznicky, Gaze, and Keating 1971).

In the hamster, the retinofugal axons may have a special affinity for the surface of the superior colliculus, but it is not clear that chemical gradients over this tectal surface are crucial to the formation of the topographic order of termination. The gradients may be primarily within the axon population. This population is distributed on the surface of the diencephalon so that different loci within the dorsoventral axis of the retina are segregated in the optic tract as it courses as a sheet of fibers over the lateral geniculate bodies (Jhaveri and Schneider 1974). The same order is maintained as the tract continues into the brachium of the superior colliculus. Thus, in each terminal region, the nasotemporal axis corresponds to the order in which the axons leave the optic tract (Jhaveri and Schneider 1974). This determination may be accomplished, at least in part, by interaxonal interactions (cf. Whitsel, Petrucelli, Ha, and Dreyer 1972).

Such a view receives some support from the analysis of topographic order in the termination of retinotectal axons on the "wrong" side of the

midbrain in hamsters with early unilateral tectum
lesions combined with removal of the ipsilateral
eye. Axons from a restricted retinal locus, having
recrossed at the tectal midline, do not all go to
an area in the remaining tectum corresponding to
their normal projection (i.e., the mirror image
position). Instead, they distribute discontinuously
to several terminal areas, some of them widely
separated from the area predicted by a chemo-
specificity hypothesis. These cases do not support
the notion of specific chemoaffinities that cause
a given axon from the retina to end on a specific
area of cells in the tectum, nor do they require
that we postulate a rostrocaudal gradient in the
tectum which influences the growth of axons
according to the nasotemporal locus of their
origin in the retina.

Recently, Ingle (1973) and Misantone and
Stelzner (1974) have reported a "rewiring" of the
undamaged tectum by regenerating axons from the
"wrong" eye in frogs consequent to unilateral
tectum ablation, with or without removal of the
ipsilateral eye. Sharma (1973) reported a similar
phenomenon in goldfish. In contrast to the hamsters with early lesions of the superior colliculus
on one side, axons from the two eyes formed
overlapping projections. Also unlike the hamster
cases was the mirror symmetry of the abnormal
retinotopic map. It is not clear in these cases
whether the mirror image maps are due to axons
which regenerate across the tectal midline, or to
axons which become re-routed at the chiasm into
the wrong optic tract. Roth (1972) and Sharma
(1973) have described such re-routing at the
chiasm after unilateral lesions of the tectum and
enucleation of the ipsilateral eye in goldfish. In
this case, the axons may behave normally except
for being on the side opposite to their normal
position. Only if they cross at the tectal
midline, as in our hamster cases, would they be
entering the tectum at an abnormal angle with
respect to the postulated gradients. If they did
this, one would expect that the map would be
abnormal (i.e., not mirror symmetric for function)
if the termination of axons were not guided by
signals from within the tectal substrate, or if
these signals were not strongly effective. A

normal map would be predicted if these substrate signals were fully determinative. The observations of 90° or 180° rotation of the retinotectal map after regeneration into pieces of goldfish tectum rotated by a corresponding amount (Sharma and Gaze 1971; Yoon 1973) appear to support the notion of a substrate gradient. However, the source of this gradient is unclear. One wonders about the possible role of the remains of the transected original axons.

Whatever gradients may exist in the tectum of the hamster, they clearly do not prevent axons which become deflected from their normal course while crossing an area of lesion from terminating at abnormal loci. This results in specific discontinuities in the retinotectal map. Thus, some kind of "mechanical" influence on axon trajectories after early lesions, effective in the determination of terminal patterns, can be suspected.

The phenomena of abnormal axonal growth or regeneration after early lesions, and the relative influence of the intrinsic and extrinsic factors which guide this growth, might be expected to vary with age. Indeed, certain neuroplasticity phenomena in mammals have been found only if the brain damage occurs within a critical period after birth. This is the case for the increase or spread of the ipsilateral retinal projections after early unilateral eye removal, which occurs in the lateral geniculate body of the cat (Kalil 1973), in the superior colliculus and the LGd of the rat (Lund, Cunningham, and Lund 1973), and in the LGv of the hamster (Schneider 1973). Critical periods for the other phenomena described for the hamster visual system have not yet been specified. Recently, Devor (1974) has reported that several specific alterations in the projections of the olfactory bulb in the hamster occur if the lateral olfactory tract is transected within a critical period after birth. Axonal growth in the hippocampus of the rat following unilateral lesions of entorhinal cortex is reported by Lynch, Stanfield, and Cotman (1973) to occur after lesions in adulthood, but a quantitatively larger effect was found after early lesions.

We have stressed four factors underlying axonal

growth following early lesions: invasion of and
competition for vacated terminal space, conserva-
tion of terminal quantity, axon-ordering, and
"mechanical" deflection leading to disordered
termination patterns. If we can learn how these
four factors interact, and how they might be
constrained by others -- e.g., cell type, age,
and chemical specificities -- then our ability to
predict and control neuroplasticity phenomena will
increase further. The four factors as here
presented can suggest many further experiments.
Beyond that, the question may now be posed: to
what extent can the developing hamster serve as a
model for effects of early injury in other
mammals, including man? For our own species, both
sparing and characteristic alterations of function
have been reported for cases of early brain injury
(references above; also, Rudel, Teuber, and
Twitchell 1966). Our experiments with hamsters
make interpretations in terms cf altered neuronal
connections seem more likely than heretofore. In
any event, these kinds of observations on rodents
underline the advantages in searching for close
correlations between specific morphological
changes and particular behavioral anomalies after
early lesions in the mammalian brain.

ABBREVIATIONS

ant comm	anterior commissure
BIC	brachium of the inferior colliculus
fx	fornix
hc	habenular commissure
HM	medial habenular nucleus
IC	inferior colliculus
L	nucleus lateralis
LGd	dorsal nucleus of lateral geniculate body
LGv	ventral nucleus of lateral geniculate body
LP	nucleus lateralis posterior
MGB	medial geniculate body
OCh	optic chiasm
po comm	posterior commissure
PoTh	nucleus posterior thalami (anterior pretectal nucleus)
PrT	pretectal area

SC   superior colliculus
sm   stria medullaris
st   stria terminalis

Acknowledgments

Financial support for previously unpublished work was provided by US Public Health Service grant EY 00126, and by a grant to the department from the Alfred P. Sloan Foundation. Additional support came from the Grant and Spencer foundations, and from NASA.
We thank D. Singer and J. Stevenson for behavioral testing; I. Winzer for help with histology; H. -L. Teuber, D.K. Morest, and M. Devor for extensive comments on the manuscript; and D. Taylor for editing and typing.

SUMMARY

Bilateral lesions of visual cortex or superior colliculus (SC) in the adult Syrian hamster have been found to cause severe and apparently permanent losses in visual pattern discrimination or visually elicited turning responses, respectively. Comparable lesions inflicted in neonatal animals caused, at maturity, only partial impairment of these functions, in some cases scarcely any obvious loss. However, the early but not the later lesions of occipital neocortex resulted in slowed learning to push through doorways and find a water reward on the testing apparatus.

The sparing of visual-pattern discrimination may depend on a retinotecto-thalamic pathway which leads to neocortex. It is worth noting, in this regard, that visual-cortex ablation, at the age of 8 days or less, causes an alteration in the laminar pattern of termination of retinotectal axons, revealed by silver staining of axons degenerating after eye removal.

The sparing of visually elicited turning movements when the superficial tectal layers are ablated at birth appears to depend on direct visual pathways to the residual SC. This conclusion is supported by a relationship between degree of functional sparing and the pattern and size of the retinotectal projection. Early tectum lesions also lead to altered retinal projections to the diencephalon, though the function of these anomalous connections is not known.

If the superficial layers of SC are destroyed unilaterally at birth, axons from the eye contralateral to the lesion not only reach the area of early damage, but also form, in most cases, an abnormal decussation, crossing the tectal midline to terminate in the undamaged colliculus. This projection to the "wrong" side of the midbrain increases greatly if the undamaged colliculus is deprived of its normal innervation by additional early removal of the contralateral eye. Hamsters with such an anomaly show turning in the wrong direction in response to stimulation in a large area of upper and temporal visual field.

Some of the factors controlling the formation of abnormal connections can be specified, based on

various neuroanatomical experiments. (1) Growing
or regenerating axons tend to invade vacated
terminal space, and compete with other axons for
occupancy, in some cases exclusive occupancy.
(2) Axons tend to conserve at least a minimum
quantity of terminal arborization, thus showing
effects of "pruning", or compensatory sprouting.
(3) The retinofugal axon population tends to
preserve its topographic order, even if it is
forced to terminate in an abnormally small area,
e.g., in the residual caudal part of SC after
ablation of superficial layers of the rostral
tectum at birth. (4) "Mechanical" influences can
cause a deflection of growing or regenerating
retinofugal axons, resulting in a disruption of
the orderly topography of their terminal distribution. These findings on topography within the SC
may help to explain several behavioral observations, such as the paradox of a full visuomotor
field with an abnormally small tectum, or the
persistent abnormalities in visually guided
orienting movements toward objects in certain
parts of an affected field.

REFERENCES

Bauer, J.H. and Hughes, K.R. (1970). Visual and non-visual behaviors of the rat after neonatal and adult posterior neocortical lesions. *Physiol. & Behav.* 5, 427-441.

Bernstein, J.J. and Goodman, D.C. (Eds.) "Neuro-morphological Plasticity", Basel: S. Karger, 1973 *(Brain, Behavior and Evolution,* 1973, 8, No. 1-2).

Bland, B.H. and Cooper, R.M. (1969). Posterior neodecortication in the rat: age at operation and experience. *J. Comp. Physiol. Psych.* 69, 345-354.

Clark, R.G. (1966). Myelinization of the central nervous system of the New Zealand (albino) rabbit and the Syrian hamster. Doctoral dissertation, The George Washington University. (University Microfilms, Inc., Ann Arbor, Michigan, No. 66-6423.)

Clark, R.G. and Telford, I.R. (1964). Myeliniza-tion of the central nervous system of the Syrian hamster. *The Anatomical Record* 148, 271.

Cunningham, T.J. (1972). Sprouting of the optic projection after cortical lesions. *The Anatomical Record* 172, 298.

Devor, M. (1974). Adjustment of olfactory bulb projections after transection of the lateral olfactory tract. *The Anatomical Record* 178, 343.

Ferm, V.H. (1967). The use of the golden hamster in experimental teratology. *Laboratory Animal Care* 17, 452-462.

Fink, R.P. and Heimer, L. (1967). Two methods for selective silver impregnation of degenerating axons and their synaptic endings in the central nervous system. *Brain Res.* 4, 369-374.

Gaze, R.M. (1970). "The Formation of Nerve Connections", New York: Academic Press.

Gaze, R.M. and Sharma, S.C. (1970). Axial differ-ences in the reinnervation of the goldfish optic tectum by regenerating optic nerve fibers. *Exper. Brain Res.* 10, 171-181.

Graybiel, A.M. (1974). Visuo-cerebellar and cerebello-visual connections involving the ventral lateral geniculate nucleus. *Exp. Brain Res.* In press.

Hall, W.C. and Diamond, I.T. (1968). Organization and function of the visual cortex in hedgehog: II. An ablation study of pattern discrimination. *Brain, Behav. & Evol.* 1, 215-243.

Hamilton, W.J., Boyd, J.D. and Mossman, H.W. (1962). "Human Embryology", 3rd ed. Baltimore: Williams & Wilkens.

Hebb, D.O. (1942). The effect of early and late brain injury upon test scores, and the nature of normal adult intelligence. *Proceedings of the American Philosophical Society* 85, 275-292.

Hicks, S.P. and D'Amato, C.J. (1970). Motor-sensory and visual behavior after hemispherectomy in newborn and mature rats. *Exp. Neur.* 29, 416-438.

Hoffmann, K.-P. (1973). Conduction velocity in pathways from retina to superior colliculus in the cat: a correlation with receptive-field properties. *J. Neurophysiol.* 36, 409-424.

Hoffmann, K.-P. and Stone, J. (1973). Central termination of W-, X- and Y-type ganglion cell axons from cat retina. *Brain Res.* 49, 500-501.

Ingle, D.J. (1973). Two visual systems in the frog. *Science* 181, 1053-1055.

Jacobson, M. (1970). "Developmental Neurobiology", New York: Holt, Rinehart & Winston.

Jhaveri, S.R. (1973). Altered retinal connections following partial tectum lesions in neonate hamsters. M.S. thesis, Department of Psychology, Massachusetts Institute of Technology.

Jhaveri, S.R. and Schneider, G.E. (1974). Retinal projections in Syrian hamsters: normal topography, and alterations after partial tectum lesions at birth. *The Anatomical Record* 178, 383.

Johnson, D.A. (1972). Developmental aspects of recovery of function following septal lesions in the infant rat. *J. Comp. Physiol. Psych.* 78, 331-348.

Kalil, R.E. (1973). Formation of new retino-geniculate connections in kittens: effects of age and visual experience. *The Anatomical Record* 175, 353.

Kennard, M.A. (1942). Cortical reorganization of motor function: studies on series of monkeys of various ages from infancy to maturity. *Arch. Neur. & Psychiat.* 48, 227-240.

Kretschmann, H.-J. (1967). Die Myelogenese eines Nestflüchters *(Acomys (cahirinus) minous*, BATE 1906) im Vergleich zu der eines Nesthockers (Albinomaus). *Journal für Hirnforschung* 9, 373-396.

Levey, N.H., Harris, J. and Jane, J.A. (1973). Effects of visual cortical ablation on pattern discrimination in the ground squirrel *(Citellus tridecemlineatus)*. *Exp. Neur.* 39, 270-276.

Lund, R.D., Cunningham, T.J. and Lund, J.S. (1973). Modified optic projections after unilateral eye removal in young rats. *Brain, Behav. & Evol.* 8, 51-72.

Lund, R.D. and Lund, J.S. (1972). Development of synaptic patterns in the superior colliculus of the rat. *Brain Res.* 42, 1-20.

Lynch, G., Stanfield, B. and Cotman, C.W. (1973). Developmental differences in post-lesion axonal growth in the hippocampus. *Brain Res.* 59, 155-168.

Meyer, R.L. and Sperry, R.W. (1973). Test for neuroplasticity in the anuran retinotectal system. *Exp. Neur.* 40, 525-539.

Milner, B. (1974). Hemispheric specialization: scope and limits. *In* F.O. Schmitt and F.G. Worden (Eds.), "The Neurosciences: Third Study Program", Cambridge: M.I.T. Press, pp. 75-89.

Misantone, L.J. and Stelzner, D.J. (1974). Competition of retinal endings for sites in doubly innervated frog optic tectum. *The Anatomical Record* 178, 419.

Nonneman, A.J. and Isaacson, R.L. (1973). Task dependent recovery after early brain damage. *Behav. Biol.* 8, 143-172.

Rosenquist, A.C. and Edwards, S.B. (1973). Projections of the lateral geniculate nucleus in the cat as demonstrated by autoradiography. *The Anatomical Record* 175, 428-429.

Roth, R.L. (1972). Normal and regenerated retino-tectal projections in the goldfish. Doctoral dissertation, Department of Anatomy, Case Western Reserve University.

Rudel, R.G., Teuber, H.-L. and Twitchell, T.E. (1966). A note on hyperesthesia in children with early brain damage. *Neuropsychologia* 4, 351-356.

Schneider, G.E. (1966). Superior colliculus and visual cortex: contrasting behavioral effects of their ablation in the hamster. Doctoral dissertation, Department of Psychology, Massachusetts Institute of Technology.

Schneider, G.E. (1967). Contrasting visuomotor functions of tectum and cortex in the golden hamster. *Psychologische Forschung* 31, 52-62.

Schneider, G.E. (1969). Two visual systems. Brain mechanisms for localization and discrimination are dissociated by tectal and cortical lesions. *Science* 163, 895-902.

Schneider, G.E. (1970). Mechanisms of functional recovery following lesions of visual cortex or superior colliculus in neonate and adult hamsters. *Brain, Behav. & Evol.* 3, 295-323.

Schneider, G.E. (1973). Early lesions of superior colliculus: factors affecting the formation of abnormal retinal projections. *Brain, Behav. & Evol.* 8, 73-109.

Schneider, G.E. Anomalous axonal connections implicated in sparing and alteration of function after early lesions. *In* D.G. Stein and E. Eidelberg (Eds.) "Functional recovery after lesions of the nervous system". *Neurosciences Research Program Bulletin* 12. In press.

Schneider, G.E. and Nauta, W.J.H. (1969). Formation of anomalous retinal projections after removal of the optic tectum in the neonate hamster. *The Anatomical Record* 163, 258.

Sefton, A.J. (1968). The innervation of the lateral geniculate nucleus and anterior colliculus in the rat. *Vision Research* 8, 867-881.

Sharma, S.C. (1972a). Reformation of retinotectal projections after various tectal ablations in adult goldfish. *Exp. Neur.* 34, 171-182.

Sharma, S.C. (1972b). Redistribution of visual projections in altered optic tecta of adult goldfish. *Proceedings of the National Academy of Sciences,* USA 69, 2637-2639.

Sharma, S.C. (1973). Anomalous retinal projection after removal of contralateral optic tectum in adult goldfish. *Exp. Neur.* 41, 661-669.

Sharma, S.C. and Gaze, R.M. (1971). The retinotopic organization of visual responses from tectal reimplants in adult goldfish. *Archives italiennes de Biologie* 109, 357-366.

Shimada, M. and Langman, J. (1970). Cell proliferation, migration and differentiation in the cerebral cortex of the golden hamster. *J. Comp. Neur.* 139, 227-244.

Snyder, M. and Diamond, I.T. (1968). The organization and function of the visual cortex in the tree shrew. *Brain, Behav. & Evol.* 1, 244-288.

Sperry, R.W. (1945). Restoration of vision after crossing of optic nerves and after contralateral transplantation of eye. *J. Neurophysiol.* 8, 15-28.

Sperry, R.W. (1963). Chemoaffinity in the orderly growth of nerve fiber patterns and connections. *Proceedings of the National Academy of Sciences* USA 50, 703-710.

Sperry, R.W. (1971). How a developing brain gets itself properly wired for adaptive function. *In* E. Tobach, L.R. Aronson, and E. Shaw (Eds.), "The Biopsychology of Development", New York: Academic Press, pp. 27-44.

Straznicky, K. (1973). The formation of the optic fibre projection after partial tectal removal in *Xenopus. J. Embryol. and Exp. Morph.* 29, 397-409.

Straznicky, K., Gaze, R.M. and Keating, M.J. (1971). The establishment of retinotectal projections after embryonic removal of rostral or caudal half of the optic tectum in *Xenopus laevis* toad. *Proceedings of the International Congress of Physiological Sciences* 9, 540.

Teuber, H.-L. (1971). Mental retardation after early trauma to the brain: some issues in search of facts. *In* C.R. Angle and E.A. Bering, Jr. (Eds.),"Physical Trauma as an Etiological Agent in Mental Retardation", Bethesda: National Institutes of Health, pp. 7-28.

Teuber, H.-L. (1974). Why two brains? *In* F.O. Schmitt and F.G. Worden (Eds.), "The Neurosciences: Third Study Program", Cambridge: M.I.T. Press, pp. 71-74.

Teuber, H.-L. and Rudel, R.G. (1962). Behavior after cerebral lesions in children and adults. *Dev. Med. & Child Neur.* 4, 3-20.

Thompson, V.E. (1970). Visual decortication in infancy in rats. *J. Comp. Physiol. Psych.* 72, 444-451.

Whitsel, B.L., Petrucelli, L.M., Ha, H. and Dreyer, D.A. (1972). The resorting of spinal afferents as antecedent to the body representation in the postcentral gyrus. *Brain, Behav. & Evol.* 5, 303-341.

Woods, B.T. and Teuber, H.-L. (1973). Early onset of complementary specialization of cerebral hemispheres in man. *Transactions of the American Neurological Association* 98, 113-117.

Yakovlev, P.I. and Lecours, A.-R. (1967). The myelogenetic cycles of regional maturation of the brain. *In* A. Minkowski (Ed.), "Regional Development of the Brain in Early Life", Oxford and Edinburgh: Blackwell Scientific Publications, pp. 3-70.

Yoon, M.G. (1971). Reorganization of retinotectal projection following surgical operations on the optic tectum in goldfish. *Exp. Neur.* 33, 395-411.

Yoon, M.G. (1972). Transposition of the visual projection from the nasal hemiretina onto the foreign rostral zone of the optic tectum in goldfish. *Exp. Neur.* 37, 451-462.

Yoon, M.G. (1973). Retention of the original topographic polarity by the 180° rotated tectal reimplant in young adult goldfish. *J. Physiol.* 233, 575-588.

CENTRAL REGENERATION AND RECOVERY OF FUNCTION: THE PROBLEM OF COLLATERAL REINNERVATION

Robert Y. Moore
The University of Chicago
Chicago, Illinois

The enigma of recovery of function is that it occurs. All of the behavioral, motor and sensory phenomena that constitute recovery of function after disruption of neural tissue are well known but, save for the events that transpire following transection of a peripheral nerve, we have little understanding of the mechanisms responsible for the recovery. Peripheral nerve lesions continue to provide the clearest model, restitution of morphologic integrity, but it is clear from the extensive studies of Cajal and others (cf. Cajal 1928; Clemente 1964, for reviews) that this form of regeneration and consequent recovery of function does not occur in the mammalian central nervous system. From this it also has come to be accepted, and stated dogmatically (cf. Das and Altman 1972, p. 233), that regeneration does not occur in the mammalian central nervous system and, consequently, cannot participate in a recovery phenomenon (cf. Stein *et al.* 1969). In this review I shall take the position that this view is too restrictive. Regeneration will be defined here as any change in the morphologic organization of the nervous system occurring in response to injury in which there is growth of neuronal processes to form new, functional synaptic contacts. It should be noted that this is a largely morphologic statement without functional implications beyond the cellular level. At the present time two types of neural regenerative response are generally recognized (Fig. 1). The first is the formation of regenerative sprouting from transected axons. The second is collateral sprouting from intact axons. Both have been studied extensively in the peripheral nervous system (cf. Edds 1953; Guth 1956; Olson and Malmfors 1970, for reviews) but only regenerative sprouting has been investigated in detail in the mammalian central nervous system (Clemente 1964). Dendritic responses to injury have received little attention. The focus of this paper will be on

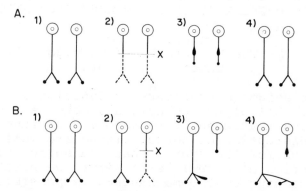

*Figure 1. Basic paradigms of regeneration in the
nervous system. (A) Regenerative sprouting. The
axons of neurons innervating a structure are
severed. The axon distal to the lesion degenerates. The proximal stumps form growth cones and
regenerate new axons and terminals. (B) Collateral
sprouting. Part of the innervation to a structure
is severed. The distal axons and terminals
degenerate and collateral sprouts form from the
remaining innervation to reconstitute a terminal
plexus. From Moore et al. 1973.*

collateral sprouting but this topic is best introduced by reviewing some recent work on regenerative
sprouting. In a broad sense the question to be
addressed at this conference concerns the capacity
of the mammalian central nervous system to respond
adaptively to injury and the mechanisms by which
this does, or might, take place. The purpose of
this paper is to prove some potential morphologic
answers to that question.

REGENERATIVE SPROUTING IN THE
MAMMALIAN CENTRAL NERVOUS SYSTEM

The capacity of severed central axons to show
regenerative sprouting similar to that occurring
in the peripheral nervous system has been shown
since the pioneering work of Cajal (1928). This
work has been confirmed in many laboratories but,
at least in mammals, there have been no instances
in which restoration of connections has occurred
within the central nervous system (Cajal 1928;

Clemente 1964; Bernstein and Bernstein 1971, 1973). The studies of Bernstein and Bernstein (1971, 1973) have suggested that this is due, at least in part, to an extensive growth and formation of synapses within the region proximal to the area of destruction. This might be taken to imply that central axons are incapable of growth beyond this area and formation of a functional terminal plexus. Recent studies on the regenerative capacity of central adrenergic neurons indicate that this is not the case. Following destruction of axons of a central adrenergic neuron, there is a rapid accumulation of amine neurotransmitter, demonstrated by the Falck-Hillarp method, in the severed axon proximal to the area of destruction (Katzman *et al*. 1971; Ungerstedt 1971). Within two to three days after the injury the proximal stumps of severed axons are seen as coarse, beaded and distorted fibers. By a week after transection of the axon regenerative sprouts appear from the proximal stump as groups of small, densely packed, delicate, varicose fibers. Between the first and third weeks following an injury these fibers develop into an abundant system which substantially fills the proximal border of the lesion (Katzman *et al*. 1971). In addition to sprouting to form a dense plexus of terminals proximal to the lesion, these axons are capable of forming a marked anomalous innervation, particularly of blood vessels and nerve roots at the base of the brain. In blood vessels, for example, a dense plexus of terminals forms across the entire wall of the vessel regardless of whether or not the peripheral, sympathetic innervation is intact (Katzman *et al*. 1971). This vigorous regenerative axonal sprouting has been observed after lesions involving the ascending adrenergic pathways in the medial forebrain bundle system and lesions involving the descending adrenergic pathways into the spinal cord (Björklund *et al*. 1971).

These observations demonstrated the capacity of central adrenergic neurons to exhibit regenerative sprouting following axonal transection but they did not show whether the sprouting fibers were capable of forming a potentially functional terminal network. To test the capacity of central adrenergic neurons to reinnervate a denervated tissue, Bjorklund and his colleagues (Björklund and

Stenevi 1971; Björklund *et al*. 1971) carried out an ingenious set of experiments in which transplants of peripheral tissues are placed within the ascending or descending pathways of brainstem adrenergic neuron systems. In each case, the transplant is denervated when it is removed from its normal position and implanted into the central nervous system. Placing the transplant into the central nervous system serves to transect the axons of the adrenergic neurons so that these studies examined regenerative sprouting responses. The most successful of these experiments involved transplantation of the iris from the anterior chamber of the eye into the medial forebrain bundle (Björklund and Stenevi 1971). As in the studies outlined above, amine accumulation appeared early in the transected axons adjacent to the transplant and subsequently regenerative sprouting of delicate varicose fibers occurred. For the first week following placement of the transplant it is free of adrenergic innervation, but by two weeks many adrenergic fibers can be traced from the transected medial forebrain bundle and nearby dorsal catecholamine bundle (Ungerstedt 1971) into the transplanted iris. In many areas this new innervation comes to have the characteristic appearance of a normally innervated iris but it is clearly innervation of central origin because a similar pattern is observed in sympathectomized animals. The transplants remain viable and innervated for as long as six months after implantation with a pattern of innervation which continues to strongly resemble the normal adrenergic innervation of the iris. These observations establish that the transected central adrenergic axons are capable of innervating a denervated tissue if it is placed in the immediate vicinity of newly forming axonal sprouts. The fact that the pattern of innervation is like that of the normal peripheral sympathetic innervation of the iris indicates that the transplanted tissue determines the organization of the new terminal plexus. This view was further supported by observations that transplanted mitral valve is also reinnervated and with a pattern quite characteristic of that seen in the normally innervated heart (Björklund and Stenevi 1971; Björklund *et al*. 1971). In contrast to this, diaphragm or uterus, which normally have little peripheral adrenergic innervation, are not innervated by central adrenergic neurons when transplanted into the ascending adrenergic fiber systems (Björklund and Stenevi 1971). Thus, it is evident that sprouting central adrenergic axons are capable of extensive growth and of reinnervation of a denervated tissue but it is not known whether this can be a functional innervation.

Other recent experiments add a further interesting dimension to these studies. Nerve growth factor (NGF) injected intraventricularly at the time of transplantation of an iris stimulates the growth of transected central adrenergic axons into the transplant (Björklund and Stenevi 1972). This effect can be very selective in that injection of the NGF directly in the vicinity of the adrenergic neurons or their ascending pathways (Bjerre *et al.* 1973) also provides a marked stimulation of an adrenergic axonal growth into the transplant but with much lower doses of NGF than are required with intraventricular injection. These observations open up many interesting possibilities for further experimentation and they certainly suggest that NGF may participate in the regenerative response of at least some neurons to injury. A further remarkable example of the capacity of central monoamine-producing neurons to exhibit regenerative sprouting is shown by the experiments of Olson and Seiger (1972). It is not known at the present, however, whether these neurons have a specialized capacity for regenerative responses or whether these observations are a function of the ease with which these neurons can be selectively demonstrated by current histochemical techniques.

COLLATERAL SPROUTING IN THE MAMMALIAN CENTRAL NERVOUS SYSTEM

Nearly all studies of central regeneration have examined the regenerative capacity of transected axons. It is evident from the observations reviewed above that axons of central adrenergic neurons are capable of a remarkable regenerative sprouting and growth following transection. The functional status of these sprouting axons is not

known and, indeed, there is only one situation in
which a functional regeneration has occurred from
regenerative sprouting. This is in the unusual
situation exhibited by hypothalamo-hypophysial
axons following transection (Adams *et al.* 1969).
In this case the regenerating axons are not
innervating other neurons and it now appears that
much of the functional regeneration depends upon
properties of blood vessels (Raisman 1973). The
phenomenon of collateral sprouting is clearly of
great potential functional significance but it
has not been extensively investigated in the
central nervous system. The available literature
is noted in Table 1. Several things are striking

TABLE 1
STUDIES OF COLLATERAL SPROUTING IN THE
ADULT MAMMALIAN CENTRAL NERVOUS SYSTEM

INVESTIGATORS	SYSTEM STUDIED	INTERPRETATION OF DATA OBTAINED
Liu & Chambers, 1958	Somatic sensory	Collateral sprouting of dorsal root fibers
Westrum & Black, 1971	Somatic sensory	Probably collateral sprouting in spinal trigeminal nucleus
Kerr, 1972	Somatic sensory	No collateral sprouting in spinal trigeminal nucleus
Goodman & Horel, 1967	Visual	Collateral sprouting of some optic tract axons
Bogdasarian & Goodman, 1971	Visual	Collateral sprouting of optic tract axons
Lund & Lund, 1971	Visual	Probable collateral sprouting in superior colliculus
Cunningham, 1972	Visual	Collateral sprouting of optic tract axons
Guillery, 1972	Visual	No collateral sprouting of optic tract axons
Ralston & Chow, 1973	Visual	Either collateral sprouting or relocation of existing terminals
Raisman, 1969 Raisman & Field, 1973	Limbic	Collateral sprouting of fornix or medial forebrain bundle axons
Lynch, *et al.*, 1973	Limbic	Collateral sprouting of septal or entorhinal axons
Moore, *et al.*, 1971, 1973 Stenevi, *et al.*, 1972	Central Adrenergic	Collateral sprouting in denervated areas
Pickel, *et al.*, 1972	Central adrenergic neurons	Collateral sprouting from collateral branches of severed axons

in the Table. The first is that there have been so
few studies of collateral sprouting and reinnervation in the central nervous system. The second is
that the first study to clearly demonstrate the
phenomenon was carried out as recently as the
1950's (Liu and Chambers 1958). The third is that,
until recently, nearly all studies had been performed on either the somatic sensory system or the
visual system. This certainly reflected the state
of our knowledge concerning the detailed anatomy
of these systems but it is remarkable that so few

116

other systems have been examined. The most
extensive studies of this phenomenon in central
structures outside of the visual and somatic
sensory systems have been carried out by Raismán
(1969b) and Raisman and Field (1973) on the
innervation of the septal nuclear complex of the
rat. The foundation for these studies was
Raisman's (1966, 1969a) demonstration that septal
neurons are innervated from two primary sources,
the hippocampus via the fornix and the brainstem
via the medial forebrain bundle and that each of
these has a characteristic pattern of termination
on septal neurons. Transection of the axons from
one source of innervation produced electron-
microscopic evidence of degenerative changes in
the appropriate set of terminals within a few days
after operation but after long intervals there were
no degenerating terminals and the synaptic
architecture of the nucleus did not differ greatly
from the normal. The major change observed was an
increase in the number of axons exhibiting multiple
synaptic contacts (Raisman 1969b). These observations indicated that the intact innervation
underwent collateral sprouting to fill denervated
synaptic sites on septal nucleus neurons. This
interpretation was confirmed in a subsequent
extensive experiment (Raisman and Field 1973).
     The septal area receives a dense adrenergic
innervation from the medial forebrain bundle and
the observations noted above suggested that these
neurons might participate in the phenomena
described by Raisman (1969b) and Raisman and Field
(1973). An experiment was designed to test this
(Moore *et al.* 1971). This was done in order to
increase our understanding of the regenerative
capacity of central adrenergic axons by showing
that they exhibit collateral sprouting. In this
study rats were subjected to unilateral section of
the fornix. Since the fornix projects almost
exclusively on the ipsilateral septal nuclei
(Raisman 1966), the contralateral side served as a
control. The distribution of adrenergic neurons
was studied in the septal nuclei using the Falck-
Hillarp method in normal animals and at postoperative survival periods of 3, 8, 15, 30, 60 and
90-100 days. At 3 to 8 days after operation the
adrenergic innervation of the denervated septum

is not significantly different from that of the
normal or control septum except that a few scattered axons exhibit large monoamine accumulations
and have the appearance of severed axons. Similar
accumulations are evident at 8 and 15 days but
thereafter they are no longer observed. Between 15
and 30 days after fornix section, there is an
evident increase in the number of adrenergic fibers
in the denervated medial and lateral septal nuclei
and this becomes stable by 30 days and is maintained through at least 100 days after operation.
There is no other area in the basal telencephalon
that exhibits a similar change. There are several
possible interpretations for this change in septal
innervation that occurs following transection of
the fornix. The most obvious of these, and the one
consonant with the observations of Raisman (1969b)
and Raisman and Field (1973), is that the histo-
chemically demonstrable increase in the density of
adrenergic innervation in the septal nuclei
represents a true increase in the number of
terminals and, thus, collateral sprouting of the
medial forebrain bundle axons innervating these
nuclei. There is an increase in norepinephrine
content in the denervated septum demonstrable by
biochemical assay (Moore *et al*. 1971), but these
data provide only indirect support for this
interpretation. The sequence of events is
demonstrated diagrammatically in Figure 2. An
alternative explanation would be that the increase
in number of adrenergic fibers represents
collateral sprouting from intact collaterals of
axons that have been sectioned (see below). Another
interpretation would be that the apparent increase
in innervation really represented accumulation of
amine in axons proximal to the transected axons,
including its collaterals (Ungerstedt 1971). This
would not appear a likely explanation in that the
changes occurred only in the medial and lateral
septal nuclei and these changes are not the only
ones receiving collaterals of medial forebrain
bundle adrenergic axons. In addition, the effect
observed is an increase in the apparent number of
fibers not in their intensity. If this were to be
attributed to accumulation of amine in collaterals
it would require that the collaterals normally not
be demonstrable in the septum and there are no data

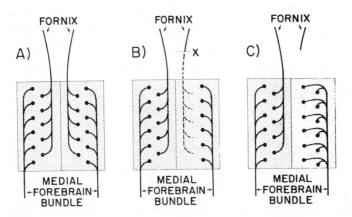

Figure 2. Collateral sprouting in the denervated septum, diagrammatically represented. (A) Normal relationship between fornix input and medial forebrain bundle input to the septal nuclei. (B) Unilateral fornix section resulting in partial denervation of the ipsilateral septal nuclei. (C) Denervated area reinnervated by the remaining, intact medial forebrain bundle adrenergic axons. From Moore et al. 1973.

to suggest that this is true. And, the time course for the accumulation of amine following transection is usually brief but the changes noted here were constant over an interval as long as 100 days.

This study represented the first in which collateral sprouting occurred from axons that have been characterized by identification of their probable neurotransmitter (Moore *et al.* 1971). Further studies were carried out to determine if this was a general phenomenon among adrenergic axons (Moore *et al.* 1973; Moore 1973; Stenevi *et al.* 1973). The results of these studies will be briefly summarized. The dorsal lateral geniculate and anteroventral nuclei of the thalamus each receives a dense adrenergic innervation. Following fornix section which removes hippocampal afferents to the anteroventral nucleus, there is an apparent increase in the adrenergic innervation of the nucleus that occurs concomitantly with that in the septal nuclei. Following removal of the retinal input to the lateral geniculate, there is no alteration in the adrenergic innervation of the

nucleus (Stenevi *et al*. 1972). After cortical
ablation, however, there is a marked increase in
the adrenergic innervation which occurs before
significant gliosis and shrinkage of the nucleus
takes place. When the reactive glial response
becomes maximal, there is marked shrinkage of the
nucleus and the adrenergic innervation is difficult
to visualize because of the other morphologic
changes. This situation would appear, then, to be
another in which collateral sprouting of adrenergic
axons occurs, in this case only when a massive
denervation is present in the nucleus due to
degeneration of dorsal lateral geniculate cell
bodies. A number of other experimental situations
have been examined and these will be mentioned
only briefly. Removal of retinal and raphe input to
the suprachiasmatic hypothalamic nucleus does not
alter its sparse adrenergic innervation. Similarly,
there is no alteration of the adrenergic innervation of the superior colliculus after ablation of
either the ipsilateral visual cortex or section of
the contralateral optic nerve, or both. Again in
this situation the adrenergic fibers to the optic
tectum are sparse and distributed principally to
deep layers of the structure whereas the retinal
and corticofugal afferents are distributed
principally to superficial layers. Amygdala
ablation with consequent degeneration of the
ventral amygdalo-fugal pathway into the lateral
hypothalamus does not produce any change in the
distribution of adrenergic fibers in this area.
Olfactory bulb ablation, in contrast, produces a
small but significant increase in the dopaminergic
innervation of the olfactory tubercle and this is
confirmed by chemical determinations (Meyer *et al*.
1973; Moore 1973). This study suggests that the
dopamine-producing fibers undergo a collateral
sprouting in response to denervation but this
requires further confirmation.

The interpretation of this series of studies
has been that the relationship between the extent
of denervation and the density of innervation by
adrenergic fibers is critical. For collateral
sprouting to take place and be recognized, it
would appear essential that the denervation of
non-adrenergic elements must be considerable. This
clearly obtains in the septal area studies, the

120

olfactory tubercle study and the lateral geniculate study. In addition there must be a minimal density of adrenergic innervation within the denervated area for it to respond and to be demonstrable by the methods employed. A corollary of this is that the adrenergic innervation should be in sufficient proximity to denervated sites to provide collateral reinnervation. The stimulus for collateral sprouting is unknown but, as in the periphery (Edds 1953), the denervated synaptic site provides the best candidate to promote growth of nearby axons.

There are two further important questions which cannot be answered at the present time. The first is whether collateral sprouting is a ubiquitous phenomenon amongst central axons or more restricted to certain groups or systems. The responses of adrenergic neurons would appear to be greater than those of some components of the visual system (Guillery 1972) or some cortical neurons (Cajal 1928; Rutledge et al. 1972) but we require additional information on this point. Second, the functional significance of collateral sprouting remains a continuing question, particularly as this is related to recovery of function. An intriguing aspect of this is raised by recent studies by Pickel et al. (1972). These authors observed apparent collateral sprouting from intact axons which were collaterals of transected adrenergic axons. This is shown diagrammatically in Figure 3. This apparent collateral sprouting is of particular interest for two reasons. First, it takes place in an intact axon which is in an area that has not undergone denervation. Thus, the sprouting axons occupy space at the expense of other elements within the neuropil of the innervated structure. Second, the phenomenon is self-limited. It appears within a few days after placement of the lesion and is gone by 6 weeks. This time course bears a close resemblance of many events of recovery of function and this phenomenon may be of great importance in determining some of the events of recovery.

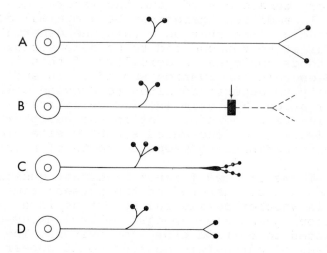

Figure 3. Collateral sprouting from collaterals of transected axons, a proposed model. (A) Normal neuron with axon with a collateral and two separate terminal fields. (B) Axon is severed and distal portion degenerates. (C) Collateral sprouting with increase in terminal field occurs from intact axon, while severed portion shows early regenerative sprouting with a restricted terminal field. (D) Regenerative sprouting produces a full size terminal field and collateral terminal field returns to normal.

CONCLUSIONS

Regenerative responses to injury occur widely in the mammalian central nervous system, both in the form of regenerative sprouting and collateral sprouting. The evidence currently available suggests that some groups of neurons have a greater capacity for regenerative responses than others but this, and a number of other parameters of the regenerative response, has not been investigated in any detail. Regenerative sprouting probably is not of great functional significance in the mammalian central nervous system. This does not imply that central axons cannot show a vigorous regenerative sprouting response not that they are unable to maintain extensive growth and the formation of an elaborate terminal innervation

plexus. Nevertheless, there is no instance known
in which restitution of anatomic integrity occurs
after destruction of central axons within the
mammalian central nervous system. For this reason,
regenerative sprouting cannot be used as a basis
for recovery of function after central lesions
although it may participate to some extent as a
component of recovery phenomena.

Collateral sprouting and reinnervation are now
known to occur in many areas of the central nervous
system in response to injury. Studies of this
phenomenon have been restricted to a few systems
and it is not known whether this is a general
response of central axons to injury. As with
regenerative sprouting the data available suggest
that collateral sprouting is more easily elicited
from some groups of neurons but this remains to be
firmly established. In addition we have not
established that collateral sprouting results in
functional contacts but the morphology certainly
suggests that this is the case. At present there
appear to be two forms of collateral sprouting.
The one most extensively studied occurs from intact
axons in response to a local denervation. This
seems to be a permanent response and results in a
reorganization of synaptic architecture in a
denervated area. The second form is collateral
sprouting from collateral branches of a transected
axon. In this situation the injured neuron
apparently attempts to maintain its terminal field
at a given size. The collateral sprouting takes
place within an intact area so that, if the newly
formed terminals make functional contacts, it is at
the expense of the terminal of other systems. This
response appears to be a temporary one with
restitution of the original organization within a
few weeks after the injury. Collateral sprouting
and reinnervation, particularly in response to
local denervation, takes place without the
morphologic handicaps that interfere with regenerative sprouting. There is only one instance
(McCouch et al. 1959) in which collateral sprouting
has been proposed to have a functional consequence.
This would appear to be because the significance of
this regenerative response has been largely
discounted or ignored. It is certainly a component
of the central nervous system's response to injury

and one which may well participate in the phenomena of recovery of function. The dogma that regeneration does not occur in the mammalian central nervous system and cannot contribute to recovery of function should be put aside in favor of further experimentation.

ACKNOWLEDGMENTS: This work was supported by grants NS-05002 and HD-04583 from the National Institutes of Health, United States Public Health Service. It was carried out in part in collaboration with Drs. Anders Bjorklund and Ulf Stenevi, Department of Histology, University of Lund, Lund, Sweden.

REFERENCES

Adams, J.H., Daniel, P.M. and Prichard, M.M.L. (1969). Degeneration and regeneration of hypothalamic nerve fibers in the neurohypophysis after pituitary stalk section in the ferret. *J. Comp. Neurol.* 135, 121-144.

Bernstein, J.J. and Bernstein, M.E. (1971). Axonal regeneration and formation of synapses proximal to the site of lesion following hemisection of the rat spinal cord. *Exper. Neurol.* 30, 336-351.

Bernstein, M.E. and Bernstein, J.J. (1973). Regeneration of axons and synaptic complex formation rostral to the site of hemisection in the spinal cord of the monkey. *Intern. J. Neurosci.* 5, 15-29.

Bjerre, B., Björklund, A. and Stenevi, U. Stimulation of growth of new axonal sprouts from lesioned monoamine neurons in adult rat brain by nerve growth factor. *Brain Res.*

Björklund, A. and Stenevi, U. (1971). Growth of central catecholamine neurons into smooth muscle grafts in the rat mesencephalon. *Brain Res.* 31, 1-20.

Björklund, A. and Stenevi, U. (1972). Nerve growth factor: Stimulation of regenerative growth of central noradrenergic neurons. *Science* 175, 1251-1253.

Björklund, A., Katzman, R., Stenevi, U. and West, K. (1971). Development and growth of axonal sprouts from noradrenaline and 5-hydroxytryptamine neurons in the rat spinal cord. *Brain Res.* 31, 21-33.

Bogdasarian, R.S. and Goodman, D.C. (1970). Axonal sprouting of intact retinofugal neurons as a consequence of opposite eye-removal: homotypic compared to heterotypic axonal sprouting. *Anat. Rec.* 166, 280.

Cajal, S.R. (1928). "Degeneration and Regeneration of the Nervous System," London: Oxford University Press.

Clemente, C.D. (1964). Regeneration in the vertebrate central nervous system. *Int. Rev. Neurobiol.* 6, 257-301.

Cunningham, J.J. (1972). Sprouting of the optic projection after cortical lesions. *Anat. Rec.* 172, 298.

Das, G.D. and Altman, J. (1972). Studies on the transplantation of developing neural tissue in the mammalian brain. I. Transplantation of cerebellar slabs into the cerebellum of neonate rats. *Brain Res.* 38, 233-249.

Edds, M.V. (1953). Collateral nerve regeneration. *Quart. Rev. Biol.* 28, 260-276.

Goodman, D.C. and Horel, J.A. (1967). Sprouting of optic tract projections in the brain stem of the rat. *J. Comp. Neurol.* 127, 71-88.

Guillery, R.W. (1972). Experiments to determine whether retinogeniculate axons can form translaminar collateral sprouts in the dorsal lateral geniculate nucleus of the cat. *J. Comp. Neurol.* 146, 407-420.

Guth, L. (1956). Regeneration in the mammalian peripheral nervous system. *Physiol. Rev.* 36, 441-478.

Katzman, R., Björklund, A., Owman, Ch., Stenevi, U. and West, K.A. Evidence for regenerative axon sprouting of central catecholamine neurons in the rat mesencephalon following electrolytic lesions. *Brain Res.*

Kerr, F.W. (1972). The potential of cervical primary afferenrs to sprout in the spinal nucleus of V following long term trigeminal denervation. *Brain Res.* 43, 547-560

Liu, C.N. and Chambers, W.W. (1958). Intraspinal sprouting of dorsal root axons. *Arch. Neurol. (Chicago)* 79, 46-61.

Lund, R.D. and Lund, J.S. (1971). Synaptic adjustment after deafferentation of the superior colliculus of the rat. *Science* 171, 804-807.

Lynch, G., Matthews, D.A., Mosko, S., Parks, T. and Cotman, C. (1972). Induced acetylcholinesterase-rich layer in rat dentate gyrus following entorhinal lesions. *Brain Res.* 42, 311-319.

Lynch, G.S., Mosko, S., Parks, T. and Cotman, C.W. (1973). Relocation and hyperdevelopment of the dentate commissural system after entorhinal lesions in immature rats. *Brain Res.* 49, 57-61.

McCouch, G.P., Austin, G.M., Liu, C.N. and Liu, C.Y. (1958). Sprouting as a cause of spasticity. *J. Neurophysiol.* 21, 205-216.

126

Moore, R.Y., Björklund, A. and Stenevi, U.
Growth and plasticity of adrenergic neurons. *In*
F.O. Schmitt and F.G. Worden (Eds.) "The
Neurosciences - Third Study Program,"
Cambridge, Mass.: M.I.T. Press. In press.
Moore, R.Y. Growth of adrenergic neurons in the
adult mammalian nervous system. *In* K. Fuxe,
L. Olson and Y. Zotterman (Eds.) "Dynamics of
Degeneration and Growth in Neurons,"
Pergamon Press. In Press.
Moore, R.Y., Björklund, A. and Stenevi, U. (1971).
Plastic changes in the adrenergic innervation
of the rat septal area in response to denerva-
tion. *Brain Res.* 33, 13-35.
Olson, L. and Malmfors, T. (1970). Growth
characteristics of adrenergic nerves in the
adult rat. *Acta Physiol. Scand. Suppl.* 348,
1-112.
Olson, L. and Seiger, A. (1972). Brain tissue
transplanted to the anterior chamber of the
eye. I. Fluorescence histochemistry of immature
catecholamine and 5-hydroxytryptamine neurons
reinnervating the rat iris. *Z. Zellforsch.* 135,
175-194.
Pickel, V.M., Krebs, H. and Bloom, F.E. (1972).
Proliferation of cerebellar norepinephrine-
containing fibers in response to peduncle
lesions. Paper presented to Society for
Neuroscience, Houston, Texas.
Raisman, G. (1966). The connections of the septum.
Brain 89, 317-348.
Raisman, G. (1969a). A comparison of the mode of
termination of the hippocampal and hypothalamic
afferents to the septal nuclei as revealed by
electron microscopy of degeneration. *Exp. Brain
Res.* 7, 317-343.
Raisman, G. (1969b). Neuronal plasticity in the
septal nuclei of the adult rat. *Brain Res.* 14,
25-48.
Raisman, G. (1973). Electron microscopic studies
of the development of new neurohaemal contacts
in the median eminence of the rat after
hypophysectomy. *Brain Res.* 55, 245-261.

Raisman, G. and Field, P.M. (1973). A quantitative investigation of the development of collateral reinnervation after partial deafferentation of the septal nuclei. *Brain Res*. 50, 241-264.

Ralston, H.J., IV and Chow, K.L. (1972). Synaptic reorganization in the degenerating lateral geniculate nucleus of the rabbit. *J. Comp. Neurol*. 147, 321-350.

Rutledge, L.T., Duncan, J. and Cant, N. (1972). Long term status of pyramidal cell axon collaterals and apical dendrites in denervated cortex. *Brain Res*. 41, 249-262.

Stenevi, U., Björklund, A. and Moore, R.Y. (1972). Growth of intact central adrenergic axons in the denervated lateral geniculate body. *Exper. Neurol*. 35, 290-299.

Stenevi, U., Björklund, A. and Moore, R.Y. Morphological plasticity of central adrenergic neurons. *Brain, Behav. Evol*. In press.

Ungerstedt, U. (1971). Stereotaxic mappings of the monoamine pathways in the rat brain. *Acta Physiol. Scand. Suppl*. 367, 1-48.

Westrum, L.E. and Black, R.G. (1971). Fine structural aspects of the synaptic organization of the spinal trigeminal nucleus (pars interpolaris) of the cat. *Brain Res*. 25, 265-287.

THE EFFECTS OF INTERFERENCE WITH THE MATURATION OF THE CEREBELLUM AND HIPPOCAMPUS ON THE DEVELOPMENT OF ADULT BEHAVIOR

Robert L. Brunner and Joseph Altman
Purdue University
West Lafayette, Indiana

Comparisons of the consequences of insults to the nervous system in infants and adults have yielded seemingly opposite results. Some treatments, such as undernutrition (Winick and Noble 1966; Altman, Das and Sudarshan 1970), hormonal treatments (Balázs, Kovács, Cocks, Johnson and Eayrs 1971; Nicholson and Altman 1972a, b) and X-irradiation (Hicks and D'Amato 1966; Altman, Anderson and Wright 1969; Altman, Anderson and Strop 1971) produce greater deficits in infants than adults. This greater vulnerability of the infant than adult brain has been related to evidence of irreversible damage produced by some of these treatments in the developing nervous system where the same insult produces no demonstrable harm or only a transient effect in the mature brain. For instance, permanent cell loss is produced in infancy by undernutrition but a recoverable reduction in cell size in adults (Winick and Noble 1966). In contrast to this great vulnerability of the immature nervous system, several brain lesion experiments (discussed in this Symposium) found more sparing or greater extent of functional recovery when operations were performed in infancy than in adulthood. The latter kind of finding is sometimes rationalized in terms of greater potential for regeneration or reorganization in the developing brain (such as sprouting of new nerve processes or the establishment of new synaptic connections) than in adults, although compelling evidence in mammals for adaptive reorganization is lacking.

The experiments to be described in this paper were not designed to compare the differential effects of early and late brain damage. Instead, the purpose was to trace the consequences of early brain damage longitudinally. This approach yielded direct information about the time course of the development of some behavior patterns in intact and brain damaged animals, and it has indirectly provided data relating to the problem of "recovery of function". Following the presentation of these data it will be argued that the longitudinal approach has many advantages in studying the problem of recovery of function after early and late brain damage because recovery at any time is essentially a developmental event and can be fully assessed only when it is so examined.

The technique that we use to produce early brain damage has been described in detail elsewhere. Multiplying cells are extremely radio-sensitive, hence X-irradiation of those brain regions with low-level X-ray in which cell acquisition is still in progress after birth results in decimation of their cell population. In the cerebellar cortex of the rat, the basket, stellate and granule cells are acquired after birth (Altman 1969) and when the cerebellum is exposed to multiple doses of low-level X-ray the acquisition of these cells can be prevented fully or in a graded fashion (Altman, Anderson and Wright 1968). Similarly, a large proportion of the granule cells of the hippocampal dentate gyrus are acquired after birth (Altman and Das 1965, 1966) and the exposure of this region results in the selective loss of granule cells (Bayer, Brunner, Hine and Altman 1973). Previous studies established that the behavioral changes produced by selective elimination of cerebellar microneurons (Wallace and Altman 1969; Altman, Anderson and Strop 1971; Brunner and Altman 1973) or hippocampal granule cells (Bayer, Brunner, Hine and Altman 1973; Haggbloom, Brunner and Bayer, in press) parallels those seen after ablation of the cerebellum or hippocampus *in toto*.

GENERAL METHOD

Subjects: Male rats bred and reared in our laboratory in litters of 6 pups were used in the present experiments. Long-Evans derived hooded rats were used in studies of cerebellar irradiation. Purdue-Wistar rats were used in studies of hippocampal irradiation. Rats were tested during one of the three general age periods, preweaning (1-21 days), young adult (2-3 months), adult (6-8 months).

Irradiation Procedure: The approximate rostral-caudal extent of the cerebellum and hippocampus had been determined in rats between 1 and 21 days of age. Treated rats were then immobilized in small sections of Tygon tubing on which the distance from the tip of the snout to the approximate caudal edge of the structure was marked. The wrapped (immobilized) pups were then slipped into a lucite and lead holder which was positioned under the X-ray source. An adjustable slit in the lead allowed only the appropriately marked portion of the pups' head to be exposed to the X-ray beam, delivered by a Maxitron 300 Kv unit. At the rate of 50 r/min, 200 r was delivered to the hippocampal region on days 2 and 3 followed by 150 r on days 5, 7, 9, 13 and 15. The cerebellum was irradiated using the same schedule beginning at 4 days of age.

Open Field Test. Open field procedures were the same in both the cerebellar and hippocampal irradiated experiments. The field consisted of an open black plastic surface (52.5 X 52.5 cm) divided into 10 cm squares by white lines and bounded by 20 cm walls. Room lights and a single 60 W bulb suspended directly over the field provided illumination. Rats were tested on 5 successive days for 3 minute periods. The number of four paw square entries and hindlimb rearing responses were tallied. Defecation scores were also determined.

Rod Crossing. Neonatal rats were trained to traverse an elevated wooden "bridge" 60 cm long and 2.5 cm wide in order to reach their littermates that were located on a platform attached to the bridge. An individual pup was placed at the end of the bridge and the time required to reach the platform, limb slips and falls was recorded. Rats were tested on the 2.5 cm wide bridge from 1 week to 3 weeks of age. Testing on a narrower (1.2 cm) pathway was done during the third week.

Adult rats were tested on two cylindrical plastic pipes (10.5 cm diameter, 3 m length) which could be rotated by means of a motor driven pulley at up to 150 RPM. One rod was roughened by applying fine grade sand to its freshly painted surface while the other remained untreated. Rats were trained to cross the rough surfaced rod for wet mash in daily sessions of 8 or more trials. After running speed reached asymptote on the stationary rod, rotation was introduced in a stepwise manner. The standard increase in speed was 5 RPM per day although particularly capable rats progressed more quickly. Every effort was made to induce each rat to perform at the top speed that it would. The criterion for failure was 2 successive days of 3 failures (falls plus refusals) at the same rotational speed. Any rat that achieved 50 RPM was terminated. After reaching best performance on the rough surfaced rod, the same training and testing procedure was used for the slippery surfaced rod.

Spontaneous Alternation. Hippocampal X-irradiated and control rats were given tests of spontaneous alternation behavior in an unpainted wood T-maze (each arm equalled 50 cm in length) covered by clear Plexiglass. Rats were tested at 2-3 months or 8 months of age. The room was semi-darkened and rats were given one test per day on two successive days. Rats that refused to make a four paw goal arm entry within 120 seconds were terminated on that particular day. Rats were gently removed from the maze immediately after making a choice and were confined to a holding cage for 30 seconds between trials.

Two-Way Active Avoidance. A fully automated shuttle box (Lafayette Instrument Co.) was used to test two-way avoidance performance in hippocampal X-irradiated and control rats at 2-3 months and 8 months of age. The rats were allowed to explore the darkened shuttle box for 10 minutes with the guillotine door opened. The number of spontaneous crossing responses during the exploration period was recorded. A white noise masking source was on continuously. Immediately following the exploration period was a single 100 trial avoidance session was initiated. A one milliamp interrupted, scrambled shock (0.5 sec. on, 2 sec. off) was administered if the rat did not cross from one compartment to the other within 8 seconds of the onset of a compound light and tone condi-

132

tioned stimulus. Shock and cues continued until the rat escaped to the opposite compartment.

RESULTS
Cerebellar X-irradiation

Histological Assessment. The extent of cerebellar retardation produced by 7 exposures between days 4 and 15 is illustrated in Fig. 1. The appreciable

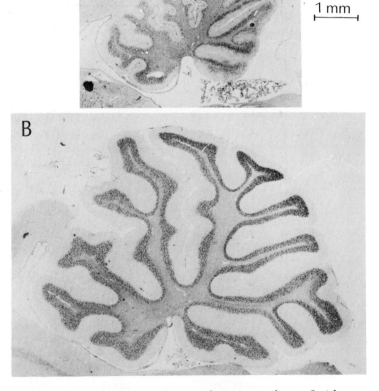

Figure 1. Low power photomicrographs of the cerebellum (A) of an X-irradiated rat and (B) of a control rat used in these experiments. Age: 8 months.

reduction in the size of the cerebellum was associated with a failure of Purkinje cells to form a monolayer, a reduction in the width of the molecular layer, and the paucity of granule cells.

Open Field Activity. Fig. 2 shows ambulation levels in terms of average square entries per rat summed across five test days. Juvenile control rats were more active than adults, an observation which has been reported previously (Livesey and Egger 1970; Brunner 1971; Bronstein 1972). Following irradiation the juvenile rats were much less active than their age-matched controls (p $<$ .05). However, the adult X-irradiated rats were at least as active as normal adults, indicating normalization of this function with age.

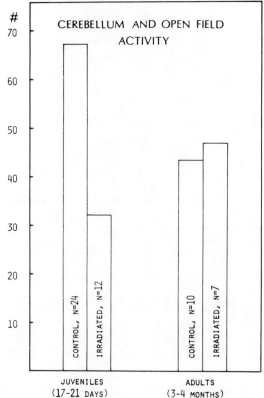

Figure 2. Mean number of squares traversed in the open field in control and cerebellar-X-irradiated juvenile and adult rats.

<u>Rearing</u>. Fig. 3 shows the average number of unsupported hindlimb responses per rat summed across five test days. Unlike ambulation, rearing frequency increases in young adults with respect to juveniles. The juvenile X-irradiated rats reared rarely and the difference with respect to the controls was significant (p < .05). Rearing frequency increased in the adult irradiated rats but did not reach the level of normal adults (p > .05 < .10).

<u>Rod Crossing</u>. Juvenile irradiated rats did poorly with respect to age-matched controls in traversing a narrow path for the reward of joining littermates (Table 1) both in terms of forelimb slips (p < .01) and hindlimb slips (p < .05) and latency of crossing responses (p < .05). Young adult rats (Fig. 4) performed equally well on rotating rods with good or poor traction. The irradiated young

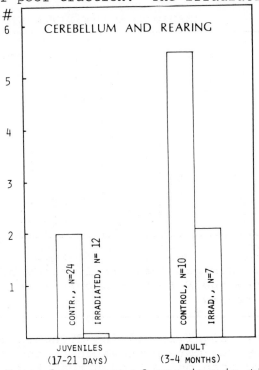

Figure 3. Mean frequency of rearing in the open field.

Table 1

TRAVERSING A NARROW PATHWAY (1.2 cm)

AGE: 17-21 days

	CONTROL	CEREBELLAR-IRRADIATED
FORELIMB SLIPS (frequency)	0.1	0.6
HINDLIMB SLIPS (Frequency)	0.8	2.3
BEST LATENCY (seconds)	7.0	16.0

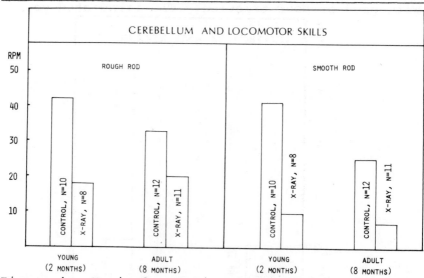

Figure 4. Maximal rotational speeds of rods mastered by the different groups when crossing for food reward.

adults were significantly handicapped and their deficiency was more pronounced on the slippery smooth rod than on the rough rod (Fig. 4). In the irradiated old (8 months) rats there was no indication of recovery of function on either the rough or the smooth rod.

Hippocampal X-irradiation

Histological Assessment: The extent of hippocampal degranulation produced by 7 exposures between days 2 and 15 is illustrated in Fig. 5. A previous quantitative study (Bayer, Brunner, Hine and Altman 1973) showed that this treatment produces an irreversible reduction of granule cells in the range of 82-85%.

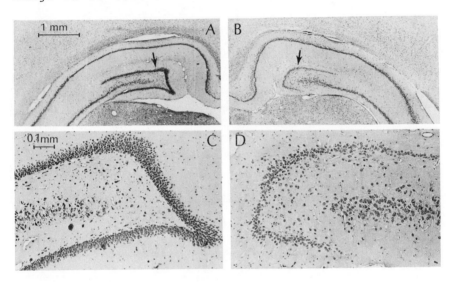

Figure 5. Photomicrograph of the hippocampus in normal (A, C) and X-irradiated (B, D) rats. Arrows in A and B point to the granular layer (C and D) of the dentate gyrus of the hippocampus.

Open Field Test. Hippocampal X-irradiated rats began showing evidence of hyperactivity, concurrently with a developmental increase in ambulation in normal animals, from day 16 onward (Fig. 6A). Activity level declined after weaning in both normal and irradiated rats but the difference between the two groups was maintained (Fig. 6B) and there was no clear indication of normalization in 240 day old animals (Fig. 6C).

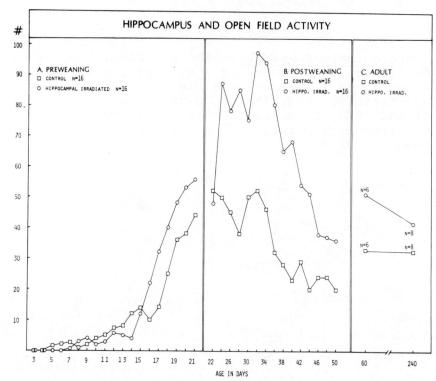

Figure 6. Mean number of squares traversed in the open field by four groups of X-irradiated and control rats of different ages.

Rearing. A similar developmental course was observed in the frequency of rearing in the open field (Fig. 7) as for ambulation. The level of activity was higher throughout the observation period in weanling (Fig. 7B) and adult rats (Fig. 7C) with some indication of convergence by 240 days. By that time rearing frequency was declining appreciably in rats not habituated to the open field.

Defecation. There was a developmental increase in defecation when rats were placed in the open field (Fig. 8). The young irradiated rats had very low bolus counts and the effect was still evident at 8 months of age.

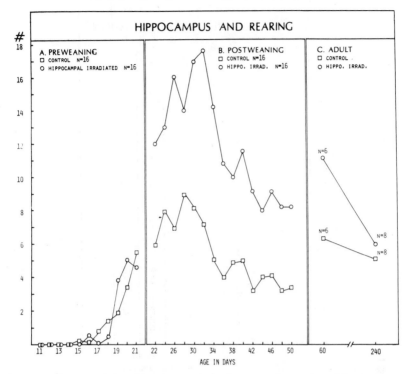

Figure 7. Mean frequency of rearing in the open field by four groups of X-irradiated and control rats of different ages.

Two-Way Active Avoidance. Irradiated young rats made substantially more avoidance in a shuttle box (Fig. 9A) than did their normal littermates. Although the magnitude of the differences declined between normal and irradiated older rats they still differed significantly (p<.05) at 8 months of age.

Spontaneous Alternation. The 2 month old control rats displayed a high alternation rate while the X-irradiated rats did not alternate significantly above chance level (Fig. 9B). Alternation was still evident in normal rats 8 months of age whereas the irradiated rats of the same age repeated turns significantly (alternation rate of 27%).

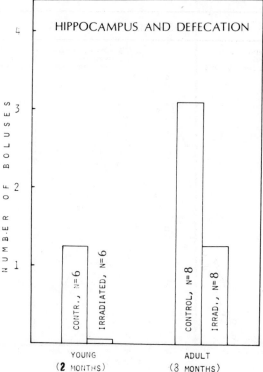

Figure 8. *Mean number of bolus counts in the open field.*

DISCUSSION

The results of this pilot study indicate normalization of at least one motor function with age following interference with the development of the cerebellum but no evidence of full restitution or any recovery in other instances. Cerebellar-irradiated juveniles displayed less ambulatory activity in the open field than their normal age-mates but at 3-4 months there was little difference in activity between controls and experimental animals. This normalization was associated with a decline in the activity of normal rats and an increase in irradiated animals. We noted such an age-dependent decline in the locomotion of normal rats in a previous study (Wallace and Altman 1969) in which the performance

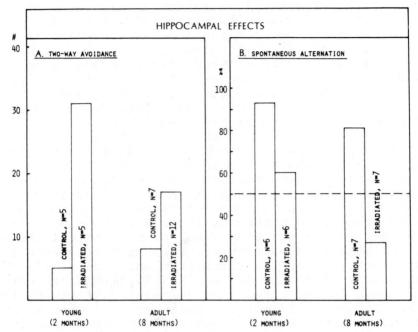

Figure 9. (A) Mean number of avoidance in the shuttle box. (B) Spontaneous alternation in a T-maze.

of 50, 100 and 150 day old rats was compared in activity wheels. The same study showed that rats irradiated with doses (8-10 X 200 r) comparable in effect to that used in this study have increased their locomotor activity with age.

Contrary to this evidence of normalization (or hypercompensation) of locomotor activity after cerebellar-irradiation, the tests that were used to assess specific motor skills indicated permanent deficits. Rearing, which requires stationary balancing on the hindlimbs, was seen less frequently in juvenile and young-adult irradiated rats than in age-matched controls. On the rotating rough or smooth rods, which is a difficult locomotor task, there was no evidence of recovery between 2 and 8 months of age. We cannot at present reconcile these seemingly contrary findings. We speculate that the increase with age in the ambulatory activity of the cerebellar-irradiated animals does not reflect recovery but rather a failure in the development of cerebellar inhibition which in normal animals becomes manifest as a decline in open field activity. Coupled with this effect, retardation of cerebellar development also produces lasting deficits in the execution of motor skills as seen in the tests described (rearing and traversing rotating rods) and in others in progress (swimming style and climbing up on rods).

Even less recovery was seen in the animals in which hippocampal development was interfered with by X-irradiation during infancy. The effect of irradiation became manifest by the beginning of the third week, when there is a spurt in locomotor activity, and it was characterized by hyperactivity with respect to controls. There were developmental changes in the activity level of the control and experimental animals with age but the relative hyperactivity of the irradiated rats was manifest as late as 8 months of age. Little normalization was seen in the irradiated animals with respect to the frequency of rearing responses by 2 months, although there were indications of convergence by 8 months of age, by which time rearing frequency diminished greatly in both groups. Defecation in the open field was also subject to developmental changes but there was no clear evidence of normalization by 8 months of age, although there was a reduction in the relative difference between the two groups. There was no clear evidence of normalization in two-way avoidance performance and an apparent deterioration with age in the irradiated animals in spontaneous alternation.

This study was not designed to compare the effects of early and late brain damage (low-level irradiation is effective only during early infancy) nor has it shed much light on the controversial question whether or not, to what extent, and under what circumstances, there is recovery of function after early brain damage. What it may have accomplished is to have highlighted the importance of the developmental or longitudinal approach in the study of the problem of recovery of function. Some of the research designs that have been used or may find usefulness in this area are summarized in Fig. 10. A distinction is made between "discrete" and "longitudinal" paradigms.

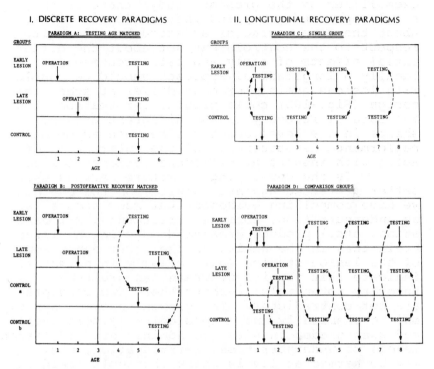

Figure 10. Research paradigms dealing with the problem of recovery of function. Broken arrows point to valid comparisons.

In the discrete paradigms (Fig. 10A, B) testing is done at one specific age. If both early and late operates are tested at the same age (Fig. 10A) then the difference in postoperative recovery time is necessarily neglected - a pitfall in design that is universally acknowledged. If both groups are tested after comparable intervals and two age-matched control groups are available (Fig. 10B) then both age and postoperative recovery time are controlled for. However, this design presumes that the pace of recovery is constant across all ages, and that requires empirical verification. In the longitudinal paradigm (Figs. 10C, D) tests are repeatedly administered and developmental trends in the behavior of normal and operated animals are compared. In one of these paradigms (Fig. 10C;

exemplified by the present study) there is only a single operated group and information is gained about the time course of affected behavior with respect to the controls but not about the differential effects of early and late treatments. Ideally a longitudinal approach should be coupled with lesions administered at different ages. This design (Fig. 10D) could provide information about the rate of recovery in the different groups, shifts in the level and the time when asymptotic performance is attained, and the interaction of aging with insults at different periods of life.

Is the developing or mature nervous system better protected against insults? On the one hand, we have compelling evidence that many agents (such as undernutrition, hormonal treatments, X-irradiation, etc.) produce greater damage in the infant brain than in the adult, on the other hand, some of the lesion studies (particularly in primates) indicate that the infant brain has greater recovery potentials. Perhaps these two concepts are not contradictory. The growing nervous system may be chemically and morphologically more labile, and when graded insults are administered (different levels of undernutrition, X-irradiation, etc.) it may be harmed at levels where the adult brain is still spared. However, when suprathreshold insults are applied to both (such as actual removal of brain tissue) then the immature brain may display its advantages as a growing system with greater capacity for reorganization. But all this is very speculative at present. We really have little evidence for adaptive reorganization in the developing nervous system. The sprouting of new nerve processes and the formation of new synaptic connections could aid or hinder recovery depending whether they lead to reorganization or disorganization. Our evidence of the harmful behavioral consequences of early interference with the organization of cerebellar fine-circuitry by X-irradiation (Altman and Anderson 1972, 1973) suggests the possibility of a disorganizing effect produced by the aberrant neural connections produced.

ACKNOWLEDGMENT: This research program is supported by the National Institute of Mental Health and the

U.S. Atomic Energy Commission. The assistance of Zeynep Kurgun, Patricia McNerney, Kiran Sudarshan and William Schoenlein is gratefully acknowledged.

REFERENCES

Altman, J. (1969). Autoradiographic and histological studies of postnatal neurogenesis. III. Dating the time of production and onset of differentiation of cerebellar microneurons in rats. *J. Comp. Neur.* 136, 269-294.

Altman, J. and Anderson, W.J. (1972). Experimental reorganization of the cerebellar cortex. I. Morphological effects of elimination of all microneurons with prolonged X-irradiation started at birth. *J. Comp. Neur.* 146, 355-406.

Altman, J. and Anderson, W.J. (1973). Experimental reorganization of the cerebellar cortex. II. Effects of elimination of most microneurons with prolonged X-irradiation started at four days. *J. Comp. Neur.* 149, 123-152.

Altman, J., Anderson, W.J. and Strop, M. (1971). Retardation of cerebellar and motor development by focal X-irradiation during infancy. *Physiol. Behav.* 7, 143-150.

Altman, J., Anderson, W.J. and Wright, K.A. (1968). Gross morphological consequences of irradiation of the cerebellum in infant rats with repeated doses of low-level X-ray. *Exp. Neur.* 21, 69-91.

Altman, J., Anderson, W.J. and Wright, K.A. (1969). Early effects of X-irradiation of the cerebellum in infant rats: Decimation and reconstitution of the external granular layer. *Exp. Neur.* 24, 196-216.

Altman, J. and Das, G.D. (1965). Autoradiographic and histological evidence of postnatal hippocampal neurogenesis in rats. *J. Comp. Neur.* 124, 319-335.

Altman, J. and Das, G.D. (1966). Autoradiographic and histological studies of postnatal neurogenesis. I. A longitudinal investigation of the kinetics, migration and transformation of cells incorporating tritiated thymidine in neonate rats, with special reference to postnatal neurogenesis in some brain regions. *J. Comp. Neur.* 126, 337-390.

Altman, J., Das, G.D. and Sudarshan, K. (1970). The influence of nutrition on neural and behavioral development. I. Critical review of some data on the growth of the body and the brain following dietary deprivation during gestation and lactation. *Devel. Psychobiol.* 3, 281-301.

Balàzs, R., Kovàcs, S., Cocks, W.A., Johnson, A.L. and Eayrs, J.T. (1971). Effects of thyroid hormone on the biochemical maturation of rat brain: Postnatal cell formation. *Brain Res.* 25, 555-570.

Bayer, S.A., Brunner, R.L., Hine, R. and Altman, J. (1973). Behavioral effects of interference with the postnatal acquisition of hippocampal granule cells. *Nature, New Biol.* 242, 222-224.

Bronstein, P.M. (1972). Repeated trials with the albino rat in the open field as a function of age and deprivation. *J. Comp. Physiol. Psychol.* 81, 84-93.

Brunner, R.L. (1971). The effects of early infant handling on the development of exploration and passive avoidance. Ph.D. Thesis, University of Cincinnati (unpublished).

Brunner, R.L. and Altman, J. (1973). Locomotor deficits in adult rats with moderate to massive retardation of cerebellar development during infancy. *Behav. Biol.* 9, 169-188.

Haggbloom, S.J., Brunner, R.L. and Bayer, S.A. (1973). Effects of hippocampal granule cell agenesis on acquisition of escape from fear and one-way active avoidance responses. *J. Comp. Physiol. Psychol.* (in press).

Hicks, S.P. and D'Amato, C.J. (1966). Effects of ionizing radiations on mammalian development. *In* D.H.M. Woollan (Ed.) "Advances in Teratology." London: Logos Press. pp. 195-250.

Livesey, P.J. and Egger, G.J. (1970). Age as a factor in open-field responsiveness in the white rat. *J. Comp. Physiol. Psychol.* 73, 93-99.

Nicholson, J.L. and Altman, J. (1972a). The effects of early hypo- and hyperthyroidism on the development of rat cerebellar cortex. I. Cell proliferation and differentiation. *Brain Res.* 44, 13-23.

Nicholson, J.L. and Altman, J. (1972b). The effects
   of early hypo- and hyperthyroidism on the
   development of the rat cerebellar cortex.
   II. Synaptogenesis in the molecular layer.
   Brain Res. 44, 25-36.
Wallace, R.B. and Altman, J. (1969). Behavioral
   effects of neonatal irradiation of the
   cerebellum. II. Quantitative studies in young-
   adult and adult rats. *Devel. Psychobiol.* 2,
   266-272.
Winick, M. and Noble, A. (1966). Cellular response
   in rats during malnutrition at various ages.
   J. Nutrition 89, 300-306.

AN ALTERNATIVE TO DEVELOPMENTAL PLASTICITY: HETEROLOGY OF CNS STRUCTURES IN INFANTS AND ADULTS

Patricia S. Goldman
National Institute of Mental Health
Bethesda, Maryland

It is now well established that central nervous system injury sustained in infancy often produces fewer and less severe aftereffects than does similar injury sustained at maturity. The milder effects of early injury have led to the view that the immature brain is endowed with mechanisms for compensatory adjustment that the adult brain partly or totally lacks. Evidence from studies in rhesus monkeys has become increasingly more difficult to reconcile with this view and, indeed much of it may be interpreted as antithetical to plasticity. The purpose of this paper is twofold - to call attention to difficulties with compensatory formulations, and to develop evidence for an alternative approach to the behavioral effects of early brain injury.

Currently, two different views of compensatory mechanisms in young animals predominate. One of these derives from the important discovery that new or unusual anatomical connections are formed following early postnatal injury and are present in animals that exhibit some measure of behavioral adaptation (Hicks and D'Amato 1970; Schneider 1970). These demonstrations of coincident anatomical restructuring and behavioral sparing are bolstered by evidence that altered anatomy (Lynch, Mosko, Parks, and Cotman 1973; Lynch, Deadwyler and Cotman 1973) or altered function (Stewart and Riesen 1972) in neonatally operated animals can be correlated with changes in electrophysiological activity. Thus, the view has arisen that behavioral sparing following early lesions may be mediated by anomalous neuroanatomical connections.

The other view of the compensatory process suggests that early-operated animals learn to get along without a given structure, not by rerouting connections, but by evolving new solutions to problems based on the intrinsic functions of residual structures. According to this view, early-operated animals employ different strategies

to solve problems than do unoperated controls and
more successful strategies than do adult-operated
animals. The strength of this approach lies
chiefly in its explanatory appeal rather than in
the empirical evidence available to support it;
even so, it cannot be dismissed.

It is both reasonable and appealing to
conceptualize the neural basis of developmental
plasticity in terms of compensatory mechanisms --
involving either new connections or new strategies.
Yet, as will be developed, neither new connections
nor new strategies can be considered as general
or final solutions to the problem of sparing.

Dorsolateral vs. Orbital Lesions in Infant Monkeys

The limitations of existing formulations about
sparing of deficits in early-operated animals are
especially apparent in dealing with the results
from studies of prefrontal lesions in infant
monkeys. These studies have established that the
functions of the dorsolateral and orbital prefrontal regions of the monkeys' frontal lobe are not
spared to the same degree following lesions
sustained at or before 50-days of age. The initial
evidence for sparing of dorsolateral function was
provided by Akert, Orth, Harlow and Schiltz (1960).
These investigators removed cortex in and around
the principal sulcus in two rhesus monkeys at five
days of age. The two monkeys failed to show the
delayed-response impairments that are characteristic for monkeys operated upon in adulthood.
Subsequently, the same phenomenon was investigated
over a wider range of conditions in closely
related studies by Harlow, Blomquist, Thompson,
Schiltz and Harlow (1968), Tucker and Kling (1967,
1969) and by Goldman (1971). Altogether in these
studies, seventeen monkeys given lesions of the
dorsolateral cortex within the first 50 days of
life were tested on delayed response. Despite
differences in the extent of the lesion within and
beyond the dorsolateral area and differences in
the procedures used to test delayed response, the
results were the same -- monkeys operated upon in
infancy, unlike those operated at maturity, were
capable of learning delayed response, and in fact,
performed as well as unoperated controls (Goldman

1971).

In contrast to the effects of dorsolateral lesions, early removals of the orbital prefrontal cortex failed to spare functions mediated by this region. The evidence for impairment of orbital function following early lesions came originally from studies of monkeys lobectomized in infancy. These monkeys with removals including both the dorsolateral and orbital cortical regions were impaired on measures of orbital function at the same time that they were unimpaired on tests of dorsolateral function (Goldman, Rosvold and Mishkin 1970a; 1970b). Later, four monkeys given lesions limited to the orbital cortex at 50 days of age were compared with monkeys given similar lesions as juveniles (Goldman 1971). The early-operated monkeys were impaired on the same tests and to the same degree as monkeys operated upon later in life. More recently, this finding has been confirmed in thirteen additional cases that underwent orbital prefrontal surgery within the first, fourth, or eighth week of life (Miller, Goldman and Rosvold 1973).

Instances of failure to find evidence of sparing are not limited to studies of the orbital cortex of the monkey. Kennard (1938) mentioned that the deviation of the head and eyes which follows unilateral lesions of the frontal eye fields in the adult monkey are no less severe and enduring in monkeys that had undergone removal of this area in infancy. Although the evidence was not entirely clear, it appeared also that placing and hopping reactions were abolished after neonatal ablation of the motor areas. In addition, while spasticity and rigidity were not immediate symptoms after early motor cortex ablation, these signs of dyskinesia became progressively more prominent as the monkeys grew older and consequently must be regarded as expressions of uncompensated pathology (Kennard 1940; 1942). The work of Lawrence and Hopkins (1970) indicates that bilateral pyramidotomy ultimately impairs individual finger movements just as much in monkeys subjected to this operation in infancy as it does in monkeys pyramidotomized as adults, and extends Kennard's finding that fine motor skills were not well developed in her otherwise remarkably

compensated monkeys. Hicks and D'Amato (1970)
although providing evidence that the stride
component of locomotion was spared following early
hemispherectomy in rats, failed to find sparing of
contralateral tactile placing, visual pattern
discrimination and visually-elicited jumping.
Bland and Cooper (1969) failed to find greater
visual function after early as compared with late
visual cortex removals in the rat. Murphy and
Stewart (1974) likewise found no difference between
adult and infant destriated rabbits on tests of
pattern discrimination. Doty (1971) has recently
concluded that sparing of visual pattern vision
can be obtained following area 17 lesions in adult
cats as well as in kittens, thus placing his
earlier report of greater sparing in kittens (Doty
1961) in a new light.

Thus, the principle that function is spared
after early lesions is not a general one, but
rather has many important exceptions that no
theory so far discussed can readily explain. For
example, the formation of anomalous connections is
thought to depend, among other things, on synaptic
space being made available when fibers degenerate
as a result of injury (Goodman and Horel 1966;
McCouch, Austin, Liu and Liu 1958; Raisman 1969;
Schneider 1970). Since synaptic space is presumably
made available in the case of all central nervous
system lesions, it would be expected that new
connections could as well be formed following
lesions that result in deficits as following those
that lead to sparing. A related issue is that of
whether new connections are formed only in the
young or are adaptive only in the young. Much of
the evidence for collateral sprouting has in fact
been obtained in studies of adult animals (Goodman
and Horel 1966; Liu and Chambers 1958; Moore,
Björklund and Stenevi 1971; and Raisman 1969).
Thus a mechanism for anatomical restructuring that
obtains both in infants and adults, and may obtain
both in animals that exhibit sparing and in those
that do not, could not easily account for
differential behavioral aftereffects following
central nervous system injury.

Similar problems are encountered when
considering an explanation of sparing in terms
of new solutions. It is difficult to comprehend,

for example, why young animals with one cortical lesion would have recourse to residual strategies while young animals with another lesion would not. It is more difficult still to envision how juvenile or young adult monkeys could be at a disadvantage in developing new solutions as compared with less experienced and less mature monkeys.

Any theory of plasticity must account for why some functions are recovered following early brain injury, while others are not. Since the factors that limit sparing in some systems following early nervous system lesions are presumably similar to those operating against sparing in the adult, the problem is at the heart of the plasticity issue. Although we are at an early phase in the evolution of ideas about sparing, neither new connections nor new strategies now provide a conceptual framework in which both behavioral deficits and behavioral sparing can be readily subsumed.

Cortical vs. Subcortical Lesions in Infancy

Much of the strongest evidence for collateral sprouting comes from studies involving lesions in subcortical structures and in fiber systems connecting subcortical structures (Moore, Björklund and Stenevi 1971; Raisman 1969; and Schneider 1970). Yet, it is precisely after subcortical lesions in infancy that behavioral sparing has been least impressive. Removal of the hippocampus in kittens results in as severe passive avoidance deficits as those found following similar removals in adults (Isaacson, Nonneman and Schmaltz 1968; Nonneman and Isaacson 1973). Amygdalectomies alter fear response patterns as much in monkeys operated upon in infancy as in monkeys operated upon as adults (Thompson, Schwartzbaum and Harlow 1969). Johnson (1972) failed to find evidence for milder effects of septal lesions in neonates than in adult rats on avoidance responding, fixed ratio responding and social behavior and it appears also that lesions of the ventromedial nucleus of the hypothalamus in weanling rats result in hyperinsulinemia and increased body fat just as they do in adult rats (Bernardis and Frohman 1971; Frohman and Bernardis 1968).

We have been studying the effects of early lesions in subcortical structures that are related both functionally and anatomically to the prefrontal cortex. The dorsolateral prefrontal cortex projects, among other places, to the anterodorsal sector of the head of the caudate nucleus (Johnson, Rosvold and Mishkin 1968; Kemp and Powell 1970). Figure 1 provides evidence that lesions of this sector in infancy produce deficits on delayed response and delayed alternation just as they do in juveniles or adults. As we have previously reported (Goldman and Rosvold 1972), the incidence and severity of the impairments is related to the extent of the lesion both in infants and in juveniles.

The caudate nucleus is a subcortical target of efferent projections from the prefrontal cortex. We have also placed lesions in the principal thalamic source of afferent projections to the prefrontal cortex -- the dorsomedial nucleus. Only a few studies have examined the effects of lesions in this structure on the delayed-response repertoire of adult monkeys, so far with inconclusive results (Chow 1954; Peters, Rosvold and Mirsky 1956; Shulman 1964). It now appears, however, that dorsomedial lesions in young adults can produce clear and consistent deficits on delayed alternation unaccompanied by deficits on problems, such as a visual pattern discrimination, that do not depend upon the integrity of frontal cortex. Figure 2 indicates that the effects of dorsomedial lesions in infancy are at least as

---

Figure 1. The effect of early and late lesions in the anterodorsal sector of the head of the caudate nucleus on three tests: DR, delayed response; DA, delayed alternation; OR, object discrimination reversal. The monkeys operated at 50 days of age were tested beginning at 1 year of age; the juvenile monkeys were estimated to be 18-24 months of age at surgery and 28-34 months old when tested. The scores of early-operated monkeys and their age-matched controls are shown in the left section of the figure; the late-operated group and their controls are shown on the right. Bars indicate trials; dots, errors.

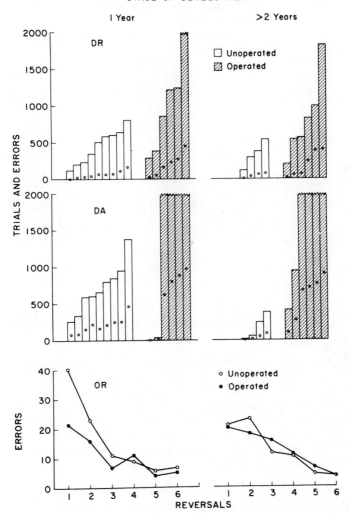

STAGE OF DEVELOPMENT

severe and selective as those of similar lesions incurred later in life.

These findings challenge us to explain why, generally speaking, sparing of function should be less following early subcortical lesions than following early cortical removals. Formulations in terms of new connections or new strategies have yet to provide a basis for expecting that these processes would be brought into play to a greater

STAGE OF DEVELOPMENT

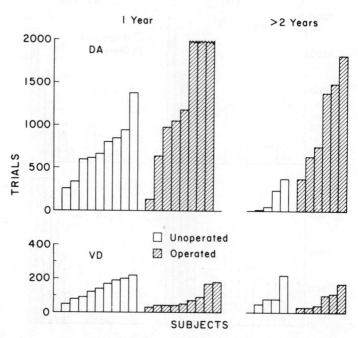

Figure 2. The effect of lesions in the dorsomedial nucleus of the thalamus on delayed alternation (DA) and on a visual pattern discrimination problem (VD). Early-operated monkeys and their age-matched controls are shown on the left; late-operated monkeys and unoperated controls are shown on the right. Age at surgery and at testing as explained in the legend to Fig. 1.

extent following cortical and to a lesser extent following subcortical lesions in infancy.

The Effects of Early Lesions at Different Stages of Development

As mentioned earlier, Kennard (1940; 1942) reported that some aspects of motor performance that were not present in the immediate post-operative period became evident as the monkeys with motor cortex lesions grew older. Similarly Lawrence and Hopkins (1970) found deficiency in

the fine control of movement as monkeys with
pyramidal tract lesions in infancy grew older.
Kling (1966) commented that when major alterations
in the social behavior of rats, cats, and monkeys
subjected to lesions of the amygdala in infancy
were noted at all, they were noted at the time the
animals reached puberty. Tucker and Kling (1967)
also reported evidence of increasing delayed-
response impairment with age when they retested
one monkey that had been given a prefrontal lesion
in infancy. When first tested at 10 months of age,
this monkey was able to attain criterion levels of
performance at delays as long as 40 seconds; when
retested at 18 months of age, however, the monkey
was not able to perform correctly at delays greater
than 5 seconds. I have previously reported that
monkeys with early dorsolateral removals did not
differ significantly from unoperated controls on
delayed alternation when the two groups were
compared at 15 months of age (Goldman 1971; 1972).
Later, however, when these same monkeys were
retested on delayed alternation at two years of
age, the operated monkeys made significantly more
errors than did the unoperated monkeys and, in
fact, there was no overlap in the error distribution of the two groups.
  We have recently obtained additional evidence
for exacerbation of deficits with advancing age in
monkeys given dorsolateral lesions in infancy. In
this experiment, the surgical removals were
performed at the same age (50 days) and the
monkeys were tested in the same way as in previous
studies. The single difference between the present
experiment and previous ones was that the testing
was deferred until the monkeys were two-years old,
rather than originating when they were one year of
age. The study is still in progress but the
results obtained on the first test of the battery,
delayed response, are available and are shown in
the middle section of Figure 3. In the left
section of the figure, the performance of monkeys
operated upon in infancy is compared with that of
unoperated controls when both groups were tested
at one year of age. Operating monkeys at 50 days
of age and testing them on delayed response ten
months later at one year of age yields a picture
of complete sparing. The section to the right

157

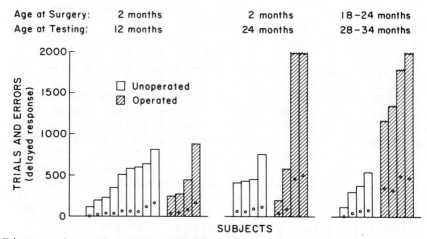

Figure 3. The effects of early and late dorso-lateral prefrontal lesions on delayed-response performance at specified times following surgery. Bars indicate trials; dots, errors.

compares the performance of monkeys operated upon as juveniles (18-24 months) with that of unoperated controls, both groups being tested at 28-34 months of age. Operating upon the monkeys as juveniles and testing them ten months later produces the classical adult pattern of complete impairment. However, operating upon monkeys at 50 days of age but postponing the testing until the monkeys were two years old produced a result intermediate to the complete sparing at the one-year stage of development and the complete impairment at 2 1/2-3 years of age (Fig. 3, middle section). Two of these early-operated monkeys exhibited complete sparing of delayed-response ability; two others exhibited total loss of the ability. It is not yet possible to offer a conclusive explanation for the bimodality of effect in the group tested at two years. A possibility that particularly interests us is that individual differences in rates of cortical development are contributing to these results and that the two monkeys that are unimpaired at this stage of the experiment will begin to evidence impairments as they advance in age. The point to be emphasized here, however, is that the two

impaired monkeys are the first cases to exhibit a
full-blown impairment on delayed response after
lesions sustained in infancy. Since all seventeen
of the cases documented in the literature were
tested either at 12 months of age (Goldman 1971)
or earlier (Akert *et al*. 1960; Harlow *et al*. 1968;
and Tucker and Kling 1967) and all were unimpaired,
we are of the view that the present results extend
previous evidence for a transformation in the
effects of early lesions at later stages of
development.

Just as there is evidence for increasing
impairment with age following dorsolateral lesions
in infancy, there is also new evidence of a
parallel phenomenon following early orbital
lesions. In previous studies, monkeys given orbital
lesions at 50 days of age were tested over a six
month period between 12 and 18 months of age.
During this time span, they were impaired on the
same tests and to the same degree as monkeys
operated upon as juveniles. In the following
experiment, monkeys were operated upon at 50 days
of age as in previous studies but instead of
delaying the testing until they were one-year of
age, testing began at 2 1/2 months of age. The
monkeys were trained on only one test -- object
discrimination reversal -- because it was necessary
to confine the testing to a restricted period of
development and to select a measure that is
discriminatively sensitive to orbital prefrontal
injury. Monkeys operated upon as juveniles,
unoperated infants and juveniles served as
controls. The results for the four groups are
presented in Figure 4. As would be expected,
monkeys operated upon as juveniles were severely
impaired. However, in contrast to all previous
studies in which monkeys with early orbital
lesions performed more poorly than controls on
object reversal, in this study, there were no
significant differences between the monkeys
operated upon in infancy and their age-matched
controls. Thus, sparing of deficits can be shown
to precede impairment of function following orbital
as well as dorsolateral lesions in infancy. The
major difference between the two systems appears
to be in the time course of effects. Following
dorsolateral lesions, impairments do not emerge

STAGE of DEVELOPMENT

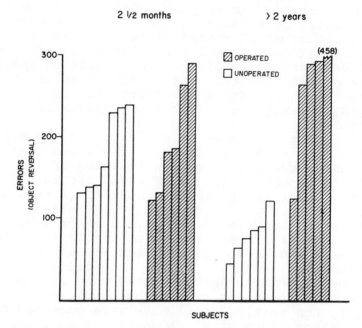

Figure 4. *The effects of orbital prefrontal lesions at 50 days of age on object reversal performance at 2 1/2 months of age are shown on the left; the effects of the same lesions in young adults are shown on thr right. The measure is the total number of errors made over six reversals.*

until at least two years of age whereas following orbital lesions, deficits appear as early as one-year of age.

There remains one more source of evidence that the consequences of early brain injury vary at different stages of development, and this source stems also from monkeys with orbital lesions. As we have previously reported (Goldman 1971; Miller, Goldman and Rosvold 1973), and as illustrated in Figure 5, monkeys given orbital lesions in infancy were severely impaired on delayed alternation when they were initially tested on this problem at about 15 months of age. However, when the same monkeys were retested at 24 months of age, all but three of them were able to solve the problem (Fig.

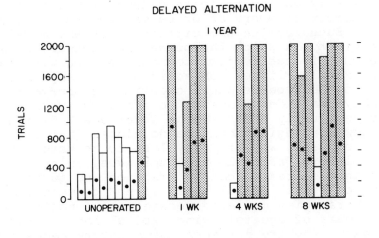

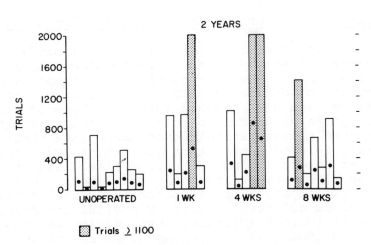

Trials ≥ 1100

Figure 5. Trials (bars) and errors (dots) on delayed alternation at different stages of development following orbital prefrontal lesions in infancy.

5, lower). Of the three, two have subsequently relearned delayed alternation in additional testing. The late learning of this subgroup may again reflect the contribution of individual differences in rates of brain development in these experiments. Nevertheless, of the original group of seventeen monkeys given orbital lesions in infancy, only one ultimately failed to learn delayed alternation and to exhibit recovery at or beyond two years of age.

Such results are difficult for any model of plasticity in which the mechanism envisioned is one that is not subject to modification with age. For example, if new connections were responsible for the delayed-response capacity of one-year old monkeys with dorsolateral lesions, why would they not be equally effective at later ages? Similarly, if new strategies could be developed in the first year of life, why are they lost to monkeys with dorsolateral removals at later ages, in spite of having been reinforced by practice and success in some cases at earlier ages? If new connections or new strategies mediated recovery of function at two years of age following orbital lesions in infancy, why are not such compensatory mechanisms available sooner?

Recent Studies on the Neural Basis of Recovery

In order to explore the neural basis for recovery in monkeys with long-standing orbital lesions six of the monkeys that had demonstrated recovery of delayed alternation ability at two years of age were studied further. Three of them were given bilateral dorsolateral lesions and then retested postoperatively once again on a number of tasks; delayed alternation (for the third time), object reversal (for the second time), and go - no go alternation (for the first time). In the juvenile or adult, performance on delayed alternation is affected equally by orbital and dorso-lateral lesions (Mishkin, Vest, Waxler and Rosvold 1969; Goldman 1971), although each region is thought to be necessary for different features of the task. Performance on object reversal and go - no go differentiation, on the other hand, is impaired only by orbital lesions (Goldman 1971; Brutkowski, Mishkin and Rosvold 1963). The three monkeys given dorsolateral lesions at this stage of the experiment were compared with three other monkeys that similarly had orbital lesions origi-nating in infancy and that had similarly recovered delayed alternation ability at two years of age. These monkeys were either left unoperated (n = 2) or given a control lesion (n = 1; in this case, tissue was removed caudal to the inferior limb of the arcuate sulcus and from the superior gyrus of the temporal lobe). The results are presented in Figures 6, 7, and 8. Superimposing dorsolateral

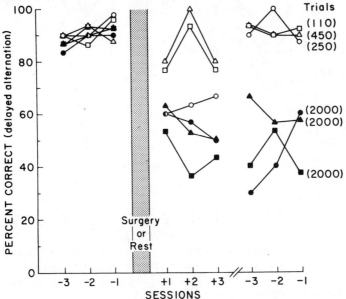

Figure 6. Delayed-alternation performance of monkeys with early orbital lesions before and after dorsolateral lesions (filled symbols) or control procedures (open symbols).

lesions after two years of age eliminated delayed alternation capacity, reducing the animals to chance levels of performance that were not improved upon in 2000 additional trials of training, but had no effect on object reversal relearning nor on go - no go acquisition. Since the pattern of results corresponds to that obtained following dorsolateral lesions in normal monkeys at this age, it provides no support for the idea that the dorsolateral cortex is involved in compensation of orbital function and, indeed, permits the direct opposite conclusion that the development of dorsolateral functions are unaltered by early orbital surgery.

The ability of monkeys with early orbital lesions to ultimately learn delayed alternation is an ability not exhibited by monkeys operated upon as adults and would appear to constitute support

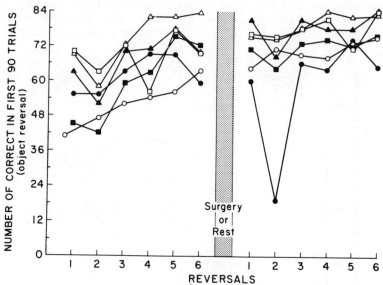

Figure 7. Object reversal performance of monkeys with early orbital lesions before and after dorsolateral lesions (filled symbols) or control procedures (open symbols).

for the idea that compensatory mechanisms operate in developing monkeys. Thinking in terms of compensatory mechanisms, it would follow that structures other than the dorsolateral cortex must be involved in the maintenance of orbital function and that it should be possible to identify these structures by a further process of elimination. Certainly, this is a logical possibility that cannot be dismissed. However, the ability of monkeys with early orbital lesions to learn delayed alternation can equally be regarded as direct evidence that delayed alternation is a task that can be solved without the orbital cortex. Given this interpretation, the question of interest then becomes that of why adult monkeys with such lesions are as impaired as they are on this task. Perhaps the profound impairments of monkeys operated upon as adults is due not to a loss in an intrinsic function of the orbital cortex as has been assumed, but rather to an indirect interference with dorsolateral function. One mechanism for such

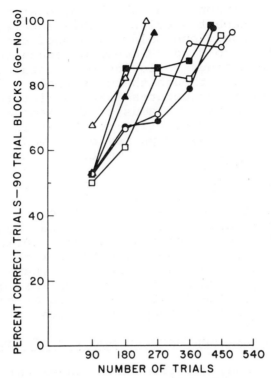

Figure 8. Go - no go differentiation performance of monkeys with early orbital lesions after dorsolateral lesions (filled symbols) or control procedures (open symbols).

interference might be related to the fact that both cortical regions project to the head of the caudate nucleus. While the dorsolateral and orbital areas project to topographically distinct locations in the caudate, there is also an area of the caudate in which the projections overlap to a considerable extent (Johnson, Rosvold and Mishkin 1968). Interestingly, these overlapping projections arise from those subdivisions of the dorsolateral and orbital prefrontal regions that are most critical for delayed alternation performance (Goldman and Rosvold 1970; Iversen and Mishkin 1970). At the locus in the caudate where these projections converge, it is possible that degenerating axons from an orbital prefrontal lesion in adulthood could impair the functional integrity of

the caudate neurons upon which dorsolateral axons
terminate. Recent studies in this laboratory
(Johnson, Rosvold and Goldman, unpublished) have
so far failed to find evidence of degeneration in
the caudate nucleus following prefrontal lesions
in infants, even though there is ample evidence of
degeneration in structures like the internal
capsule and dorsal thalamus of the same brains.
The absence of argyrophilic reactions in infant
cortico-striatal pathways may be viewed as an
index of their functional immaturity (Leonard
1973) and could provide a basis for the protection
of striatal mechanisms. The advantage to a monkey
with an orbital prefrontal ablation in infancy
would be that dorsolateral projections to the
caudate could escape the transneuronal consequences
of orbital injury, and could develop normally.

Thus, while it is possible to view the recovery
of delayed alternation ability at 2 years of age
as evidence for compensatory mechanisms, other
alternatives, relating to the status of the
nervous system in infancy, are no less plausible.

A Developmental Approach to Sparing of Function

The many questions and issues raised in
preceding sections of this paper have been upper-
most in our minds as we have been considering:
(1) the contrasting effects of dorsolateral and
orbital lesions at any given point in time,
(2) the evidence for greater sparing of ability
following cortical as compared with subcortical
lesions within the same neurobehavioral system,
(3) the changing consequences of early injury at
different stages of ontogenetic development, and
(4) the lack of positive evidence for central
nervous system reorganization in monkeys with
orbital injuries.

The picture that emerges from the many studies
referred to above is that in the six-month
period between 12 and 18 months of age, the losses
in behavior caused by lesions in infancy of the
orbital cortex, the anterodorsal sector of the
head of the caudate nucleus and the dorsomedial
nucleus of the thalamus are as selective and as
severe as those caused by similar injuries in
young adulthood. During the same six-month period,

monkeys deprived of the dorsolateral cortex in infancy fail to exhibit deficits on tests that the same lesions later in life will impair profoundly. While compensatory mechanisms may be invoked to explain these differential effects, an alternative explanation for these findings is that the orbital prefrontal cortex, the caudate nucleus, and the dorsal thalamus are functionally mature by one year of age whereas the dorsolateral cortex is not. According to a developmental perspective, dorsolateral lesions do not impair delayed response at that age because the dorsolateral cortex does not play a role in delayed-response behavior at that age, i.e., the dorsolateral cortex is functionally heterologous rather than homologous in infants and adults. Compensatory pathways or strategies would be superfluous for the simple reason that the neural substrate normally responsible for delayed-response behavior at this stage of development would be intact in operated and unoperated monkeys alike.

Further, if compensatory mechanisms were responsible for the sparing of dorsolateral function at the one-year stage of development, it might be supposed that these processes would sustain the monkeys as they grew older and performance on delayed-response tasks would be as preserved at one stage of development as at another. In contrast, if the sparing of dorsolateral function were related to the functional immaturity of the dorsolateral cortex at that age, then deficits should be increasingly more apparent as the animal matures and the dorsolateral cortex normatively becomes more essential for delayed-response behavior. The results of several experiments now lend some support to this possibility. When monkeys given dorsolateral lesions in infancy were tested on delayed alternation for a second time at 24 months of age, they exhibited deficits on this task for the first time (Goldman 1971). The present report contains evidence for emergent and full-blown deficits on delayed response at two years of age in previously untrained monkeys with dorsolateral lesions, even though these lesions were sustained in infancy.

If the phenomenon of sparing in monkeys with dorsolateral lesions is dependent on the normative

maturity of the brain at the time behavior is
assessed, then it should be possible to obtain
results indicative of sparing or of impairment in
monkeys with other central nervous system lesions
simply by testing them at different stages of
development for the particular function in
question. Testing early-operated monkeys with
dorsolateral lesions well beyond one year of age
brought out impairments. Testing monkeys with
orbital lesions well before one year of age should
diminish impairments. Indeed, the evidence
obtained when monkeys with orbital lesions were
tested at 2 1/2 months of age indicates that these
monkeys are, at that age, functionally equivalent
to unoperated controls. Although the orbital
cortex is necessary for object discrimination
reversal learning in adults, it would appear that
structures other than the orbital cortex mediate
such learning in infants.

Thus, the maturational status of the central
nervous system enters into the explanation of
spared functions after early injury in at least
two ways. First, there is the matter of the degree
to which the damaged substrate would normally
participate in a given function at a given age.
Functions will appear preserved when the neural
substrate is removed in infancy and animals are
evaluated at prefunctional stages for the development of the substrate. Indeed, functions will
appear to have been compensated when, in fact,
they had not been lost. Thus, monkeys with dorsolateral lesions appear normal or nearly so at
one year of age; monkeys with orbital lesions
appear normal at two and one-half months of age.
These operated monkeys may in fact be normal for
their age. However, they are not normal for age
when they are assessed at terminal stages for the
development of the substrate. In the case of
dorsolateral injury, evidence of abnormality first
begins to emerge at two years of age while in the
case of orbital injury such evidence is already
present by one year of age. In both cases, however,
the monkeys exhibit arrest of normal development
for the particular function in question.

The second way developmental factors may affect
behavior following early lesions concerns the
maturational status of intact structures that the

brain-injured animal can fall back upon. The maturational condition of these structures also varies at different stages of development. At one year of age, the orbital cortex, the caudate nucleus and the dorsomedial nucleus of the thalamus are all functionally mature. These structures may subserve delayed-response behavior before the dorsolateral cortex develops, both in normal one-year old monkeys and in those with dorsolateral lesions. At the same time, monkeys with orbital lesions would appear to have only the subcortical frontal-lobe structures to rely upon if, as the evidence suggests, the dorsolateral cortex is pre-functional at the one-year stage of development. At two years of age, however, when the dorsolateral cortex appears to become committed to its own functions, the monkeys with orbital removals in infancy demonstrate the ability -- absent at the earlier stage -- to solve delayed alternation.

Conclusion

In spite of the momentum given by many lines of research to the concept of central nervous system reorganization as a basis for recovery or sparing of function in cases of early brain damage, it is most unlikely that the full range of mechanisms underlying cerebral plasticity has yet been catalogued. The evidence and arguments presented here may justify adding still another category to the inventory of potential mechanisms. Behavioral evidence obtained in monkeys with early central nervous system injury may be regarded as definitive for the proposition that the brain operated upon in infancy is not entirely homologous to the brain operated upon at maturity. Immature and mature brains may well differ in their potential for collateral sprouting and for developing strategies but they may differ also in the extent to which their functions and connections have been established and consequently in the extent to which lesions may affect these functions and connections.

REFERENCES

Akert, K., Orth, O.S., Harlow, H.F. and Schiltz, K.A. (1960). Learned behavior of rhesus monkeys following neonatal bilateral prefrontal lobotomy. *Science* 132, 1944-1945.

Bernardis, L.L. and Frohman, L.A. (1971). Effects of hypothalamic lesions at different loci on development of hyperinsulinemia and obesity in the weanling rat. *J. Comp. Physiol. Psychol.* 141, 107-115.

Bland, B.H. and Cooper, R.M. (1969). Posterior neodecortication in the rat: age at operation and experience. *J. Comp. Physiol. Psychol.* 69, 345-354.

Brutkowski, S., Mishkin, M. and Rosvold, H.E. (1963). Positive and inhibitory motor conditioned reflexes in monkeys after ablation of orbital or dorsolateral surface of the frontal cortex. *In* E. Gutman (Ed.) "Second Symposium on Peripheral and Central Mechanisms of Motor Functions." Liblice, Czechoslovakia: Czechoslovakian Academy of Sciences.

Chow, K.L. (1954). Lack of behavioral effects following destruction of some thalamic association nuclei in monkeys. *Arch. Neurol. Psychiat.* 71, 762-771.

Doty, R.W. (1961). Functional significance of the topographical aspects of the retino-cortical projection. *In* R. Jung and H. Kornhuber (Eds.) "The Visual System: Neurophysiology and Psychophysics." Heidelberg: Springer-Verlag. pp. 228-245.

Doty, R.W. (1971). Survival of pattern vision after removal of striate cortex in the adult cat. *Comp. Neurol.* 143, 341-370.

Frohman, L.A. and Bernardis, L.L. (1968). Growth hormone and insulin levels in weanling rats with ventromedial hypothalamic lesions. *Endocrinology* 82, 1125-1132.

Goldman, P.S. (1971). Functional development of the prefrontal cortex in early life and the problem of neuronal plasticity. *Exptl. Neurol.* 32, 366-387.

Goldman, P.S. (1972). Developmental determinants of cortical plasticity. *Acta Neurobiologiae Exp.* 32, 495-511.

Goldman, P.S. and Rosvold, H.E. (1972). The effects of selective caudate lesions in infant and juvenile rhesus monkeys. *Brain Res.* 43, 53-66.

Goldman, P.S. and Rosvold, H.E. (1970). Localization of function within the dorsolateral prefrontal cortex of the rhesus monkey. *Exp. Neurol.* 27, 291-304.

Goldman, P.S., Rosvold, H.E. and Mishkin, M. (1970a). Evidence for behavioral impairment following prefrontal lobectomy in the infant monkey. *J. Comp. Physiol. Psychol.* 70, 454-463.

Goldman, P.S., Rosvold, H.E. and Mishkin, M. (1970b). Selective sparing of function following prefrontal lobectomy in infant monkeys. *Exp. Neurol.* 29, 221-226.

Goodman, D.C. and Horel, J.A. (1967). Sprouting of optic tract projections in the brain stem of the rat. *J. Comp. Neurol.* 127, 71-88.

Harlow, H.F., Blomquist, A.J., Thompson, C.I., Schiltz, K.A. and Harlow, M.K. (1968). *In* R. Isaacson (Ed.) "The Neuropsychology of Development." New York: Wiley. pp. 79-120.

Hicks, S.P. and D'Amato, C.J. (1970). Motor-sensory and visual behavior after hemispherectomy in newborn and mature rats. *Exp. Neurol.* 29, 416-438.

Isaacson, R.L., Nonneman, A.J. and Schmaltz, L.W. (1968). Behavioral and anatomical sequelae of damage to the infant limbic system. *In* R. Isaacson (Ed.) "The Neuropsychology of Development." New York: Wiley. pp. 41-78.

Iversen, S.D. and Mishkin, M. (1970). Perseveration interference in monkey following selective lesions of the inferior prefrontal convexity. *Exptl. Brain Res.* 11, 376-386.

Johnson, David A. (1972). Developmental aspects of recovery of function following septal lesions in the infant rat. *J. Comp. Physiol. Psychol.* 78, 331-348.

Johnson, T.J., Rosvold, H.E. and Mishkin, M. (1968). Projections from behaviorally defined sectors of the prefrontal cortex to the basal ganglia. septum, and diencephalon of the monkey. *Exptl. Neurol.* 21, 20-34.

Kemp, J.M. and Powell, T.P.S. (1970). The cortico-striate projection in the monkey. *Brain* 93, 525-546.

Kennard, M.A. (1938). Reorganization of motor function in the cerebral cortex of monkeys deprived of motor and premotor areas in infancy. *J. Neurophysiol.* 1, 477-496.

Kennard, M.A. (1940). Relation of age to motor impairment in man and in subhuman primates. *Arch. Neurol. and Psychiat.* 44, 377-397.

Kennard, M. (1942). Cortical reorganization of motor function: studies on series of monkeys of various ages from infancy to maturity. *Arch. Neurol. and Psychiat.* 47, 227-240.

Kling, A. (1966). Ontogenetic and phylogenetic studies on the amygdaloid nuclei. *Psychosom. Med.* 28, 155-161.

Kling, A. and Tucker, T.J. (1967). Effects of combined lesions of frontal granular cortex and caudate nucleus in the neonatal monkey. *Brain Res.* 6, 428-439.

Lawrence, D.G. and Hopkins, D.A. (1970). Bilateral pyramidal lesions in infant rhesus monkeys. *Brain Res.* 24, 543-544.

Leonard, C.M. (1973). A method for assessing stages of neural maturation. *Brain Res.* 53, 412-416.

Liu, C.N. and Chambers, W.W. (1958). Intraspinal sprouting of dorsal root axons. *Arch. Neurol. and Psychiat.* 79, 46-61.

Lynch, G., Deadwyler, S. and Cotman, C. (1973). Post-lesion axonal growth produces permanent functional connections. *Science* 180, 1364-1366.

Lynch, G., Mosko, S., Parks, T. and Cotman, C. (1973). Relocation and hyperdevelopment of the dentate gyrus commissural system after entorhinal lesions in immature rats. *Brain Res.* 50, 174-178.

McCouch, G.P., Austin, G.M., Liu, C.N. and Liu, C.Y. (1958). Sprouting as a cause of spasticity. *J. Neurophysiol.* 21, 205-216.

Miller, E.A., Goldman, P.S. and Rosvold, H.E. (1973). Delayed recovery of function following orbital prefrontal lesions in infant monkeys. *Science* 182, 304-306.

Mishkin, M., Vest, B., Waxler, M. and Rosvold, H.E. (1969). A reexamination of the effects of frontal lesions on object alternation. *Neuropsychologia* 7, 357-364.

Moore, R.Y., Bjorklund, A. and Stenevi, U. (1971). Plastic changes in the adrenergic innervation of the rat septal area in response to denervation. *Brain Res.* 33, 13-35.

Murphy, E.H. and Stewart, D.L. (1974). The effects of neonatal and adult striate lesions on visual discrimination in the rabbit. *Exptl. Neurol.* 42, 89-96.

Nonneman, A.J. and Isaacson, R.I. (1973). Task dependent recovery after early brain damage. *Behav. Biol.* 8, 143-172.

Peters, R.H., Rosvold, H.E. and Mirsky, A.F. (1956). The effect of thalamic lesions upon delayed response-type tests in the rhesus monkey. *J. Comp. Physiol. Psychol.* 49, 111-116.

Raisman, G. (1969). Neuronal plasticity in the septal nuclei of the adult rat. *Brain Res.* 14, 25-48.

Schneider, G.E. (1970). Mechanisms of functional recovery following lesions of visual cortex or superior colliculus in neonate and adult hamsters. *Brain, Behav. & Evol.* 3, 295-323.

Shulman, S. (1964). Impaired delayed response from thalamic lesions. *Arch. Neurol.* 11, 477-499.

Stewart, D.L. and Riesen, A.H. (1972). Adult Versus Infant Brain Damage: Behavioral and Electrophysiological Effects of Striatectomy in Adult and Neonatal Rabbits. *In* G. Newton and A.H. Riesen (Eds.) "Advances in Psycho-biology." New York: Wiley - Interscience. Volume 1, pp. 171-211.

Thompson, C.I., Schwartzbaum, J.S. and Harlow, H.F. (1969). Development of social fear after amygdalectomy in infant rhesus monkeys. *Physiol. & Behav.* 4, 249-254.

Tucker, T.J. and Kling, A. (1967). Differential effects of early and late lesions of frontal granular cortex in the monkey. *Brain Res.* 5, 377-389.

Tucker, T.J. and Kling, A. (1969). Preservation of delayed response following combined lesions of prefrontal and posterior association cortex in infant monkeys. *Exptl. Neurol.* 23, 491-502.

DIFFERENTIAL CHANGES IN THE ACQUISITION
OF DEVELOPMENTAL SKILLS IN CHILDREN
WHO LATER BECOME DYSLEXIC

A THREE YEAR FOLLOW-UP

Paul Satz
Janette Friel and Fran Rudegeair
University of Florida
Gainesville, Florida

The results of the present study provide a unique opportunity to compare changes on a number of motor, perceptual, cognitive and language skills in a group of elementary school boys, some of whom three years later became severely disabled readers. One of the long-term objectives of this longitudinal project (MH 19415) is to examine prognosis and recovery processes in this disorder over time. The present paper, however, is addressed to the developmental precursors of this disorder before the child begins formal reading (i.e. kindergarten) and changes in these developmental skills some three years later (Grade 2) at which time independent reading measures were also administered.

This research departs from more traditional studies which have investigated recovery processes following acute brain lesions in the laboratory animal and following naturally-occurring brain lesions in humans ("experiments of nature"). The present study, in contrast, is addressed to a disorder which involves no acute or demonstrated trauma to the CNS nor, by definition, any evidence of symptom reduction, vicarious function, substitution or reorganization. Such terms including diaschisis and collateral sprouting, are used to explain the reinstatement of function following acute lesions to the infant and adult brain. The focus of the present paper is addressed to a lag mechanism in brain maturation which is postulated to underlie and forecast the later onset of dyslexia (Satz and Van Nostrand 1973). Consequently, the recovery process in this framework is restricted to a more basic investigation of acquisition rather than of re-acquisition following acute trauma to the CNS.

The process of acquisition has been given little attention in the recovery literature, except for the childhood aphasias. Lenneberg (1967) has reported that cerebral trauma during infancy (ages 2-3) will render the patient totally unresponsive, sometimes for weeks at a time; however,

> ... when he becomes cognizant of his environment again, it becomes clear that whatever beginning he had made in language before the disease is totally lost, but soon he will start on the road toward language acquisition, traversing all stages of infant vocalization, perhaps at a slightly faster pace, beginning with babbling, single words, primitive two-word phrases, etc., until perfect speech is achieved. In the very young, then, the primary process in recovery is acquisition, whereas the process of symptom-reduction is not in evidence (pp. 146, 150).

Theory. The theory guiding the present research is that developmental dyslexia (which is defined as a severe retardation in reading and writing in children who otherwise have at least average intelligence, educational opportunity and freedom from gross neurological, sensory or cultural handicap) is due to a lag in the maturation of the cerebral cortex (primarily the left hemisphere). This lag mechanism, which is unobservable and thereby treated as a hypothetical construct, is postulated to delay the acquisition of certain developmental skills which are in primary ascendancy during pre-school years and which are crucial to the early phases of reading (e.g., perceptual-mnemonic-somesthetic sequencing skills). The lag mechanism is meant to be distinguished from a brain lesion or insult which, in adults, is associated with a loss or impairment in function. In other words, the theory attempts to conceptualize the reading disorder within the framework of a developmental model rather than a disease model and postulates that the underlying lag in brain maturation (unobservable event) causes a delay in the rate or acquisition of developmental skills rather than a loss or impairment in corresponding skills. However, the fact that the child goes through consecutive stages of thought during development, each of which incorporates the processes of the preceding stage into more complex operations, suggests that the process of this disorder should vary as a function of the stage and/or chronological age of the child (Satz and Van Nostrand 1973; Bruner 1968; Hunt 1961). Thus, it is predicted that those children, during pre-school, who are delayed developmentally in skills which are in primary ascendancy at this stage, will eventually fail in acquiring reading proficiency. It is predicted, however, that these children will eventually "catch-up" on these earlier-developing skills but will then lag on those more cognitive-linguistic skills which have a slower and later ontogenetic development (Thurstone 1955; Bloom 1964; Satz and Van Nostrand 1973). These later developing operations are assumed to represent a more complex integration of preceding stages which involve pre-conceptual and sensori-motor components (Bruner 1968; Hunt 1961).

The theory, in brief, conceptualizes developmental dyslexia as more than a reading disorder *per se*. That is, the disorder is explained as a delay in those crucial early sensori-motor and later conceptual-linguistic skills which are intrinsic to the acquisition of reading and which are triggered by a lag in the maturation of the cerebral cortex. In other words, dyslexia is seen as a disorder in central processing, the nature of which varies with the age and developmental stage of the child. This delay in central processing is not meant to imply damage, loss of function or impairment. Such terms are more compatible with a disease model which too often implies a static developmental-acquisition course. In the present framework, the older dyslexic child is developmentally like a normal younger child. However, if the retarded reader fails to "catch-up" on those more cognitive-language skills which develop in later childhood (i.e., when the brain is reaching full maturation), then more permanent delays in language and reading skills are predicted (Satz and Van Nostrand 1973).

Study. The present paper is addressed to a comparison of developmental changes between two groups of elementary school children, a dyslexic group and a control group of average-superior readers, both of whom were tested at the beginning of Kindergarten in 1970 and at the end of Grade 2 in 1973. Both groups of children were selected in 1973 on the basis of independent reading measures administered to the larger total population of white male children who have been followed longitudinally since 1970 in Alachua County, Florida (Satz and Friel 1973; Satz and Friel 1974, in press; Satz 1974, in press). The dyslexic group was selected from the larger group of disabled readers in this population by being retarded in reading on all three criterion reading measures administered at the end of Grade 2: (1) Iota Word Recognition ≥ 7 months, (2) Gates-McGinitie Vocabulary ≥ 7 months, and (3) classroom reading level (First Grade Reader or below). In addition, the child had to have a Peabody IQ of 90 or above and no evidence of gross neurological, sensory or emotional handicap. The fact that the children were all white males largely from an urban middle class community further excluded the influence of cultural deprivation in this endeavor to select children defined as developmental dyslexics. Sixty children were identified who met these exclusive selection criteria.

A control group of children were then rigorously and individually matched with each of the 60 disabled readers. They were initially selected from the much larger population of average readers and had to be reading at grade level or above on each of the criterion reading measures. From this group individual matching was conducted in the following sequence: (1) chronological age within one month or less, (2) socioeconomic level the same and (3) rural school vs. county school the same. Whenever more than one child met similar matching characteristics, random sampling was employed. No attempt was made to match on IQ or level of reading proficiency. Thus, it was possible that some control children could have lower IQ scores or very advanced levels of reading proficiency.

The results of this selection and matching procedure can be seen in Table 1. The dyslexic group was severely retarded in reading on each of

TABLE 1

Group Means and Standard Deviations
on the Criterion Reading Tests, Age and IQ

Groups

	Dyslexic (N = 60)		Control (N = 60)	
	x̄	s.d.	x̄	s.d.
Age[a]	92.6	4.3	92.4	4.1
PPVT IQ[b]	99.8	8.3	114.3	13.8
Iota[a]	-12.6	4.1	16.6	9.4
Gates Vocab.[a]	-12.2	2.5	13.5	7.0
Classroom Reading[c]	4.18	0.9	7.5	0.9

[a]Score in months
[b]PPVT = Peabody Picture Vocabulary Test
[c]Range (0-9) with 4 = Primer and 7 = Second Reader, Book 2

the criterion measures with a mean lag of greater than 12 months on both the Iota and Gates. The mean of 4.18 on Classroom Reading placed this group at approximately the Primer Level. By contrast, the control group obtained advanced reading and word recognition scores on the Iota (X̄ = +16.6 mos.), the Gates (X̄ = +13.5 mos.) and Classroom Reading (X̄ = 7.5). The latter score falls between Second Reader (Book 2) and Third Reader (Book 1) which is just slightly above the expected normal reading level for the end of Grade 2. Inspection of Table 1 also shows that while both groups of children had mean IQ's at least within the normal range (Dyslexic IQ = 99.8, Control IQ = 114.3), the dyslexic group was substantially lower. In fact, the IQ scores ranged from 90-127 in the dyslexic group and from 84-145 in the control group. In contrast, both groups were nearly identical in mean age (Dyslexic = 92.6 mos., Control = 92.4 mos.).

The preceding selection procedure therefore identified two carefully dichotomized groups on reading level (i.e., between Ss) who otherwise were nearly identical in racial, ethnic, cultural, age and sex comparisons. Moreover, all children in the dyslexic group had at least average (although lower) intelligence. Within subjects, the children were identical with initial testing available in Year 1 (Kindergarten) and repeat testing in Year 3 (Grade 2). This research design, which is based in part on a longitudinal follow-up, represents one of the most powerful paradigms for assessing between-subject and within-subject effects. In addition, the initial testing administered at the beginning of Kindergarten (Year 1, 1970), before formal reading, provides a rare opportunity to examine and evaluate the developmental precursors postulated to underly this disorder (Satz and Van Nostrand 1973). Finally, the readministration of the developmental tests on the same Ss in Year 3, at the end of Grade 2, provides an equally unique opportunity to evaluate the nature of developmental changes postulated to occur in this disorder (Satz and Van Nostrand 1973). One particular problem, however, in the current study is that the interval between test (1970) and retest (1973) was not long enough to assess the primary cognitive and linguistic delays postulated to occur in the older dyslexic child (i.e., ages 10-12). More rigorous test of this hypothesis will not be possible for three more years (1976).

Test Battery and Previous Results (Early Detection). A description and rationale for the test battery is given in some detail in an earlier study (Satz and Friel 1973). Briefly, the predictive tests (N = 16) comprise a number of developmental and neuropsychological measures (non-reading) which assess a variety of fine motor, perceptual (visual/auditory), perceptual-motor, somatosensory and cognitive-language skills. Factor analysis of the total test battery (N = 20; Satz and Friel 1973) revealed four primary

independent factors which were defined as follows:
Factor 1 (Somatosensory-perceptual-mnemonic),
Factor II (Teacher Evaluations), Factor III
(Conceptual-verbal) and Factor IV (Fine Motor).
Preliminary evaluation of the predictive validity
of these tests to end of Kindergarten achievement
(Year 1) and to end of Grade 1 reading level
(Year 2) are presented in two separate studies
(Satz and Friel 1973; Satz and Friel 1973, in
press). The predictions to end of Grade 1 reading
level (Satz and Friel 1974, in press) were
extremely high. The tests correctly predicted over
91 percent of the total population ($\underline{N}$ = 473).
Based on discriminant function composite scores,
the tests correctly identified 100 percent of the
severely handicapped readers within the High Risk
group and 95 percent of the superior readers
within the Low Risk group. Virtually all of the
misclassification errors were confined to the
mildly retarded and average reading subgroups.
Similar results (unpublished) were recently
found in predictions to Grade 2 reading level
(Year 3).

Of theoretical significance was the finding
that in the last two follow-up studies (Years 2
and 3), the stepwise regression analyses ranked
the Factor I tests higher in terms of predictive
discriminability. These variables represent the
type of earlier developing skills which are in
rapid ascendancy during pre-school years and which
are postulated to be crucial to the early phases
of reading (Gibson 1968). The Finger Localization
Test, Recognition-Discrimination Test, Alphabet
Recitation and Beery Developmental Test of Visual-
Motor Integration have consistently ranked high in
these and related prediction studies.

Current Results. The analyses were divided
into two phases. The first phase was addressed to
the predictive efficiency of the tests administered
during Kindergarten ($\underline{N}$ = 16) in 1970 (Year 1) to
the criterion groups (dyslexic and control)
identified in the Spring of 1973 (Year 3). A two-
group discriminant function and stepwise
regression analysis were computed (Fisher 1936).
The results are presented in Table 2 for the 60 $\underline{Ss}$
in each criterion group. Based on the optimal
composite cutting-line established by the computer

Table 2

Predictive Classification and Ranking of Tests
on Normal and Disabled Reading Groups
in Year Three

TESTS	DYSLEXIC	CONTROL	TOTAL
Positives (+)	49	7	56
Negatives (-)	11	53	64
TOTAL	60	60	120

Stepwise Regression Rank

Variable	Hit
1. Finger Localization	75.8%
2. Alphabet	79.1%
3. Recognition-Discrimination	83.3%
4. Total Battery	85.0%

(Bi-Med Program), the tests correctly classified
102 of the total 120 Ss (H_T = 85%); they also
correctly predicted 49 of the 60 dyslexics (Valid
Positive Rate = 82%) and misclassified only 7 of
the 60 controls (False Positive Rate = 11.7%).
     Stepwise regression analysis again confirmed
the high discriminability of the Factor I tests.
In fact, the Finger Localization, Alphabet and
Recognition-Discrimination Tests accounted for
virtually 98% of the total predictive accuracy
(i.e., 83.3% vs. 85%). These tests represent
measures of pre-reading skills which are postulated to be in rapid ascendancy during pre-school
and which are crucial to the early phase of
reading (Satz and Van Nostrand 1973). The theory
is further strengthened by virtue of the lower
predictive ranking of the verbal-cognitive
(Factor III) and fine-motor (Factor IV) tests in

the present and preceding predictive studies (Years 1 and 2).

The second phase in the analyses was addressed to a comparison between the developmental-neuropsychological tests administered at the beginning of Kindergarten (Year 1, 1970) and readministered at the end of Grade 2 (Year 3, 1973) on the same Ss in each group. A 2 by 2 analysis of variance (repeated measures) was computed on each of the tests with groups (dyslexic and control) representing the between-subjects factor, and age (Years 1 and 3) representing the within-subjects factor. The first three analyses were computed on the three Factor I tests which in Table 2 revealed the highest predictive ranking (Finger Localization, Alphabet and Recognition-Discrimination). The results of Finger Localization can be seen in Figure 1. There was a highly significant between-subjects effect ($F = 51.97$, $df = 1$, 118, $p \leq .001$), within-subjects effect ($F = 267.77$, $df = 1$, 118, $p \leq .001$) and group by age interaction ($F = 45.34$, $df = 1$, 118, $p \leq .001$). In other words, the performance of the dyslexic children was much lower than the control children on this test, but only during Year 1 before formal reading had commenced. By Year 3 (Grade 2) the dyslexic children had caught-up on this developmental skill.

Similar results were found for Alphabet Recitation (Figure 2). There was a highly significant between-subject effect ($F = 52.94$, $df = 1$, 118, $p < .001$), within-subjects effect ($F = 65.88$, $df = 1$, 118, $p \leq .001$) and group by age interaction ($F = 46.42$, $df = 1$, 118, $p \leq .001$). Figure 2 shows that in Year 1 (Kindergarten) there was a striking delay in this skill for those children who later became dyslexic. However, by Year 3 (Grade 2) the dyslexic group had essentially caught-up with respect to the control group. In contrast, the control children, by Kindergarten, had essentially mastered this earlier-developing mnemonic skill.

Performance on the Recognition-Discrimination Test revealed a similar pattern between and within subjects (Figure 3). There was a highly significant between-subjects effect ($F = 40.21$, $df = 1$, 118, $p \leq .001$), within-subjects effect ($F = 203.57$, $df = 1$, 118, $p \leq .001$) and group by

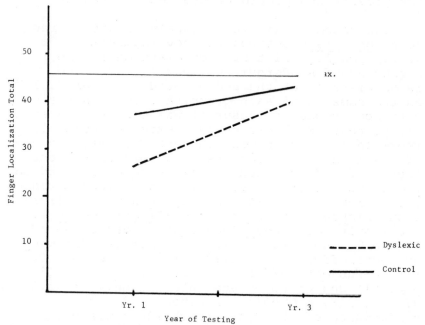

Figure 1. Mean raw scores (correct) on Finger Localization Test for years and groups.

age interaction ($F = 12.09$, $\underline{df} = 1$, 118, $\underline{p} \leq .001$). Again, the major difference between groups was due to the striking lag in the younger children (Year 1) who later became dyslexic. However, by Year 3 (Grade 2) the dyslexic group had substantially but not completely caught-up with their matched controls on this earlier-developing skill.

Each of the preceding tests, in summary, revealed a striking delay in those pre-school children who by the end of Grade 2 developed severe problems in reading. Moreover, performance on these tests, during pre-school, was shown to forecast with high accuracy these later reading handicaps. An interesting point is that although the dyslexic children eventually caught-up on these developmental, non-reading predictive skills, they were still severely deficient in reading by the end of Grade 2. An equally interesting observation is that the dyslexic children, by Grade 2, attained performance levels on these tests comparable to their matched

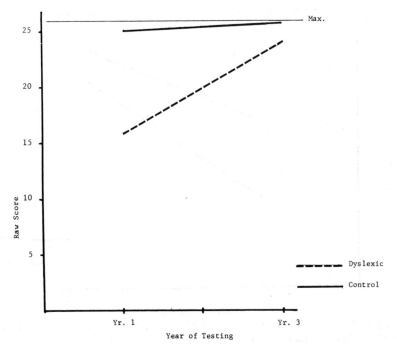

Figure 2. *Mean raw scores (correct) on Alphabet Test for years and groups.*

controls although a 14-point IQ discrepancy prevailed between groups in Grade 2 (Dyslexic IQ = 99.83, Control IQ = 114.33). Discussion and interpretation of these points are deferred to the conclusion section of this chapter.

The following analyses are based on those tests which revealed a lower discriminative ranking in the stepwise regression analysis (Table 1). Additional Factor I tests are presented first. The results of the Auditory Discrimination Test (ratio scores) revealed a significant between-subjects effect (F = 26.10, df = 1, 118, $p \le .001$) and a robust within-subjects effect (F = 141.14, df = 1, 118, $p \le .001$). There was no age by group inter-action. Inspection of Figure 4 reveals differences between groups at both ages with the dyslexic children delayed almost a year and a half on this task even by the end of Grade 2. It should also be stressed that the lag persisted despite significant

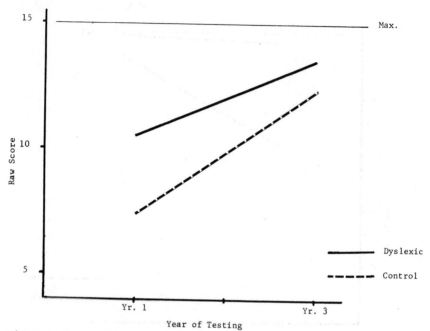

Figure 3. Mean raw scores (correct) on Recognition
Test for years and groups.

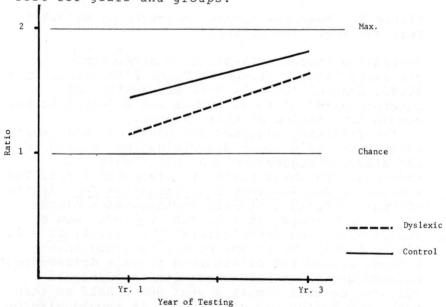

Figure 4. Mean ratio scores (correct) on Auditory
Discrimination Test for years and groups.

developmental gains on this skill in both groups over time.

Similar results were also found on the Right-Left Discrimination Test (Body Schema). There was a significant between-subjects effect (F = 27.86, df = 1, 118, $p \leq .001$) and a within-subjects effect (F = 41.84, df = 1, 118, $p \leq .001$). No age by group interaction was demonstrated. Inspection of Figure 5 reveals differences between groups at both ages. In fact, in Year 1 the children who later became dyslexic performed at only chance level and still lagged behind their matched controls in Year 3 (Grade 2) despite the fact that both groups made significant strides on this developmental skill over time.

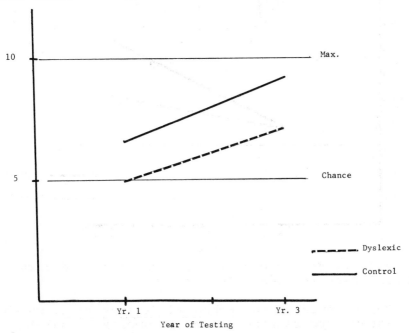

Figure 5. Mean raw scores (correct) on Right-Left Discrimination Test (Body Schema) for years and groups.

Significant differences were also found between groups on the Auditory-Visual Integration Test, but only in Year 3 (Grade 2). There was a significant between-subjects effect (F = 21.46, df = 1, 118, $p \leq .001$), a robust within-subjects

187

effect ($\underline{F}$ = 184.58, $\underline{df}$ = 1, 118, $\underline{p} \leq$ .001) and an age by group interaction ($\underline{F}$ = 31.68, $\underline{df}$ = 1, 118, $\underline{p} \leq$ .001). Inspection of Figure 6 reveals that performance on this task was too difficult for both groups in Year 1 and that the major differences occurred only in Year 3. This lag in the dyslexic group again persisted despite significant gains in both groups over time. However, the rate of developmental acquisition of this skill in the dyslexic group was slower than for their matched controls.

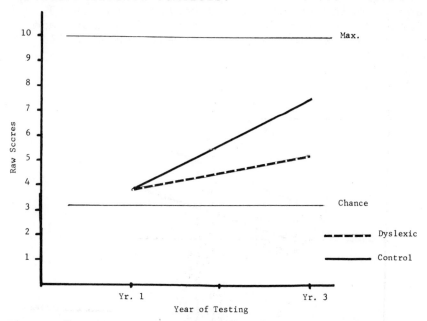

Figure 6. Mean raw scores (correct) on Auditory-Visual Test for years and groups.

Performance on the Embedded Figures Test, which is assumed to represent a more complex visual-perceptual skill, resulted in significant differences between groups at both ages (Years 1 and 3). There was a significant between-subjects effect ($\underline{F}$ = 43.59, $\underline{df}$ = 1, 118, $\underline{p} \leq$ .001) and a robust within-subjects effect over years ($\underline{F}$ = 372.60, $\underline{df}$ = 1, 118, $\underline{p} \leq$ .001). There was no age by group interaction. Inspection of Figure 7 reveals a persistent lag in the dyslexic group in both years despite the fact that both groups again

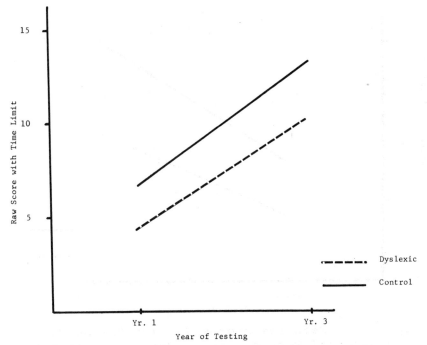

Figure 7. Mean raw scores (timed/correct) on Embedded Figures Test for years and groups.

made significant developmental strides on this skill over time.

Performance on the Beery Developmental Test of Visual-Motor Integration also revealed differences between groups although the delay in the dyslexic group substantially increased between Years 1 and 3 (Figure 8). There was a significant between-subjects effect (F = 52.67, df = 1, 118, $p \leq .001$), within-subjects effect (F = 315.44, df = 1, 118, $p \leq .001$) and age by group interaction (F = 10.80, df = 1, 118, $p \leq .005$). Performance on this test, based on equivalent age in months, revealed a 10 month lag in Year 1 in the children who later became dyslexic which increased to an 18 month lag by the end of Grade 2 (Year 3). By contrast, the control group's performance (in months) almost identically matched their mean chronological age in both years!

The following two analyses are based on tests which loaded highly on Factor IV (Fine Motor

189

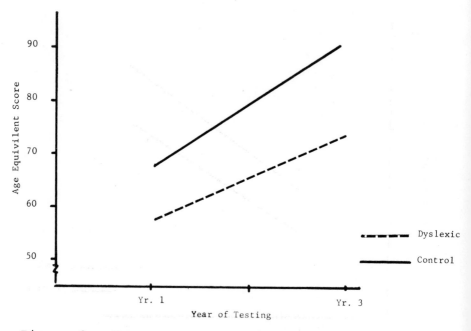

Figure 8. Mean age scores (in months) on Beery Developmental Test of Visual-Motor Integration for years and groups.

Skill). Results of the Finger Tapping Test can be seen in Figures 9 and 10 (Preferred and Non-Preferred Hand, respectively). Significant differences in both analyses were only found for within-subjects: Preferred Hand ($\underline{F}$ = 59.00, $\underline{df}$ = 1, 118, $\underline{p} \leq .001$) and Non-Preferred Hand ($\underline{F}$ = 136.23, $\underline{df}$ = 1, 118, $\underline{p} \leq .001$). The higher within-subjects effect in the latter analysis merely indicates that the subjects in both groups demonstrated more substantial gains over time with the non-preferred hand. It is interesting to note that this measure, which involves no assessment of conceptual or pre-conceptual processing, revealed similar scores between-subjects (i.e., groups) in both years.

The final three analyses are based on those tests which loaded highly on Factor III (Verbal-

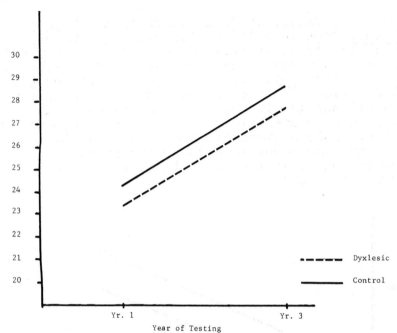

Figure 9. Mean raw scores of preferred hand on Finger Tapping Test for years and groups.

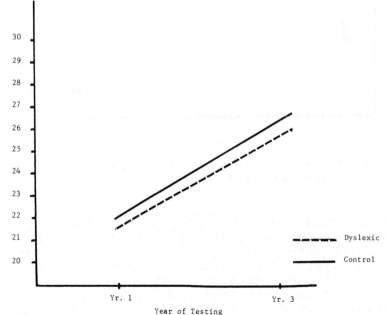

Figure 10. Mean raw scores of nonpreferred hand on Finger Tapping Test for years and groups.

Cognitive Skills).* Performance on the Verbal
Fluency Test revealed a significant between-
subjects effect ($F = 23.54$, $df = 1$, 118, $p \leq .001$),
and a robust within-subjects effect ($F = 119.12$,
$df = 1$, 118, $p \leq .001$). There was no age by group
interaction. Inspection of Figure 11 reveals a
significant lag in the children in Year 1 who
later became dyslexic which persisted through the
end of Grade 2 (Year 3). The results again show
that the lag occurred despite significant
developmental strides on this skill in both
groups over time.

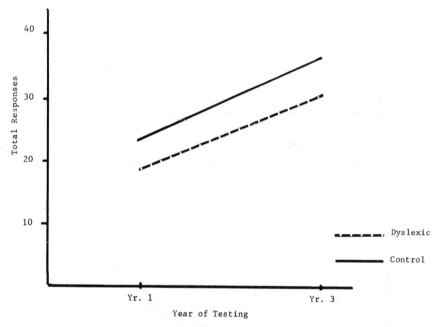

*Figure 11. Mean raw scores on Verbal Fluency
Test for years and groups.*

*The results of the Dichotic Listening Test are
excluded pending further analyses, particularly
regarding factor loadings. Preliminary analyses of
the ear asymmetry revealed no between-subject
(i.e., group) differences at either age (Years 1
and 3), although the magnitude of the ear
asymmetry showed a significant increase in both
groups over time (within-subjects).

Similar results were found on the Peabody Picture Vocabulary Test (Raw Scores). There was a significant between-subjects effect (F = 31.87, df = 1, 118, $p \leq .001$) and a robust within-subjects effect (F = 358.25, df = 1, 118, $p \leq .001$). There was no age by group interaction. Figure 12 reveals a significant lag in the children in Year 1 who later became dyslexic which persisted through the end of Grade 2 (Year 3). The results again show that the lag occurred despite significant developmental strides on this skill in both groups over time.

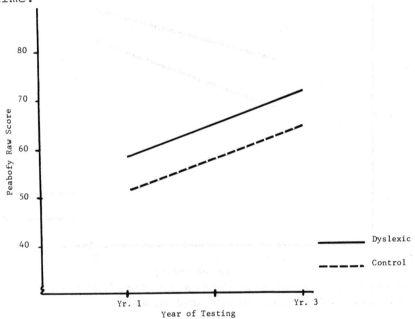

Figure 12. *Mean raw scores on Peabody Picture Vocabulary Test for years and groups.*

Performance on the Similarities subtest of the Wechsler Intelligence Scale for Children (WISC) revealed a significant between-subjects effect (F = 41.08, df = 1, 118, $p \leq .001$), a robust within-subjects effect (F = 168.15, df = 1, 118, $p \leq .001$) and an age by group interaction (F = 4.05, df = 1, 118, $p \leq .05$). These results can be seen in Figure 13. Again a lag is demonstrated in those children in Year 1 who later became dyslexic which persisted through the end of Grade 2

(Year 3). However, the age by group interaction indicates that the lag was slightly greater in Year 1. The results also show that the lag persisted despite significant developmental strides on this verbal-cognitive skill in both groups over time.

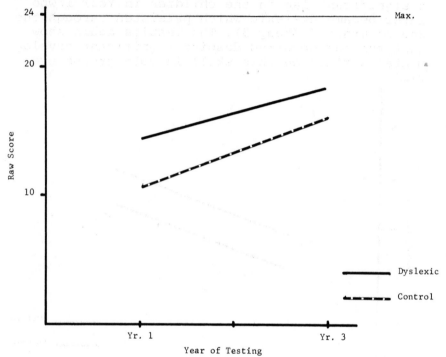

Figure 13.   Mean raw scores in Similarities Subtest (WISC) for years and groups.

Discussion

The preceding results provide additional insights into the nature of this disorder called developmental dyslexia. First, there are precursors which exist at least by five and a half years of age which, if objectively assessed, can forecast the level of reading proficiency in the child some three years later. These precursors, which in the present study were identified before the children were exposed to formal reading (i.e., Kindergarten), were all based on pre-reading measures of perceptual and

194

cognitive skill. Some of these precursors, moreover, were shown to have greater predictive
discrimination for reading achievement at the end
of Grade 2 (Year 3). The step-wise regression
analysis (Table 2) revealed that the more
discriminating tests (Finger Localization,
Alphabet Recitation and Recognition-Discrimination), which accounted for virtually 98 percent of
the predictive accuracy, all loaded on Factor I.
This factor, in previous research (Satz and Friel
1973), has been identified as a general measure of
somatosensory-perceptual-mnemonic ability.
Variables which load highly on this factor are
felt to represent those earlier-developing skills
which are in rapid ascendancy during pre-school
years and which are postulated to be crucial to
the early phases of reading (Satz and Van Nostrand
1973).

Studies which have investigated the nature of
the reading process have recognized that this
process unfolds in an orderly and developmental
sequence. Gibson (1968) and Luria (1966) have
shown that the early phases of reading depend
largely on perceptual discrimination and analysis.
In this early phase (i.e., ages 5-7 years) the
child must discriminate the distinctive features
of letters (e.g., break vs. close, line vs. curve,
rotation and reversal) before he can proceed to
later phases which require more complex visual-
phonetic mapping and still later linguistic
analysis of words and meaning (i.e., ages 10-12
years). This schema is, in fact, quite similar to
those developmental theories which postulate that
the child goes through consecutive stages of
thought during childhood, each of which incorporates the processes of the preceding stage into
more complex modes of operation (Piaget 1926;
Hunt 1961; Bruner 1968). Bruner (1968) has
advanced three distinct stages which unfold in an
orderly sequence in the child's cognitive
development. He constructs models of his world
through action (enactive representation), through
imagery (iconic representation) and through
language (symbolic representation). "Their
appearance in the life of the child is in that
order, each depending upon the previous one for
its development, yet all of them remaining more or

195

less intact throughout life" (p. 478). According to Bruner, the transition to symbolic representation (i.e., ages 10-12 years) marks the final and most important stage in cognitive development. This stage frees the child from dependence upon the concrete and immediate aspects of perceptual representation and, through language internalization, facilitates a so-called second-signal system (Luria 1966) in which experience can be both represented and transformed.

In the present study, those children who were destined to severe reading failure at the end of Grade 2 (Year 3) were those who were lagging in these crucial early modes of perceptual and cognitive representation during Kindergarten. Conversely, those children who were destined to superior levels of reading proficiency at the end of Grade 2 (Year 3) revealed a higher level of perceptual and cognitive organization during this earlier stage of development.

Thus, it appears that a lag mechanism, expressed in terms of a delay in developmental readiness, can forecast a delay in the later acquisition of reading skills. But does this developmental lag persist in later years when reading competency can be independently assessed (e.g., end of Grade 2)? The results of the second phase of the analyses (test-retest) revealed that the dyslexic children continued to lag on the majority of the developmental skills which were re-assessed two and a half years later (Year 3). In fact, these children "caught-up" on only three of the developmental skills which, incidentally, comprised the highest predictive estimates of later reading proficiency (i.e., Finger Localization, Alphabet Recitation and Recognition-Discrimination, respectively). One possible explanation of this finding is that each of the tests represent measures of earlier-developing skills which, while perceptually and cognitively less complex, are nevertheless in rapid ascendancy or growth during the pre-school years (i.e., ages 5-6). Bloom (1964) has already shown that variations in the environment have their greatest quantitative effect on a characteristic at its most rapid period of change and the least effect at the least rapid period of change. One

196

might therefore conclude that variations in the
CNS (e.g., brain maturation lag) might similarly
affect those skills which are experiencing rapid
change during this period in development (Satz and
Van Nostrand 1973).

Although the dyslexic children eventually
"caught-up" on those skills which were more
predictive of later problems in reading, they
still lagged in reading two and a half years
later. Moreover, they continued to lag on all of
the developmental skills which required more
complex perceptual, cognitive and verbal
mediation. This latter finding further suggests
that the more predictive tests may have been less
complex in terms of perceptual and cognitive
processing. If so, does this mean that those
skills which involve more complex cognitive and
verbal processing will reveal an increasing
developmental lag in the next three years?
Unfortunately, this question cannot be answered
within the context of the present time span (i.e.,
Kindergarten to Grade 2). But the suspicion is
that the nature of the developmental lag will
change as the child maturates into puberty. The
theory advanced by Satz and Van Nostrand (1973)
postulates that those skills which during childhood develop ontogenetically earlier (e.g.,
visual-perceptual and cross-modal integration)
are more likely to be delayed in younger children
who are maturationally immature. Conversely,
those skills which during childhood have a later
or slower rate of development (e.g., language and
formal operations) are more likely to be delayed
in older children who are maturationally
immature. While support for this theory largely
rests on cross-sectional studies at present, it
clearly suggests that the nature of the disorder
varies dramatically with age (Satz 1974, in press;
Satz and Van Nostrand 1973). The nature of the
disorder, in the older dyslexic child (ages 10-12),
largely reflects a problem in language processing
whereas the younger dyslexic child (ages 7-8)
reveals a lag in visual-perceptual integration.
The fact that this differential pattern of
disturbance parallels the unfolding process of
cognitive development in the child (Bruner 1968;
Hunt 1961) provides additional though indirect

support for the developmental changes postulated
to occur in this disorder. Yet, the matter is not
that simple. Many of the language skills (Factor
III tests) were shown to be delayed in those
kindergarten children who later became disabled
readers (Grade 2). Furthermore, the delay on
these verbal skills did not reveal an increasing
lag in the time interval used in this study
(Kindergarten to Grade 2). However, one might
argue that the time interval was too brief or that
it involved a phase in which pre-conceptual or
iconic representation was in primary development
(Bruner 1968). It is apparent that these discrepancies cannot be resolved within the limited
time span of the present study. A more definitive
answer to these questions must await the outcome
of the next retest phase in Year 6 when the
children are nearing puberty.

Although questions still remain concerning
possible changes in the developmental course of
this disorder, the present results were shown to
be encouraging vis-a-vis the precursors or
developmental antecedents of specific reading
disability. They also provide additional information on the nature of this disorder called
dyslexia. Namely, the problem is more than a
reading disability *per se*. Support for this
statement rests on that fact that: (1) the disorder
can be forecasted from developmental measures of
non-reading skill at the beginning of Kindergarten
(ages 5-6) and (2) the majority of these skills
continue to be depressed in dyslexic children at
the end of Grade 2 (ages 7-8). Thus, it is
apparent that a more basic disorder probably
underlies the reading disorder which, in the
present context, involves a number of central
processing functions. The question as to whether
this disorder in central processing reflects a lag
in the maturation of the brain cannot at the
present time be determined. However, the concept
of a developmental lag, expressed in the temporal
acquisition of skills, is partially supported by
the present results. It was shown that the
dyslexic children continued to make significant
strides in the acquisition of these developmental
skills even though a lag persisted some three
years later. These results thus tend to discredit

the concept of a disease model which often
implies the loss or impairment of a function
rather than acquisition.

However, one might argue that despite the
developmental strides that the dyslexic children
made, they still continued to lag behind their
matched controls on most of the tests. Moreover,
in terms of psychometric intelligence, the
dyslexic children revealed a mean depression of
approximately 14 IQ points compared to the control
group. These findings might therefore suggest that
the observed differences between groups could be
explained more parsimoniously in terms of a defect
in cognitive-intellectual capacity. To answer this
question, 32 Ss from each group of children were
identically matched on psychometric intelligence
and a separate analysis of variance (repeated
measures) was again computed for groups (dyslexic
and control) and age (Years 1 and 3) for each of
the developmental tests. The results were
identical to the preceding analyses. That is, the
dyslexic children still lagged behind their
matched controls in Years 1 and 3 on the same
developmental measures. In similar fashion, they
showed the same initial lag during Kindergarten
on Finger Localization, Alphabet Recitation and
Recognition-Discrimination which disappeared by
the end of Grade 2 (Year 3). These results are
therefore incompatible with an intellectual defect
hypothesis.

It is apparent from the preceding discussion
that many questions still remain to be answered on
the nature and course of this disorder. Identification of the precursors before the reading
handicap is clinically evident does not prove or
disprove the mechanism postulated to underlie the
disorder (i.e., brain maturation lag). Nor does
it prove that a developmental lag concept provides
the most parsimonious account of the nature of the
disorder. The concept of a developmental lag,
while compatible with the present results, must be
evaluated within the context of a longer test-
retest interval. Only then can one determine
whether the course of this disorder follows a
differential temporal acquisition of developmental
skills. The present chapter represents the initial
approach to this more relevant longterm problem.

ACKNOWLEDGMENTS: Research supported in part by funds from the National Institute of Mental Health, Behavioral Sciences Research Branch (MH 19415) and by the National Institute of Neurological Diseases and Stroke (NS 08208). The authors also wish to acknowledge the statistical and conceptual input of Ms. Ann Altman and Dr. Harry Van der Vlugt in the preparation of this manuscript.

REFERENCES

Bloom, S. (1964). "Stability and Change in Human Characteristics," New York: John Wiley and Sons, Inc.

Bruner, J.S. (1968). The course of cognitive growth. *In* N.S. Endler, L.R. Boulter and H. Osser (Eds.), "Contemporary Issues in Developmental Psychology," New York: Holt, Rinehart and Winston, Inc. pp. 476-494.

Fisher, R.A. (1936). "Statistical Methods for Research Workers," 6th edition. Edinburgh: Oliver and Boyd.

Gibson, E.J. (1968). Learning to read. *In* N.S. Endler, L.R. Boulter and H. Osser (Eds.), "Contemporary Issues in Developmental Psychology," New York: Holt, Rinehart and Winston, Inc. pp. 291-303.

Hunt, J. McV. (1961). "Intelligence and Experience" New York: Ronald Press.

Lenneberg, E.H. (1967). "Biological Foundations of Language," New York: John Wiley and Sons.

Luria, A.R. (1966). "Higher Cortical Functions in Man," New York: Basic Books, Inc.

Piaget, J. (1926). "The Language and Thought of the Child," London: Routledge and Kegan Paul Ltd.

Satz, P. (1974). Learning disorder and remediation of learning disorders. Research Task Force, National Institutes of Mental Health, Section on Child Mental Illness and Behavior Disorders, In press.

Satz, P. and Friel, J. (1973). Some predictive antecedents of specific learning disability: A preliminary one year follow-up. *In* P. Satz and J.J. Ross (Eds.), "The Disabled Learner: Early Detection and Intervention," Rotterdam, The Netherlands: Rotterdam University Press. pp. 79-98.

Satz, P. and Van Nostrand, G.K. (1973). Developmental dyslexia: An evaluation of a theory. *In* P. Satz and J.J. Ross (Eds.), "The Disabled Learner: Early Detection and Intervention," Rotterdam, The Netherlands: Rotterdam University Press. pp. 212-248.

Satz, P. and Friel, J. (1974). Some predictive antecedents of specific reading disability: A preliminary two-year follow-up. *J. Learning Disabilities* In press.

Thurstone, L.L. (1955). "The Differential Growth of Mental Abilities," Chapel Hill, North Carolina: University of North Carolina Psychometric Laboratory, #14.

DETERMINANTS OF CEREBRAL RECOVERY

M.S. Gazzaniga
State University of New York
Stony Brook, New York

There seems to be, presently, a swingback, in part, to older views of basic central nervous system maintenance and growth principles. Prior to Sperry's truly stunning long series of studies emphasizing the presence of a high degree of neurospecificity, the wildest claims had been made about the extent of functional recovery possible, following either central or peripheral nerve damage (Sperry 1965). For years, it was these studies, as well as Harlow's (1971) at a psychological level, that put a halt to the runaway interpretation that function precedes form. Recently research has again focused attention on the question of the degree of plasticity in the CNS - for example, the work on visual deprivation (Hirsch and Spinelli 1971; Blakemore and Cooper 1970). These studies have shown us how discrete visual experience during rearing modifies the basic organization of the primary visual system. Along with this work, of course, are the studies of Schneider (1973), Raisman (1969), Moore (1971) and others which detail the extent to which neural growth is possible following central neural lesions. As a result, the idea in everyone's mind is that we may now have a handle on the physical basis of recovery in the CNS - not to mention the insights such work affords us on the broader question of the physical basis of learning and memory.

Indeed, Hirsch and Jacobson (1974) have recently argued that adaptive behavior, in general, is the product of changes in the microneurons or Type II cells of Golgi. These cells, it is believed, remain adaptive while the long axon cells responsible for the major transmission of information into and out of the CNS are under early, and exacting, genetic control and specification. How long this state of flexibility obtains for the microneurons is not known. It supposedly extends into the teens, which thereby allows for the speculation that it is a process involved in the

203

kind of speech and language recovery seen in the
rehemispherization of these processes following
early brain damage. It simultaneously could
explain why the relocalization of speech and
language rarely occurs after twelve years of age.
In this regard, it is worth noting the studies of
Nottebohm (1970) on the bird-song of canaries. He
has shown that up to the age of one year, the song
can be taught to birds deprived of hearing the
song. Birds deprived for longer periods can not be
so trained. Yet, if the birds are castrated when
young, thus altering the testosterone level, they
are able to learn the song well into the second
year. Here we see an exciting model for the
experimental manipulation of how and why the CNS
at some time "wires out" adaptive changes in
communicative behavior.

In my view, however, all of this fascinating
basic work in neural development does not
directly bear on the question of recovery of
function in the CNS as the term is normally used
in a clinical sense. Before proceeding, however,
let us look at the stature of clinical functional
recovery.

Clinical Recovery: There are a variety of
claims on the mechanisms and extent of nervous
system recovery. Luria feels that temporarily
depressed areas can be "disinhibited" both by
training and with the aid of pharmacological agents
such as atropine and neostigmine. Yet most
neurologists are skeptical of applying these
methods to patients and, in general, believe the
extent of long term recovery from a lesion is a
function of the individual's capacity to realize
repair and has little to do with external therapy.
For example, in studies examing the value of
rehabilitation on motility and other sensory-motor
functions on stroke patients, it has been concluded
that no more improvement is forthcoming than if the
patient had been left alone (Stern *et al*. 1971).
The same case can be made for speech and language
rehabilitation following stroke (Sarno *et al*.
1970). Indeed, in the clinical setting it is hard
to improve upon von Monakow's concept of
diaschisis, where recovery is viewed as the
reestablishment of temporarily impaired neural
systems - not the vast reorganization of neural

systems through substitution, retraining or as the result of new growth. There have been, in recent years, both physiological and metabolic studies that support von Monakow's ideas. Recordings from cortical areas distant from cerebral lesions, for example, find the areas transiently depressed followed by return to normal levels of firing (Kempinsky 1958). In stroke, it is observed that there is a marked transient decrement in metabolic rate in the brain areas opposite the lesions (Hoedt-Rasmussen 1964).

Yet, even if the basic ideas of von Monakow prove correct, some clinical instances of recovery involving the higher cognitive processes following massive brain damage probably come about through other mechanisms and involve neither disinhibition or actual structural changes. In what follows, I will show instances of recovery of function which can be brought about quickly after a brain lesion or by prelesion prophylactic measures; it will also be demonstrated that recovery can be obtained by the use of proper behavioral training routines long after diaschistic processes are thought to be active.

In general, all of the data I will report leads me to the view that recovery in the adult, arising from nonphysiological improvement, is the result of preexisting behavioral mechanisms not necessarily previously routinely involved in a particular act now covering for the mental activity under question. For instance, I believe that the implicit functional syntactic mechanism present and active in decoding a meaningful pictorial array is probably able to come to the assistance of the organism when the syntactic mechanism for language has been destroyed through stroke or lesion. But before getting into the clinical work, let me lay a broader base for this view with recent work of ours in animals.

Animal Research: We believe that the behavioral dysfunction supposedly resulting from discrete lesions in the brain can frequently be quickly circumvented by changing environmental or behavioral contigencies (Gazzaniga et al. 1973). We recently pursued this idea in one of the most exhaustively studied systems in physiological psychology, the lateral hypothalamic area.

Bilateral lesions here, of course, produce an adipsic animal who will neither drink nor eat, and if left alone postoperatively, would die. Such animals are nursed for an extended period of time and with enough coaxing some will eventually be able to sustain life postoperatively. We, however, observed that within a few days after the lesions, most rats will have a higher probability of running than they have of drinking. Thus the adipsic rat will show essentially no probability of taking a lick from a water spout but within a half hour period will run between one hundred and one hundred and fifty seconds. We then made these two behavioral events contingent such that if the animal wanted the opportunity to run, he had to drink, which in turn released a brake on a wheel that allowed the animal to run. Dramatically, the adipsic rats immediately began to drink in order to have the opportunity to run.

Now let us consider the infero-temporal lobe syndrome in monkeys where it has been repeatedly shown lesions in this area dramatically impair learning and performance in visual discriminations (Clark and Gazzaniga 1974). Clark and I (1974) have recently extended the kind of insight afforded in the preceding experiment into this area where discrimination problems are trained to monkeys undergoing infero-temporal lesions. In the beginning we assumed caged monkeys were like rats and would relish the opportunity to run in a similar type of apparatus. Instead, we seemed to have discovered the phylogenetic origin of "don't rock the boat". Here, when the animal has the opportunity to run, a preferred response turned out to be to adopt a vertical spread-eagle position so as to minimize movement in the wheel. This required a change in contingencies such that if the monkey made a correct choice, the wheel would be locked so no movement was possible.

Specifically, three monkeys were trained on a pattern discrimination for food reward using a discrimination panel that was placed inside of a large activity wheel. When the discrimination was learned, an added contingency was introduced. The wheel, driven by a motor, would automatically start to turn at the onset of the stimulus. As described, if the correct choice was made, the wheel locked during the intertrial interval. The animals, under these conditions, decreased their latency in making their responses and immediately made a perfect score even after all food reward was withdrawn.

All animals then underwent bilateral infero-temporal ablation. To our great surprise, the animals were instantly able to perform perfectly the discrimination to a food reward alone, as well, of course, as to the not-to-run contingency. Our expectation, of course, was that we would see a dissociation of performance between the food condition and the not-to-run contingency.

It would appear from the foregoing that the training of a visual task with two explicitly different kinds of rewards insulates the organism from showing the classic impairment following bitemporal lesions. It was as if the preoperative dual training encouraged the organism to use a number of conceptual strategies to solve the problem. These strategies then may have created a cerebral redundancy such that impairment to one part of the brain could in no way do exclusive damage to all of the paths used in problem solution. Indeed, the well known beneficial effects of preoperative overtraining has on postoperative scores may be the result of a similar mechanism. During the long overtraining period, the animals may well decide to solve the problem through a different kind of strategy than the one originally used. This, of course, could never be delineated by the present experimental design. At the same time, the strategy substitution interpretation is commonplace in complex discrimination training in humans. Here it has been shown, using other testing methods, that both children and adults are constantly changing their hypotheses along the way as they learn a particular visual discrimination (Levine 1966). In short, the old analysis of learning phenomena which urged simple behavioristic interpretations with the corresponding simplistic neurological models won't do anymore for the data are giving way to the view that distinctly separate mental processes are active during even the simplest kind of discrimination training.

Cognition Following Stroke: The problem of determining the amount and kind of cognitive

function remaining after severe brain damage to the
left dominant hemisphere is difficult. In the past,
little credit has been given to what the
remaining, largely undamaged, right hemisphere is
capable of in this regard. Encouraged by our
earlier studies on the cognitive capacity of the
right hemisphere (Gazzaniga *et al*. 1965; 1967;
Gazzaniga and Sperry 1967; Gazzaniga 1970) we
commenced a series of studies on the severely
left brain damaged patient in efforts to determine
what, in fact, the cognitive limits were. We
predicted that, with the right behavioral testing
technique, much more extensive behavioral capacity
would be evident than is usually claimed and this
has indeed been our experience. Using Premack's
(1970) language training system developed for the
chimp, we ran a series of tests on global aphasic
patients and quickly discovered these patients
could learn to perform many language-like operations.

Before beginning language training, a viable
social relationship must be established between
the patient and the trainer. The importance of this
phase can not be overemphasized for if the
motivational setting is inappropriate, no learning
will occur. In psychological parlance, if a
patient is emotionally flat and shows no preference, then it is impossible to arrange a
contingency where manipulating and learning X will
produce desired reward Y. Indeed, it would seem
fair to say that all too frequently neuropsychological assessment procedures ignore this factor.
Tests are designed, norms are established on a
normal population, and the relation all this has to
testing a brain damaged patient who surely is in a
complex ever changing motivational state is
frequently remote.

Using paper cut-out symbols, errorless
training procedures were administered in the
initial training. For example, in teaching "same
versus different", two similar objects, say two
erasers, were placed on a table in front of the
patient. Placed in between was another symbol, a
question marker, which comes to mean "missing
element". The subjects learned to slide the
question marker out from between the two test
objects and insert in its place the symbol meaning

"same". At first, this is the only response allowed. Subsequently, an eraser and a screwdriver are placed in front of the patient and the patient must remove the question marker and insert the symbol meaning "different". Following this training, the two symbols are both available on each trial and the subject must now make the correct response to the two varying, "same" or "different", stimuli. When the stimuli used in training are then changed, it is observed that the subjects can use the symbols correctly no matter what test objects are used by the examiner.

These procedures than enable one to teach any of a number of language operations to the global aphasic patient. The negative, yes, no, the question, and simple sentences were all successfully trained. Before teaching the sentences, the patients' lexicon was increased by teaching them a few nouns, verbs and personal names. Each of these words was taught by associating a symbol with an object, action or agent in the context of a simple social transaction. An object was placed before the patient along with the symbol for the object and the patient was required to place the symbol on the writing surface, after which he was given the object.

It is of interest to note that the training of symbols referent to actions (verbs) was consistently much more difficult than training in symbols referent to nouns. Noun symbols were learned in a few trials whereas verbs sometimes took weeks to learn. To some extent, of course, this is not too surprising. To know a verb is to know a whole context, subject and object, whereas to know a noun is simply to know a single object. The difficulty we experienced in training symbols referent to actions is also reminiscent of the finding that the right hemisphere of the split-brain patient was unable to process natural language verbs.

In a second series of cases examined on a whole battery of language tests, as well as a host of other cognitive tasks, artifical language training proved possible in most of the patients (Glass 1973). In those that failed, a series of simple cognitive assessment tests demonstrated that these patients did not possess to a normal extent, even the rudimentary aspects of cognitive life, such as a short term memory capability. In these tests, a pea placed under one of two different objects would not be reliably retrieved after a short delay. Without short term memory, it would seem very unlikely that the artificial language system could be learned.

These demonstrations of logical cognitive functions encourage one to examine more closely other dimensions of the cognitive content of the severely brain damaged individual. In all of the foregoing tests as well as those described in the following, the only criterion for accepting a global aphasic patient in the test was that he be alert and bright-eyed and in general, responsive to reward contingencies. With such a group, it has now been shown that a distinct cognitive capacity is remaining (Zangwill 1966). These tests, which are still preliminary in nature by and large, took a different approach from the standard tests which frequently require patients to manipulate symbols freshly presented at the time of testing. In our tests, pictures were used of common everyday objects or scenes. The patients were required to order them in a logical sequence or to complete a logical equation developed and posed solely with familiar pictorial material.

These studies clearly suggest that the severely left brain damaged patient can perform a wide variety of conceptual tasks. Because of the large extent of left damage, it would seem likely the intact right hemisphere is surely involved in many of these tasks. We know from other studies that the right hemisphere has enormous cognitive power (Gazzaniga and Sperry 1967; Bogen and Gazzaniga 1965; Levy, Trevarthen and Sperry 1972; Milner and Taylor 1972) and, indeed, the imagery mechanism associated with language behavior appears to be a right hemisphere process (Seamon and Gazzaniga 1973).

In these studies, use was made of Sternberg's (1966) serial processing model of short term memory processes. In brief, he found that as a memory set increased in size - for example, from one item to three items - a "probe word" examining whether that word was part of the set took longer to yield an answer the larger the memory set size.

Seamon reasoned that if the instructions to a subject were varied, different response patterns would be evident. Instead of instructing the subject to rehearse verbally the material, as is usually the case in the Sternberg design, he told them to create with the memory set words an interactive image, where all the words in the set "touched" one another in the image (Seamon 1962). Thus "tree" and "bird" should find the bird in the tree, not flying by it. Changing the instructions in this way found equivalent response times no matter how large the memory set.

This remarkable observation encouraged us, of course, to examine the possibility that there may be a left-right difference in hemisphere specialization for imagery processes. For years we had felt that it was the right hemisphere that was specialized for handling the visual abilities of mental life and, in this context, we examined whether different response times would be functioning as a feature of both our instructions for encoding the original material and the visual-field-hemisphere first receiving the probe.

Results of the study clearly showed it is the right hemisphere that is specialized in the image process and the left for verbal directions. For present purposes, these studies indicate how a cognitive system working in parallel with the language system might well come to the aid of a patient following severe left brain damage. In addition, and perhaps more importantly, we see how by manipulating the encoding instructions, wholly different brain systems are called upon to process information. In a sense, then, the idea here is that one can "shunt" around a brain lesion by setting up the environmental contingencies differently and thereby requiring a different part of the brain to be used in the solution of a problem.

Summary: For the present, we are faced with the problem of how to account for clinical improvement in terms of recovery of function. Does it reflect a process where the central and dominant language processing systems have repaired to the extent of allowing the observed behavior? Or, are these cognitive talents the product of other existing behavioral strategies that are capable of

handling the job but have previously been involved
in other more supportive roles? With the latter
view, the recovery period becomes more the time
needed to allow for the realignment of these
cognitive processes than the time needed for
physical repair.

While it is still too soon to say for sure, my
guess is that once the motivational state of a
brain damaged patient is defined and analyzed,
correct manipulation of these variables will
maximize the extent of recovery possible. Just as
the adipsic rat will drink to run - the bright-eyed
aphasic patient will learn an appropriate meta-
language system in order to communicate
meaningfully with the environment.

REFERENCES

Blakemore, C. and Cooper, G.F. (1970). Development of the brain depends on the visual environment. *Nature (London)* 228, 477-478.

Bogen, J.E. and Gazzaniga, M.S. (1965). Cerebral commissurotomy in man: Minor hemisphere dominance for certain visual-spatial functions. *J. Neurosurgery* 23, 394-399.

Clark, E. and Gazzaniga, M.S. (1974). Preventing visual discrimination defects in monkeys with infero-temporal lesions (in preparation).

Gazzaniga, M.S. (1970). "The Bisected Brain", New York: Appleton-Century-Crofts.

Gazzaniga, M.S., Bogen, J.E. and Sperry, R.W. (1967). Dyspraxia following division of the cerebral commisures in man. *Arch. Neurol.* 16, 606-612.

Gazzaniga, M.S. and Sperry, R.W. (1967). Language after section of the cerebral commisures. *Brain* 90, 131-148.

Gazzaniga, M.S., Szer, I. and Crane, A. (1974). Modifying drinking behavior in the adipsic rat. *Exp. Neur.* (in press).

Gazzaniga, M.S., Velletri, A.S. and Premack, D. (1971). Language training in brain-damaged humans. *Fed. Proc. Abs.* 30(2), 265.

Glass, A.S., Gazzaniga, M.S. and Premack, D. (1972). Artificial language training in global aphasics. *Neuropsychologia* 11, 95-103.

Glass, A.S. (1973). Cognition following stroke. Thesis, New York University.

Harlow, H. (1971). "Learning to Love", San Francisco: Albion.

Hirsch, H.V.B. and Jacobson, M. (1974). The Perfect Brain. *In* M.S. Gazzaniga and C.B. Blakemore (Eds.), "Fundamentals of Psychobiology", (in press). New York: Academic Press.

Hirsch, H.V.B. and Spinelli, D.N. (1971). Modification of the distribution of receptive field orientation in cats by selective visual exposure during development. *Exp. Brain Res.* 12, 504-527.

Hoedt-Rasmussen, R. and Skinhoj, E. (1964). Transneuronal depression of the cerebral hemispheric metabolism in man. *Acta Neurol. Scand.* 40, 41-46.

Kempinsky, W.H. (1958). Experimental study of distant effects of acute focal brain injury. *Arch. Neurol. and Psychiat.* 79, 376-389.

Levine, M. (1966). Hypothesis behavior in humans during discrimination learning. *J. Exp. Psychol.* 71, 331-338.

Levy, J. Trevarthen, C. and Sperry, R.W. (1972). Perception of bilateral chimeric figures following hemispheric deconnexion. *Brain* 45, 61-78.

Luria, A.R., Nayden, V.L., Tsvetkova, L.S. and Vinarskaya, E.N. (1969). Restoration of higher cortical function following local brain damage. *In* P.J. Winken and G.W. Bruyn (Eds.), "Handbook of Clinical Neurology", vol. 3. Amsterdam: North Holland Pub.

Milner, B. and Taylor, L. (1972). Right-hemisphere superiority in tactile pattern-recognition after cerebral commissurotomy: Evidence for nonverbal memory. *Neuropsychologia* 10, 1-16.

Moore, R.G., Björklund, A. and Stenevi, U. (1971). Plastic changes in adrenergic innervation of the rat septal area in response to denervation. *Brain Res.* 33, 13-35.

Nottebohm, F. (1970). Ontogeny of bird song. *Science* 167(3920), 950-956.

Premack, D. (1966). Reinforcement Theory. *In* M.R. Jones (Ed.), "Nebraska Symposium on Motivation," Lincoln: University of Nebraska Press.

Raisman, G. (1969). Neuronal plasticity in the septal nuclei in the rat. *Brain Res.* 14, 25-48.

Robinson, M. (1971). Factors influencing stroke rehabilitation. *Stroke* 2, 213-218.

Sarno, M.T. (1970). Speech therapy and language recovery in severe aphasia. *J.S.H.R.* 13, 607-625.

Schneider, G. (1973). Early lesions of the superior colliculus: Factors affecting the formation of abnormal retinal projections. *Brain, Behavior and Evolution.* (in press).

Seamon, J. (1972). Imagery codes and human information retrieval. *J. Exp. Psych.* 96, 468-470.

Seamon, J. and Gazzaniga, M.S. (1973). Coding strategies and cerebral laterality effects. *In* "Cognitive Psychology", (in press).

Sperry, R.W. (1966). Embryogenesis of behavioral nerve nets. *In* DeHaan and Ursprung (Eds.), "Organogenesis", pp. 161-183.

Stern, P., McDowell, F., Miller, J.M. and Robinson, M. (1971). Factors influencing stroke rehabilitation. *Stroke* 2, 213-218.

Sternberg, S. (1966). High-speed scanning in human memory. *Science* 153, 652-654.

Zangwill, O. (1964). Intelligence in aphasia. *In* A.V.S. de Rauk and M. O'Connor (Eds.), "Ciba Foundation Symposium on Disorder of Language", London: Churchill, Ltd.

Aided by USPHS Grant # MH 17883-04

RECOVERY OF FUNCTION FOLLOWING LESIONS OF THE SUBCORTEX AND NEOCORTEX

Patricia Morgan Meyer
The Ohio State University
Columbus, Ohio

My interest in the problems of recovery of function after damage to the central nervous system (CNS) began while I was still a graduate student at The Ohio State University. In fact, my first scientific publication (King and Meyer 1958) and my doctoral dissertation (Meyer 1963) both dealt with that topic. Since that time my husband and I and our students have continued our investigations in an attempt to understand how it is that neural mechanisms compensate for functional impairments. We have utilized several techniques, such as sequential surgeries, drug injections, neonatal surgeries and manipulation of stimulus parameter, in an attempt to recover performances lost as a consequence of previous brain damage. Most of our observations have been concerned with visual tasks, i.e., brightness discrimination and edge detection problems following neocortical ablations, but we have also been interested in how subcortical structures interact with each other in both learned and unlearned behaviors.

RECOVERY AND FLUX DETECTION PROBLEMS

One of the first observations of the program was a finding by Meyer, Isaac and Maher (1958). Rats were trained on a conditioned avoidance response (CAR) using light as the CS. After learning, some of the animals received bilateral visual decortication, while others received successive unilateral occipital ablations. If the rats were housed in the dark between successive surgeries, or if they were subjected to one-stage bilateral lesions, the habit was not retained. Only those rats that had undergone two successive surgeries and had been housed in the light during that interval retained the habit. These data indicated that recovery of the CAR was not spontaneous, but depended upon some kind of visual stimulation, probably elicited by changes in room illumination.

Neural reorganization was occurring somewhere in the CNS, but it was not clear whether the reorganization was taking place in a different area of the brain, or was the substitution of a similar but different function, or was a return of nonspecific inputs to areas spared. Nevertheless, soon after the Meyer *et al.* study (1958) Isaac and his co-workers (Isaac 1964; Cole, Sullins and Isaac 1967) found that other manipulations between successive removals of the visual cortex also reinstated the CAR. The habit was spared when the animals were housed during the interoperative interval in the light with noise, in the light with quiet, and in the dark with noise, but not in the dark with quiet. If, however, the dark-quiet group received injections of d-amphetamine between the two surgeries, they showed retention of the habit. Consequently, reinstatement of the CAR seemed to depend upon the general state of arousal of the CNS, and was not specifically dependent upon visual stimulation.

Nonetheless, sequential operations combined with non-specific stimulation during the interoperative interval between surgeries does not yield sparing of all visual habits. Thompson (1960) and Petrinovitch and Carew (1969) trained rats on a black-white discrimination in a Thompson-Bryant apparatus. They found that the habit was lost if the animals were housed in the light between successive radical ablations of the occipital cortex, but that the habit was spared if the rats were trained during the interoperative interval.

Since the latter findings seem to be discrepant from those of Meyer *et al.* (1958) and of the Isaac studies (Isaac 1964; Cole, Sullins and Isaac 1967), Kircher, Braun, Meyer and Meyer (1970) performed the following experiment. We trained rats on a black-white discrimination habit in the Thompson-Bryant apparatus, and, after the habit was initially acquired, we subjected them to serial, two-stage ablations of the posterior neocortex. During the interoperative interval, the animals were housed in the dark and received saline injections, were housed in the dark and received amphetamine injections, were housed in the light and received injections of saline, or were housed in the light and received injections of amphetamine. None of these procedures, although some had been shown to be highly effective in protecting CAR's, facilitated the ultimate retention of the black-white discrimination. We concluded, therefore, that CAR's and black-white habits have different neural substrates, and that this was the basis for the differences between Thompson's findings and our own.

A general consensus had thus been reached that black-white habits are completely lost following either simultaneous bilateral or serial ablations of the posterior neocortex provided that the lesions are relatively large, as suggested by Petrinovitch and Bliss (1966). In addition, it was also established that the habit could be spared if the rats with serial removals of the posterior neocortex were retrained between successive surgeries. Why retraining is effective is still unresolved, but three major theories deal with that issue. The vicariation theory says that the visual cortex mediates the black-white habit under normal conditions, but after its removal, other systems in the brain become able to subsume the same function. The diaschisis theory suggests, on the other hand, that the same mechanisms are involved in the recovery before and after aurgery, but are temporarily depressed after the operation because of their traumatic disconnection from the visual neocortex. And, finally, the substitution theory states that black-white habits can be learned in two ways. Destruction of the visual neocortex eliminates one of the two different mechanisms, and the relearning of the black-white habit is accomplished by the still intact system.

The substitution concept, as applied to black-white habits, involves the supposition that the habit is learned by normal rats as a visual pattern habit, and then, following removal of the visual neocortex, is relearned as a flux discrimination. This idea stems from Lashley's finding (1931) that rats with visual lesions fail pattern discriminations, but learn a flux discrimination as rapidly as normal animals (1921). The best modern evidence in favor of the concept is Bauer and Cooper's finding (1964) that rats given training on a black-white problem while wearing translucent occluders, suffer less impairment after posterior cortical

ablations than animals with similar lesions that
are trained preoperatively on the same problem, but
can see details in the cues.

Although perceptual changes appear to play a
role in losses of the black-white habit, our own
results indicate that recovery of these habits take
place, in part, by means of processes that permit
access to engrams that are not destroyed when the
posterior neocortex is removed (Meyer 1972).

First, in an experiment by Braun, Meyer and
Meyer (1966), we found that injections of amphetamine facilitate recovery of a previously learned
black-white habit by rats with lesions of the
visual cortex. In contrast, rats with no preoperative training, which were given the same doses of
amphetamine, learned the black-white habit at about
the same rates as normal control animals. Since
amphetamine treatments facilitated relearning, but
not original learning, it appeared that the engrams
established in rats prior to surgery were not
completely destroyed as the advocates of the
substitution theory would presume.

The Braun *et al.* experiment did not inform us
as to what kind of engram had been spared. One
possibility was that the black-white habit was
originally learned via edge or contour cues, and
that the amphetamine injections brought about a
reinstatement of detail vision. To test this idea,
Jonason, Lauber, Robbins, Meyer and Meyer (1970)
trained rats on a visual-pattern discrimination,
subjected them to lesions of the visual cortex, and
then retrained the animals while they were under
the influence of amphetamine. The drug had no
effect upon the performance of the task, and,
therefore, we concluded that the Braun *et al.*
result was due to reinstatements of access to flux-
related engrams that were formed at the time the
rats originally learned the task as normal animals.

More recently, a study by LeVere and Morlock
(1973) has offered strong support for this
conclusion, These investigators trained rats on a
black-white habit, and then subjected all of them
to large bilateral posterior neocortical ablations.
Subsequently, some of the rats were retrained on
the black-white task, while others were retrained
on reversals of the black-white problem. LeVere and
Morlock found that rats which were retrained on the

reversal problems took significantly more trials to re-reach criterion than those rats which were retrained on the original problems. Thus, removal of the posterior neocortex did not destroy all traces of the habit. Prior work of Lashley, which showed that rats with visual lesions learn the black-white task at the same rate that rats with visual lesions relearn the habit, would not have predicted the sparing that LeVere and Morlock found. The fact that the rats which were trained on reversals were slower to learn after surgery than the nonreversal group indicated that the animals had retained something from their preoperative training.

It is, therefore, evident that black-white relearning by rats with visual cortical ablations is not a simple case of recovery that can be interpreted in terms of substitution. LeVere and Morlock's data show that the preoperative engram is, to some extent, intact, and that the loss of the habit is a failure of access to the engram. The fact that amphetamine can reinstate the habit suggests that this retrieval is due to diaschisis, and that the drug facilitates recovery by acting upon the damaged, but partially-intact system. However, the fact that practice given between successive surgeries or after simultaneous ablations can restore the habit, suggests that vicariation also has a role in reinstating the habit. Therefore, it appears that each of the major theories of recovery has merits in explaining recovery of black-white habits (Meyer 1973).

When Lashley first observed that the black-white habit can be relearned by rats with visual lesions, he asked if the recovery was mediated by the remaining anterior neocortex (Lashley 1935). We also have asked the same question. Horel, Bettinger, Royce and Meyer (1966) trained rats on a black-white discrimination, removed either the anterior or posterior neocortex, and then retrained the animals on the task. Both groups were impaired, the posterior more so than the anterior, but the animals with anterior ablations also were slower to relearn than normal rats.

In the same investigation, rats were prepared with either anterior or posterior ablations, were trained on the habit, and then were subjected to

221

either posterior or anterior neocortical removals, respectively. Subsequently, they were retrained on the flux problem. Rats with pre-existing anterior lesions relearned the habit after posterior lesions at the same rate that rats with only posterior lesions relearned the task. Similarly, rats with pre-existing posterior lesions relearned the problem after anterior lesions at the same rate that rats with only anterior lesions relearned the task. Hence, both anterior and posterior removals do retard the relearning of a brightness discrimination, but in different and independent ways.

In the studies of Horel *et al.*, the anterior ablations did not encroach upon the prefrontal analogs recently described by Leonard (1969). Instead, the extent of the ablation included the rat's homologs of the precentral and postcentral gyri of non-human primates (Woolsey, Settlage, Meyer, Spencer, Hamuy and Travis 1950).

Recently, we have shown that cats with lesions of the anterior sigmoid gyri, the area homologous to precentral motor I and somatic I of primates, also are impaired in relearning a black-white habit (Meyer, Dalby, Glendenning, Lauber and Meyer in press). The nature of these deficits in rats and cats caused by anterior cortical lesions and their subsequent recoveries is still obscure, but they may arise from the fact that the regions in question are zones of termination of the pericruciate polysensory pathways described by Thompson, Johnson and Hoopes (1963).

RECOVERY AND EDGE DETECTION OBSERVATIONS

A decade ago, I trained cats with almost complete removals of the neocortex on a strip vs. check discrimination in a Yerkes-Watson apparatus (Meyer 1963). The animals failed to learn the pattern problem within 450 trials, but they, nonetheless were able to discriminate between the shallow and the deep sides of a Gibson-Walk (1960) visual cliff. This result has since been confirmed by Meyer, Anderson and Braun (1966) and by Dalby, Meyer and Meyer (1970), and shows very clearly that cats which are deprived of their geniculostriate mechanisms see something more than intensity differences in some kinds of visual displays.

Wetzel (1969) also found that cats with posterior lesions failed the same striped-check discrimination used by Meyer (1963). He then trained his animals in a horizontal adaptation of the visual cliff using the same Yerkes-Watson box. The discriminanda were located at the end of the runway. One of the stimuli was a checked panel, and the other was a black and white checked box that looked like the deep side of a Gibson-Walk cliff. Under these conditions the operated animals learned the three-dimensional discrimination. Subsequent discrimination problems involving two-dimensional patterns that were equated for flux led him to conclude that cats with occipital ablations can discriminate between visual patterns provided the targets differ substantially in the amount of edge or contour. These latter observations were highly reminiscent of Kluver's finding that one of his occipitally lesioned monkeys (1941) could discriminate a square from a pattern containing 76 circles, but failed to detect a square from a cross of equal area.

The proof that rats, also, are not completely form-blind after posterior cortical ablations has since been supplied in a recent experiment by Mize, Wetzel and Thompson (1971). They observed that rats with visual lesions could discriminate between a large equilateral triangle and five small equilateral triangles. The stimulus panels which were used in the study were equated with respect to total flux, and the positions of the triangular forms which were displayed upon the panels were changed in a systematic manner so that the animals could not solve the discrimination on the basis of local flux cues due to S-R spatial contiguity effects (Meyer, Treichler and Meyer 1965).

Having been convinced that visual preparations are not simply flux discriminators, we have since systematically explored the question as to what cats see without their visual cortex. In one of these experiments, Dalby, Meyer and Meyer (1970) trained cats prepared with visual cortical removals to discriminate between small- and large-checked patterns and between small- and large-circle patterns. We concluded, one again, that decorticated cats respond to cues related to differential edges or contour, and that differences in the number of corners within the stimulus patterns were of little importance to the animals' discrimination performance.

Previous equal-flux unequal-contour investigations had used patterns that contained differences in the total number of enclosed spatial figures per pattern. For example, in the large-check vs. small-check discrimination, the latter stimulus contained more squares than the former. Thus, it seemed possible that cats without their visual cortex still have mechanisms for discriminating whether visual space contained few objects vs. many objects, and that they were not utilizing the contour cue at all. In a study just completed, but not yet reported, Ritchie, Meyer and Meyer have found that cats with occipital ablations utilize contour to solve pattern discriminations, but were unable to solve the problem when the contour cues were equated and the number of objects within each stimulus panel varied.

The foregoing studies have illustrated that the animals with geniculostriate ablations can solve pattern discriminations, if contour is varied and flux is equated, but when both flux and contour are equated the problems become virtually unsolvable. Such is not the case, however, when cats are tested in adulthood after having been subjected to perinatal visual cortical ablations. Wetzel, Thompson, Horel and Meyer (1965) found that animals that had sustained the operation as infants learned an equal-contour equal-flux pattern habit as well as normal adult cats, whereas adult cats with comparable amounts of cortical removals were severely retarded.

In brain research, however, there are very few absolute statements that can be safely made. For example, we once thought that cats were color blind (Meyer, Miles and Ratoosh 1954), but later discovered (Meyer and Anderson 1965) that such animals, after several thousand trials, slowly learned a hue discrimination. Although they could detect colors, their ability to discriminate them was very poor. This same conclusion can be extended to pattern perception. Spear and Braun (1969) found that cats with visual lesions can learn equal-flux, equal-contour problems, but only if their training is extended over thousands of trials. Such is not the case if the cortical ablations are carried out parinatally (Wetzel et al. 1965).

Except for the variable of age at the time of removal of the visual cortex, we have not found any procedures that facilitate visual pattern learning. Pattern discrimination, however, is not the only test of edge detection that is impaired following surgery. Visual placing, for example, is typically lost after the visual cortex is removed and shows no spontaneous recovery after many post-operative months (Bard and Brooks 1934).

Many years after the Bard and Brooks findings, Meyer, Horel and Meyer (1963) reported that cats with occipital ablations had not lost the neural mechanisms to place visually. If such preparations were treated with injections of dl-amphetamine, visual placing was reinstated, but once the effects of the drug subsided, so did the ability to place. Once again, the deficit was a problem of retrieval or access to a spared mechanism.

Recently, in studies that have not yet been published, Meyer, Meyer and Ritchie have confirmed the observations reported by Meyer, Horel and Meyer. Nine cats with long-chronic lesions intend-ed to remove the lateral and posterior lateral gyri, the middle and posterior suprasylvian gyri, the Clare-Bishop area, and the visual gyri on the medial walls of each hemisphere were tested for visual placing after 12 months of postoperative recovery, but injections of d-amphetamine reversed these impairments. Initially, the drug depressed the cats and no placing was observed for periods of several hours. After that phase, placing was restored and then, as in the Meyer et al. (1963) experiment, it disappeared as the effects of the drug subsided.

We have also been exploring recoveries of visual function as measured by perimetric tests modeled after Sprague's and Meikle's (1965) and Sprague's (1966) studies of visual field defects and subsequent recoveries following visual cortical and superior collicular lesions in the cat. In our study, which used hooded rats, Kirvel, Greenfield and Meyer (in press) unilaterally lesioned one visual cortex or in combination with destruction of either the ipsilateral or contralateral superior colliculus.

Our findings were similar to Sprague's and Sprague's and Meikle's in that we observed that colliculectomies produced profound multimodal neglects of visual, olfactory and cutaneous stimuli presented to the side of the body opposite to the colliculectomy. More germane to the problem of induction of recovery of function was the fact that unilateral posterior decortication by itself caused a contralateral visual neglect to a small moving target. If, however, this lesion were combined with a simultaneous contralateral superior colliculect- omy, the visual neglect was prevented on the side contralateral to the posterior lesion. Thus, the Sprague effect was confirmed in a different species and by simultaneous cortical-subcortical operations as opposed to sequential cortical-subcortical surgeries.

It is clear that there are a number of procedures for restoring certain aspects of vision after neocortical ablation. It is also clear that the various techniques such as sequential surgeries, drug injections or neonatal operations are not appropriate for reinstating all losses following surgery. Even though our research efforts have provided us with mere glimpses as to the functioning of the brain's many neural networks, some light has been shed upon recovery of function, and we are encouraged to proceed.

We have long been interested in the vertical relationships between the brain's integrative networks and cortical and subcortical interactions, hence, our interest in the Sprague effect. Although the greater majority of our experiments have dealt with visual phenomena, our primary interest is how one can recover lost functions. Consequently, we have investigated additional CNS regions and their roles in reinstatement of functions.

RECOVERY AND SUBCORTICAL-CORTICAL INTERACTIONS

One example of recovery following sequential subcortical lesions is provided by King and Meyer (1958). We found that the hyperemotionality first noted by Brady and Nauta (1953) following lesions of the septal forebrain in rats could be attentuat- ed by a subsequent ablation of the amygdala, and that the increased emotionality could be dampened, to a lesser degree, if the amygdaloid lesion preceded removal of the septum. This attentuation, or recovery, was not observed in animals whose second operation involved removals of comparable amounts of tissue in the cingulate cortex. The implications from these data suggested that the syndrome arises from imbalances between specific and reciprocally related mechanisms between the septum and amygdaloid complex.

In our experience, the hyperreactivity of septal rats declines as a function of handling or as a function of time over days, which suggests that other CNS mechanisms compensate for the amygdaloid release following septal lesions. Yutzey, Meyer and Meyer (1964) found that the neocortex was involved in this attentuation. Rats with simultaneous removal of the septum and the neocortex exhibited the septal syndrome following a three week recovery interval, but rats with solely cortical or solely septal lesions approached normal emotionality levels. Furthermore, ablation of either the anterior or posterior neocortex or the supracallosal limbic cortex in conjunction with a lesion of the septal forebrain was sufficient for maintaining the hyperemotionality, but this behavior could not be attributed to removal of a specific cortical locus (Yutzey, Meyer and Meyer 1964; Yutzey, Meyer and Meyer 1967; Clark, Meyer, Meyer, Yutzey 1967; Srebro and Divac 1972).

We next turned to more cognitive measures in our investigations of septal and neocortical interactions. At the time we found that amphetamine could facilitate recovery of a black-white habit (Braun et al. 1966), we were looking for additional procedures that would reinstate that habit. Accordingly, we studied the effects of simultaneous ablations of the septum and visual neocortex upon retention of a black-white discrimination in the hope that the septal release phenomenon would facilitate relearning of the habit (Meyer, Yutzey, Dalby and Meyer 1968). We were quickly disabused of this hypothesis after observing that septal-posterior ablations were as severely impaired as complete removals of the neocortex, and concluded that septal lesions had absolutely no effect whatsoever on recovering flux

227

mechanisms.

More recently, however, we discovered that our idea did have some merits. In a study carried out by Meyer, Johnson and Vaughn (1970), we first replicated the well-known findings of King (1958) that rats with lesions of the septum show facili- tated acquisition of a CAR. Next, we established that rats with complete removals of the neocortex rarely learned the problem within 300 training trials. Finally, we showed that rats with simulta- neous removals of the neocortex and septum learned the CAR even faster than normal control animals. Thus, removal of the septum can compensate for some depressions following cortical removals, and we concluded that the mechanisms involved in facili- tated shuttle-box avoidance learning in rats with lesions of the septal forebrain were via subcorti- cal routes and not via neocortical mechanisms.

We have also been using the combination surgical technique to explore changes in social behavior. In one study by Jonason and Enloe (1971), it was found that septal lesions markedly enhance the amount of time that pairs of rats spend in contact with each other when both are placed together in a circular open field. A complementary study using cats with septal lesions (Glendenning 1972) showed that the social effect was not peculiar to rats despite the fact that the two species express social interests in different ways. Cats spend more time looking at each other postoperatively, and rats spend more time in contact with each other postoperatively.

Jonason and Enloe noted, in addition, that rats with amygdaloid ablations spend less time in contact with each other than normal pairs of rats. The fact that septal pairs show high contact times, that normal pairs show intermediate contact times and the fact that amygdaloid pairs exhibit low contact times suggested a reciprocity between the septum and amygdala and prompted the following experiment by Jonason, Enloe, Contrucci and Meyer (1973). Rats were tested in the open field after having been prepared with either simultaneous or successive lesions of the septum and amygdala. Animals with only septal lesions showed the typical rise in contact times and animals with only amygdaloid lesions showed the reduction in social cohesiveness following surgery. However, the increased cohesiveness in the septal group and the decreased cohesiveness of the amygdaloid group were attentuated by subsequent lesions in the amygdala and septum, respectively. In addition, simultaneous septal-amygdaloid preparations also approached normal contact times. These data, therefore, are supportive of the view that the septum and amygdala are reciprocally involved in mediating social cohesiveness in the open field.

The social effect produced by lesions of the septum has proved to be persistent over weeks, and contrasts with the transitory nature of septal hyperreactivity. Furthermore, Johnson (1972) has demonstrated that adult rats who received septal lesions as neonates also show the same increased cohesiveness as adult-lesioned animals do. There is thus a remarkable rigidity of organization of limbic mechanisms that contrasts with the apparent plasticity of some of the systems of the cerebral cortex.

Finally, a recent dissertation project of Enloe has assessed the social cohesiveness effect following lesions placed in several well-established diencephalic and mesencephalic zones of convergence pathways from the septum and the amygdala. Disruptions in terms of lower than normal contact times were observed only after lesions were placed in the hypothalamus, particularly in the anterolateral hypothalamus (LHA) and in the ventromedial zone (VMH). Low contact times between the two groups were qualitatively different. The LHA animals showed no interest in social interaction, but the VMH animals fought and consequently actively avoided each other. Thus, there is a suggestion that increased conspecific interactions and suppressions of aggressions are normally mediated by different neural sites in the hypothalamus.

SUMMARY

While pursuing these studies we have come to believe that behavior resulting from brain damage is rarely permanent. We also believe that a specific cerebral ablation has more than one important consequence. Thirdly, we have found that brain-damaged subjects are not necessarily made worse by an additional ablation. The question as to whether the surgical outcome represents an improvement is subject to debate, but there is no doubt that normalizing results can be obtained in some cases. There are, of course, perils, for ablations that correct one problem will create others. Finally, it is our sincere hope that there is a bright future for pharmacological approaches in the treatment of some forms of brain damage.

The foregoing experiments have illustrated some of the procedures we have used in an attempt to reinstate performances or to prevent impairments following damage to the central nervous system. In some cases we have been successful and in some cases we have failed. Nevertheless, in all cases, we have tried to understand, one experiment at a time, how it is that neural mechanisms compensate for functional deficits.

REFERENCES

Bard, P. and Brooks, C.M. (1934). Localized cortical control of some postural reactions in the cat and rat together with evidence that small cortical remnants may function normally. *Assoc. Res. Nerv. Ment. Dis.* 13, 107-157.

Bauer, J.H. and Cooper, R.M. (1964). Effects of posterior cortical lesions on performance of a brightness-discrimination task. *J. Comp. Physiol. Psych.* 58, 84-92.

Brady, J.V. and Nauta, W.J.H. (1953). Subcortical mechanisms in emotional behavior: Affective changes following septal forebrain lesions in the albino rat. *J. Comp. Physiol. Psych.* 46, 339-346.

Braun, J.J., Meyer, P.M. and Meyer, D.R. (1966). Sparing of a brightness habit in rats following visual decortication. *J. Comp. Physiol. Psych.* 61, 79-82.

Clark, S.M., Meyer, P.M., Meyer, D.R. and Yutzey, D.A. (1967). Emotionality changes following septal and neocortical ablations in the albino rat. *Psychonomic Science* 8, 125-126.

Cole, D.D., Sullins, W.R. and Isaac, W. (1967). Pharmacological modification of the effects of spaced occipital ablations. *Psychopharmacol.* 11, 311-316.

Dalby, D.A., Meyer, D.R. and Meyer, P.M. (1970). Effects of occipital neocortical lesions upon visual discriminations in the cat. *Physiol. Behav.* 5, 727-734.

Enloe, L.J. Mediation of septal-amygdaloid social reciprocity by some midbrain and diencephalic structures. Ph.D. Dissertation, The Ohio State University, 1973.

Gibson, E.J. and Walk, R.D. (1960). The visual cliff. *Sci. Amer.* 202, 46-71.

Glendenning, K.K. (1972). Effects of septal and amygdaloid lesions on social behavior of the cat. *J. Comp. Physiol. Psych.* 80, 199-207.

Horel, J.A., Bettinger, L.A., Royce, G.J. and Meyer, D.R. (1966). Role of neocortex in the learning and relearning of two visual habits by the rat. *J. Comp. Physiol. Psych.* 61, 66-78.

Isaac, W. (1964). Role of stimulation and time in the effects of spaced occipital ablations. *Psych. Rep.* 14, 151-154.

Johnson, D.A. (1972). Developmental aspects of recovery of function following septal lesions in the infant rat. *J. Comp. Physiol. Psych.* 78, 331-348.

Jonason, K.R. and Enloe, L.J. (1971). Alterations in social behavior following septal and amygdaloid lesions in the rat. *J. Comp. Physiol. Psych.* 75, 286-301.

Jonason, K.R., Enloe, L.J., Contrucci, J. and Meyer, P.M. (1973). Effects of simultaneous and successive septal and amygdaloid lesions on social behavior of the rat. *J. Comp. Physiol. Psych.* 83, 54-61.

Jonason, K.R., Lauber, S., Robbins, M.J., Meyer, P.M., and Meyer, D.R. (1970). The effects of dl-amphetamine upon discrimination behaviors in rats with cortical lesions. *J. Comp. Physiol. Psych.* 73, 47-55.

King, F.A. (1958). Effects of septal and amygdaloid lesions on emotional behavior and conditioned avoidance in the rat. *J. Nerv. Ment. Dis.* 126, 57-63.

King, F.A. and Meyer, P.M. (1958). Effects of amygdaloid lesions upon septal hyperemotionality in the rat. *Science* 128, 655-656.

Kircher, K.A., Braun, J.J., Meyer, D.R. and Meyer, P.M. (1970). Equivalence of simultaneous and successive neocortical ablations in production of impairments of retention of black-white habits in rats. *J. Comp. Physiol. Psych.* 71, 420-425.

Kirvel, R.D., Greenfield, R.A. and Meyer, D.R. (In Press). Multimodal sensory neglect in rats with radical unilateral posterior isocortical and superior collicular ablations. *J. Comp. Physiol. Psych.*

Klüver, H. (1941). Visual functions after removal of the occipital lobes. *J. Psych.* 11, 23-45.

Lashley, K.S. (1921). Studies of cerebral function in learning. II. The effects of long-continued practice upon cerebral localization. *J. Comp. Psych.* 1, 453-468.

Lashley, K.S. (1931). The mechanism of vision IV. The cerebral areas necessary for pattern vision in the rat. *J. Comp. Physiol. Psych.* 53, 419-478.

Lashley, K.S. (1935). The mechanism of vision: XII. Nervous structures concerned in habits based on reactions to light. *Comp. Psych. Monographs* 11, (2, whole No. 52).

Leonard, C.M. (1969). The prefrontal cortex of the rat. I and II. *Brain Res.* 12, 321-343.

LeVere, T.E. and Morlock, G.W. (1973). Nature of visual recovery following posterior neodecortication in the hooded rat. *J. Comp. Physiol. Psych.* 83, 62-67.

Meyer, D.R. (1972). Access to engrams. *Amer. Psych.* 27, 124-133.

Meyer, D.R. and Anderson, R.A. (1965). Colour discrimination in cats. *In* G.E.W. Wolstenholme and J. Knight (Eds.) "Ciba Symposium of Physiology and Experimental Psychology of Colour Vision," London: J. and A. Churchill Ltd.

Meyer, D.R., Isaac, W. and Maher, B. (1958). The role of stimulation in spontaneous reorganization of visual habits. *J. Comp. Physiol. Psych.* 51, 546-548.

Meyer, D.R., Miles, R.C. and Ratoosh, P. (1954). Absence of color vision in cats. *J. Neurophysiol.* 17, 289-294.

Meyer, D.R., Treichler, F.R. and Meyer, P.M. (1964) Discrete trial training techniques and stimulus variables. *In* A.M. Schrier and H.F. Harlow (Eds.) "Behavior of Nonhuman Primates," New York: Academic Press.

Meyer, P.M. (1963). Analysis of visual behavior in cats with extensive neocortical ablations. *J. Comp. Physiol. Psych.* 56, 397-401.

Meyer, P.M. (1973). Recovery from neocortical damage. *In* G.M. French (Ed.) "Cortical Functioning in Behavior," Palo Alto: Scott, Foresman and Co.

Meyer, P.M., Anderson, R.A. and Braun, M.G. (1966). Visual cliff preferences following lesions of the visual cortex in cats and rats. *Psychonomic Science* 4, 269-270.

Meyer, P.M., Horel, J.A. and Meyer, D.R. (1963).
Effects of dl-amphetamine upon placing responses
in neodecorticate cats. *J. Comp. Physiol. Psych.*
56, 402-404.

Meyer, P.M., Johnson, D.A. and Vaughn, D.W.
(1970). The consequence of septal and neocortical ablations upon learning a two-way
conditioned avoidance response. *Brain Res.* 22,
113-120.

Meyer, P.M., Meyer, D.R. and Ritchie, G.D.
(Unpublished). Recovery of temporary maintenance
of placing responses following amphetamine
treatments in cats with lesions of the occipital
cortex.

Meyer, P.M., Yutzey, D.A., Dalby, D.A. and Meyer,
D.R. (1968). Effects of simultaneous septal-
visual, septal-anterior and anterior-posterior
lesions upon relearning a black-white
discrimination. *Brain Res.* 8, 281-290.

Meyer, P.M., Dalby, D.A., Glendenning, K.A.,
Lauber, S.M. and Meyer, D.R. (In Press).
Behavior of cats with lesions of the septal
forebrain or the anterior sigmoid gyrus. *J.
Comp. Physiol. Psych.*

Mize, R.R., Wetzel, A.B. and Thompson, V.E. (1971).
Contour discrimination in the rat following
removal of posterior neocortex. *Physiol. Behav.*
6, 861-867.

Petrinovitch, L. and Bliss, D. (1966). Retention
of a learned brightness discrimination
following ablations of the occipital cortex in
the rat. *J. Comp. Physiol. Psych.* 61, 136-138.

Petrinovitch, L. and Carew, T.J. (1969). Interaction of neocortical lesion size and interoperative experience in retention of a learned
brightness discrimination. *J. Comp. Physiol.
Psych.* 68, 451-454.

Ritchie, G.D., Meyer, P.M. and Meyer, D.R.
(Unpublished). The nature of residual pattern
vision in cats following removal of the visual
cortex.

Spear, P.D. and Braun, J.J. (1969). Pattern
discrimination following removal of visual
neocortex in the cat. *J. Exper. Neurol.* 25, 331-
348.

Sprague, J.M. (1966). Interaction of cortex and superior colliculus in mediation of visually guided behavior in the cat. *Science* 153, 1544-1547.

Sprague, J.M. and Meikle, T.H. (1965). The role of the superior colliculus in visually guided behavior. *Exper. Neurol.* 11, 115-146.

Srebro, B. and Divac, I. (1972). Successive position reversals in rats with septal and/or frontal-polar lesions. *Physiol. Behav.* 9, 269-272.

Thompson, R. (1960). Retention of a brightness discrimination following neocortical damage in the rat. *J. Comp. Physiol. Psych.* 53, 212-215.

Thompson, R.F., Johnson, R.H. and Hoopes, J.J. (1963). Organization of auditory, somatic sensory and visual projection to association fields of cerebral cortex in the cat. *J. Neurophysiol.* 26, 343-364.

Wetzel, A.B. (1969). Visual cortical lesions in the cat: A study of depth and pattern discrimination. *J. Comp. Physiol. Psych.* 68, 580-588.

Wetzel, A.B., Thompson, V.E., Horel, J.A. and Meyer, P.M. (1965). Some consequences of perinatal lesions of the visual cortex in the cat. *Psychonomic Science* 3, 381-382.

Woolsey, C.N., Settlage, P.H., Meyer, D.R., Spencer, W., Hamuy, T.P. and Travis, A.M. (1950). Patterns of localization in precentral and "supplementary" motor areas and their relation to the concept of a premotor area. *Patterns of Organ. in the Central Nerv. Syst.* 30, 238-264.

Yutzey, D.A., Meyer, D.R. and Meyer, P.M. (1967). Effects of simultaneous septal and neo- or limbic-cortical lesions upon emotionality in the rat. *Brain Res.* 5, 452-458.

Yutzey, D.A., Meyer, P.M. and Meyer, D.R. (1964). Emotionality changes following septal and neocortical ablations in rats. *J. Comp. Physiol. Psych.* 58, 463-465.

RECOVERY AFTER SOMATOSENSORY FOREBRAIN DAMAGE

Stanley Finger
Washington University
St. Louis, Missouri

Much of the literature on experimental brain damage in laboratory animals has reflected attempts to delineate the functions of morphologically-distinct cortical and subcortical areas of the brain. Many earlier investigators were of the opinion that structure-function relationships could not be modified over the lifetime of the organism, and the data collected in some of their studies resulted in a variety of mechanistic and connectionistic interpretations of brain function (Dawson 1973).

The experiments of Margaret Kennard (1936, 1938, 1940, 1942) in the late nineteen-thirties and early nineteen-forties challenged some of these beliefs by bringing considerable attention to the fact that brain lesions in young animals may have effects different from those in more mature subjects. Specifically, she noted that the behavioral consequences of motor cortex damage were directly related to age at the time of surgery, and that large lesions of Brodmann areas 4 and 6 in animals operated upon in infancy led to considerably less severe impairments in posture and locomotion than in monkeys that underwent surgery later in life. Although some exceptions to this "rule" have been observed (e.g., Bland and Cooper 1969; Glassman, in press; Goldman 1971; Teuber and Rudel 1962), many later reports on the age variable have been in agreement with those of Kennard (Isaacson 1968).

More recently it has been emphasized that, under some conditions, expected deficits may not always be observed after well-defined lesions in adult animals. Some of the factors affecting the appearance, the time course, and the topologies of behaviors associated with given lesions have been described in recent reviews by Chow (1967) and Rosner (1970). For example, different behavioral patterns among animals with lesions have been observed after electrolytic, radio-frequency and aspirative damage (Douglas and Isaacson 1964;

237

Reynolds 1965), following preoperative administration of chemical agents such as nerve growth factor and α-methyl-p-tyrosine (Berger, Wise and Stein 1973; Glick and Greenstein 1972), and with early environmental enrichment and deprivation (Hughes 1965; Schwartz 1964).

This paper summarizes recent data on the effects of variables such as these on tactile discriminative performance of the rat after damage to the somatosensory forebrain.

GENERAL PROCEDURES

The surgical and behavioral testing procedures employed in these investigations have been described in detail in recent publications (e.g., Finger 1972; Finger, Cohen and Alongi 1972). Briefly, enucleated albino rats with and without brain lesions were required to discriminate between two aluminum surfaces extending from the choice point in a T-maze to each goal box. One of the plates was always smooth, and the other contained milled grooves between ridges. Five ridge-smooth discriminations, ranging from a relatively easy problem to a very difficult one, were presented in most experiments, although some studies dispensed with the three easier problems in the battery. Figures 1 and 2 show the apparatus and discriminanda, respectively.

T-MAZE

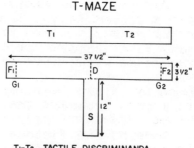

Ti-T2 TACTILE DISCRIMINANDA
S   START AREA
Fi-F2 FOOD CUPS
D   GUILLOTINE DOOR
Gi-G2 RETRACTABLE WIRE GATES

Figure 1. T-maze used for tactile discriminative testing (From Finger and Frommer 1968b)

RIDGED PLATES IN CROSS SECTION

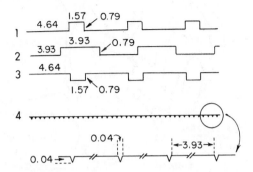

Figure 2. Four ridged tactile discriminanda. These four surfaces, and a "rough" aluminum plate (Problem 1, not shown), were paired with a smooth aluminum surface in the two wings of a T-maze. Dimension in millimeters (From Finger 1972)

An *a priori* criterion of not more than one error in two consecutive days (5 trials/day) with a perfect score on the third day defined learning in every study except one dealing with overtraining. Perfect scores on two successive days were required in the latter study. All experiments utilized strict controls for odor trails, olfactory cues from food reward, position cues and other accessory cues which may have been available to the animals.

The cortical lesions were accomplished by aspiration and were based on electrophysiological maps of the somatosensory areas (Woolsey 1958; Zubek 1951a) such as the one shown in Figure 3. Thalamic lesions were placed stereotaxically in the ventrobasal thalamus (Emmers 1965) on the basis of anatomical coordinates (König and Klippel 1963) which were confirmed with electrophysiological recordings in some studies. The lesions of all of the animals in our investigations have been verified histologically and have been found to approximate those shown in Figure 4.

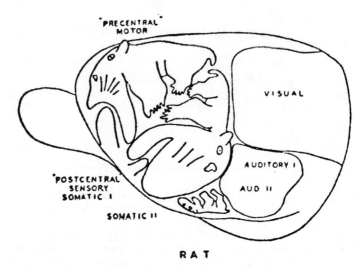

Figure 3. Diagram of rat cortex, showing general arrangement of somatic sensory areas I (SI) and II (SII), the "precentral" motor area (MI), and the gross positions of the visual and auditory areas. (From Woolsey 1958)

CORTICAL LOCALIZATION OF SOMESTHETIC TASKS

The finding that lesions in the electro-physiologically-defined somatosensory cortex of the rat can markedly impair acquisition of roughness discriminations is reasonably well documented. Zubek (1952a) observed this after lesions in the primary projection zone (SI), and with bilateral lesions in both projection zones (SI+II), but not after lesions restricted to the second somatic projection area (SII). Finger and Frommer (1968a) presented further evidence for impaired acquisition of rough-smooth habits with bilateral lesions centered in SI.

Acquisition of our series of ridge-smooth tactile form discriminations also may be impaired with lesions involving the somatosensory areas of the rat cortex. This was noted in an investigation in which the ablations involved both somatic projection zones in each hemisphere (Finger and Frommer 1968b). A more recent experiment on young adult rats has shown that acquisition deficits can appear on these problems after bilateral damage to

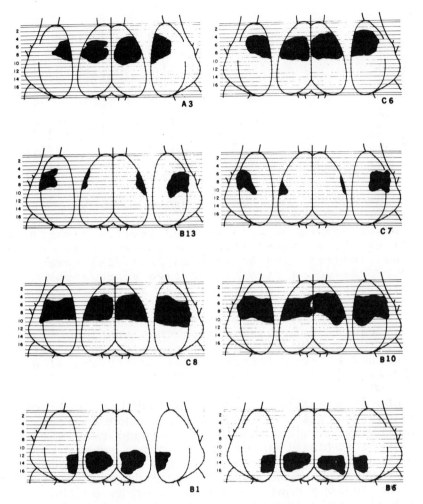

Figure 4. Reconstructions of representative cortical lesions. Rows 1, 2 and 3 show lesions of SI, SII, and SI+II, respectively. Row 4 shows a control lesion (occipital cortex) that was used in some of the studies. (After Finger, Cohen and Alongi 1972)

SI or to SII (Finger, Cohen and Alongi 1972). Figure 5 shows the relative severity of the lesion effects in the latter study.

Since these studies can be viewed as a sort of

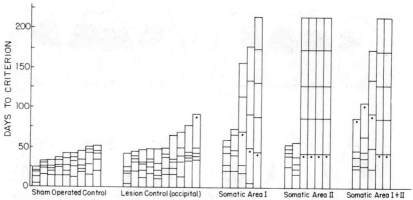

Figure 5. Performance of two control and three lesion groups on a battery of tactile discriminations. Each column shows the scores of an individual subject, and horizontal lines indicate performance on each of the five successive problems. A dot signifies that a problem was not mastered within the a priori time limit for learning. The maximum scores above such markers are based on the assumption that problems more difficult than the one not mastered would not be learned either. (After Finger, Cohen and Alongi 1972)

a baseline against which data have been collected on the significance of various methodological manipulations, it should be stressed that the tactile acquisition deficits do not appear to reflect broad performance decrements which might be attributable to general cortical damage. Rats with large lesions confined to other areas of the cortex (including frontal cortex, occipital cortex, and, in some cases, all non-somatosensory neocortex) could not be distinguished from sham operated control animals in these experiments. In addition, somatosensory cortical lesions identical to those described in the tactile discrimination studies do not retard learning reliably when rats are tested for temperature discriminative abilities, even on two-choice problems of less than 2°C. difference (Downer and Zubek 1954; Finger and Frommer 1970; Finger, Scheff, Warshaw and Cohen 1970).

METHODOLOGICAL CONSIDERATIONS

A. Postoperative Recovery Period

Behavioral impairments resulting from brain lesions frequently appear to diminish with time (Russell 1945). Cowey (1967) noted that monkeys exhibiting visual field defects after striate cortex lesions improved significantly over months of testing, even when such testing was initiated three and one-half years after surgery. Recovery also has been described by Chow (1952) in monkeys with temporal neocortical damage, by Thompson and Rich (1961) in rats with interpeduncular lesions, and by Glassman (1971) who recently correlated motoric and electrophysiological measures in an elegant experiment examining cats in the first few weeks after sensorimotor cortex damage.

Since the temporal course for tactile recovery had not been examined in the rat, Finger and Reyes (in progress) recently ablated the somatosensory cortices of a large number of rats and began testing the animals in different acquisition groups at periodic intervals after surgery. Although some groups of animals still are being evaluated, data are available on rats with SI+II lesions who were permitted 6 months in their home cages before being introduced to our battery of five ridge-smooth tactile discriminations. Examination of the learning scores in Figure 6 shows that these rats were as impaired as animals with similar lesions that were tested two weeks or five weeks after being operated upon. In all cases, the rats with bilateral somatosensory cortical lesions performed more poorly than control animals; a finding which parallels at least one early observation (Harlow 1939) and which suggests that spontaneous recovery, if it does occur after SI+II lesions in the rat, proceeds very slowly under these conditions.

B. Developmental Status

The effects of making somatosensory cortical lesions in infant and adult cats have been investigated by Benjamin and Thompson (1959). These investigators found that cats operated upon

243

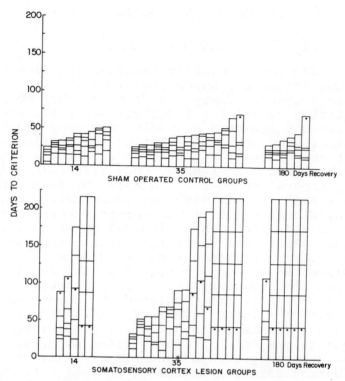

Figure 6. Graph showing tactile learning as a function of the length of the recovery period after surgery. Each column shows the scores of an individual subject, and horizontal lines indicate performance on each of the five successive problems. A dot signifies that a problem was not mastered within the a priori time limit for learning. The maximum scores above such markers are based on the assumption that problems more difficult than the one not mastered would not be learned either.

on the sixth day of life were indistinguishable from control animals in acquiring all but the most difficult tactile discriminations. In contrast, cats operated upon in adulthood, and given matching six month recovery periods, did not do well on even the simplest discriminations. Interestingly, the operated infants proved to be as deficient as the operated adults in tactile placing reflexes.

Analogous research has not been conducted on

the cortex of the one week old rat. However, as a part of a larger study, Walbran (in preparation for press) has operated upon juvenile (30 days old), mature (270 days old), and old (570 days old) rats and has tested them on the two most difficult ridge-smooth discriminations in our battery. Her findings, based on a constant recovery period of 34 days, were that: (1) all three groups of animals with SI+II lesions performed more poorly than control animals matched for age, (2) the three lesion age groups did not differ from each other, and (3) the three control age groups did not differ from each other. It still remains to be determined whether differential lesion effects have been obscured in this experiment by the use of an *a priori* time limit for learning. Walbran removed animals from testing if a problem was not mastered within three times the control group mean, and, as can be seen in Figure 7, many animals with lesions did not reach criterion within the allotted time.

C. One-stage vs. Serial Surgery

Lesions which evolve slowly often have less severe behavioral consequences than lesions which evolve rapidly in humans. This was noted in aphasic individuals by Marc Dax in a memoir dated 1836 (Joynt and Benton 1964), and, after Hughlings Jackson (1879), this phenomenon has sometimes been referred to as "the effect of momentum of lesion" (Joynt 1970). The importance of lesion momentum has been investigated under controlled conditions in laboratory animals by making successive unilateral lesions or by enlarging incomplete lesions in two or more operations (Finger, Walbran and Stein in press).

Serial lesion effects have been demonstrated in a variety of infra-human organisms including mice (Glick and Zimmerberg 1972), rats (Stein, Rosen, Graziadei, Mishkin and Brink 1969), cats (Adametz 1959), and monkeys (Travis and Woolsey 1956). Seemingly normal behaviors have appeared after successive lesions centered in the reticular formation (Chow and Randall 1964), the limbic system (McIntyre and Stein 1973), association cortex (Rosen, Stein and Butters 1971), motor cortex (Ades and Raab 1946), and sensory neocortex (Ades 1946).

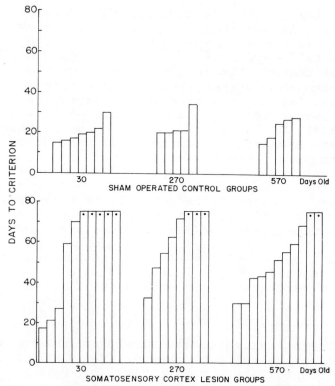

Figure 7. Graph showing tactile learning on a difficult discrimination (Problem 4) as a function of age at time of surgery. Each column shows the scores of an individual subject, and a dot indicates that the problem was not mastered within the a priori time limit for learning.

The effects of making serial lesions in rat somatosensory cortex have been studied systematically in two experiments from our laboratory (Finger, Marshak, Scheff, Cohen, Trace and Neimand 1971). Four groups of rats were compared in the first study: (1) one-stage bilateral lesions of both somatosensory areas of the cortex; (2) successive unilateral lesions of the same cortical areas with 35 days between operations; (3) one-stage sham operations; and (4) two-stage sham operations. The data collected in this experiment are presented in Figure 8. Statistical analyses revealed that the animals with two-stage lesions did not differ

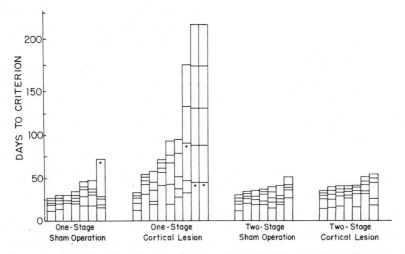

Figure 8. *Performance of rats with successive and simultaneous lesions of the somatosensory cortex on a battery of tactile discriminations. Each column shows the scores of an individual subject, and horizontal lines indicate performance on each of the five successive problems. A dot signifies that a problem was not mastered within the a priori time limit for learning. The maximum scores above such markers are based on the assumption that problems more difficult than the one not mastered would not be learned either. (After Finger, Marshak, Scheff, Cohen, Trace and Neimand 1971)*

significantly from the two-stage sham operates, and that the subjects with serial lesions learned statistically faster than the rats with one-stage lesions. The animals in the latter group performed more poorly than the one-stage sham operated animals, and the two groups without brain damage did not differ from each other in acquiring any of the five ridge smooth discriminations.

The second experiment differed from the first in that the animals with serial lesions now had small bilateral ablations of SI+II that were enlarged to full size in a second operation. These animals again learned faster than subjects with matched somatosensory cortical ablations produced in a single operation. However, although the serial animals compared favorably to control subjects on individual problems, the animals with two-stage lesions learned significantly more slowly than control animals when scores on all five tactile discriminations were pooled.

In both of these somatosensory cortical studies, the one-stage animals were operated upon at the time the serial rats received their second operation, and both groups were tested 30 days later. The bias inherent in this procedure was discussed in a recent review (Finger, Walbran and Stein, in press) in which it was claimed that a stronger case could be made for serial sparing if the one-stage animals have a recovery period measured from the time of the first surgery of the two-stage operates. The recovery period data previously described (Finger and Reyes, in progress) showing severe one-stage lesion effects 6 months after surgery is important here. The fact that the one-stage animals continued to perform poorly long after surgery can be considered strong evidence for the position that these serial lesion findings cannot be attributed to the "extra" recovery time given to the two-stage rats.

Since serial surgery appeared to minimize acquisition deficits after cortical lesions in the somatosensory system, rats with successive unilateral lesions centered in the thalamic ventrobasal nuclear homologue (Vb) recently were compared to animals with one-stage lesions in the same loci on the two most difficult tactile discriminations in our battery (Reyes, Finger and Frye 1973). Earlier studies had shown that bilateral thalamic lesions centered in Vb may impair tactile performance in rats, especially on difficult problems (Finger 1972; Finger and Frommer 1968a). In the latest study, the animals with two-stage thalamic lesions were as impaired as the rats with one-stage lesions (and an appropriate recovery period) in acquiring both ridge-smooth tactile discriminations, and both groups performed significantly worse than one-stage and two-stage sham operated and lesion control groups. These results are summarized in Figure 9.

Although the Reyes *et al.* findings raise the possibility that serial lesion effects are limited to some forebrain structures and not to others,

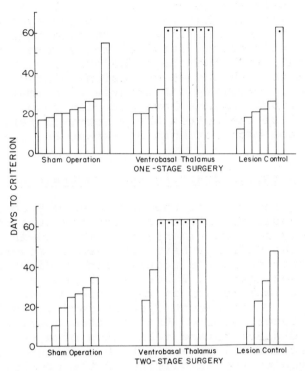

Figure 9. Performance of rats with successive and simultaneous lesions centered in the ventrobasal thalamus on a difficult tactile discrimination (Problem 4). Each column shows the scores of an individual subject, and a dot indicates that the problem was not mastered within the a priori time limit for learning. (After Reyes, Finger and Frye 1973)

the interlesion interval used in this investigation was 21 days, as compared to 35 days in the somatic cortex experiments. Other factors which could account for the differences between the cortical and thalamic results are (1) the absence of testing experience on easier problems prior to exposure to the two difficult discriminations in the thalamic study, and (2) the fact that the subcortical lesions rarely were discrete and could have damaged areas adjacent to Vb that theoretically might have contributed to a recovery process (Rosner 1970). Although the lesions appeared to be equivalent in

terms of size and locus in the two groups of
thalamic animals that were tested by Reyes *et al.*
(1973), it may be of interest to note that
sifnificantly better survival rates were found in
the animals with two-stage thalamic lesions than
in the rats with one-stage lesions placed in the
same loci. Mortality differences with small,
circumscribed lesions have not been reported at
the level of the cortex where survival rates
usually are high for both one-stage and two-stage
animals.

D.   Preoperative Training and Overtraining

        The role of the somatosensory cortex in
tactile habit retention has been the subject of
relatively few experiments on rats, and in
general the deficits have not been as severe as
those reported in the acquisition studies. In one
early investigation, Zubek (1951b) noted only
transient impairments in relearning when he tested
animals on rough-smooth discriminanda. Zubek
(1952b) later reported that somatosensory cortical
lesions did not retard relearning of a tactile
form discrimination; a negative finding which he
attributed to the simplicity of the problem which
he presented.
        The same five ridge-smooth tactile plates
that were used in our acquisition experiments also
were used in a retention study (Finger, Lennard,
Hammer and Ehrman 1971). Most rats with bilateral
lesions of SI, SII or SI+II rapidly relearned the
simple as well as the difficult discriminations in
the battery, and statistical analyses on the
difference and savings scores did not reveal
retrieval deficits in any of the lesion groups.
        Training beyond a reasonable criterion for
learning defines "overtraining", and both human
verbal learning and animal conditioning experiments
have shown that under some conditions overtrained
habits may be retained better than those trained to
criterion (Hall 1966). For example, good retention
of visual discriminations following temporal cortex
ablations in monkeys (Chow and Survis 1958; Orbach
and Fantz 1958), and of avoidance responses
following amygdaloid lesions in rats (Lukaszewska
and Thompson 1967), has been observed after

preoperative overtraining, but not with training to criterion.

Weese, Neimand and Finger (1973) hypothesized that the normal retention scores observed by Finger *et al.* (1971) after somatosensory cortex damage may have been due to overtraining since their animals had been preoperatively trained on five problems graded along a single dimension, and since the rats often showed perfect scores when transferred from one problem to another in the learning situation. In an attempt to find support for this hypothesis, an experiment was designed in which rats were trained to criterion on one ridge-smooth tactile discrimination and then either operated upon or given 100 percent additional training on the same problem before undergoing SI+II lesions or control surgery. Animals having no training prior to surgery also were tested to permit additional statistical comparisons within a single study.

The results of this experiment are presented in Figure 10. Statistical analyses revealed that

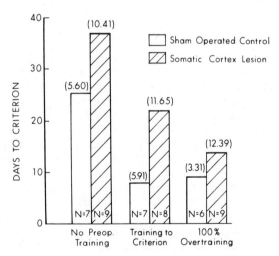

Figure 10. Graph showing means (Columns) and standard deviations (In brackets above columns) for three lesion groups and three control groups on a single tactile discrimination (Problem 4) as a function of testing experience prior to surgery. (After Weese, Neimand and Finger 1973)

overtrained rats with somatosensory cortical lesions did not differ from animals with sham operations and overtraining in relearning the original problem. However, in the case where rats were not overtrained, i.e., when the problem was learned to criterion, the rats with lesions did perform statistically worse than matched control animals. In addition, the SSI+II rats without any training performed more poorly than their control group. Although the lesion groups with preoperative training and overtraining did not differ from each other, both of these groups performed much better than animals with lesions that received no training prior to surgery. Examination of individual scores in this study showed that six of nine rats with bilateral somatosensory cortical lesions in the overtraining condition performed within one standard deviation of their respective sham operated group mean. These data show that some performance deficits can decrease as preoperative training increases on a given problem.

CONCLUSIONS

The data collected in the various acquisition and retention experiments show that under some conditions rats with somatosensory forebrain lesions may perform poorly on tactile discriminations, while under other conditions animals possessing similar lesions can learn tactile problems as rapidly as sham operated control subjects. Serial surgery and preoperative overtraining appear to minimize somatosensory cortical lesion effects, although testing experience prior to encountering a difficult problem also may relate to behavioral sparing on tactile discriminations. Varying developmental status at the time of surgery from 30 to 570 days of age, and extending the postoperative recovery period from 14 days to six months, did not significantly diminish lesion effects in the present experiments. However, these may not be general findings: Benjamin and Thompson (1959) did observe age effects when cats operated upon in the six postnatal day were compared to adult animals on a battery of tactile tasks. Since any of a number of factors (including age and species) could account for such differences, these variables will have to be examined in greater detail before more definitive statements can be made about them.

The functions of the somatosensory areas of the cortex remain unclear, and while it can be argued that these lesions reflect only what the remaining brain structures can do, it is apparent that the picture is considerably more complex than previously had been believed. Although better performance by rats in the retention paradigm than in the acquisition paradigm would suggest that somatosensory cortical areas may, under some conditions, be involved in laying down tactile engrams that are at least in part localized elsewhere (Finger, Lennard, Hammer and Ehrman 1971), alternative interpretations stressing factors such as learning how to respond in a given situation must be given careful consideration.

Glassman (1970), Norrsell (1971) and Dobrzecka, Konorski, Stepień and Sychowa (1972) reported disturbances in appreciating passively applied tactile stimuli after lesions of SII, but not after lesions of SI, in cats and dogs, respectively. Further, more severe motoric impediments after lesions of SI than after damage to SII have been described in the cat (Glassman 1970). Although neither of the above experimenters was primarily concerned with the concepts of information storage and retrieval, differences in active vs. passive touch (Schwartzman and Semmes 1971; Semmes 1969; Wall 1970), together with some of the rat data (e.g., Zubek 1952a), would argue against the hypothesis that the two somatosensory areas of the cortex merely reflect redundancy in the somatic afferent system. In fact, the different interpretations in the various tactile lesion experiments would raise the interesting theoretical possibility that some elements in the somatosensory system can serve more than one function. The hypothesis that the various functions associated with a given structure should be weighted in accordance with both the experiential history and genetic endowment of each subject should be fully explored.

Although the observation that animals with somatosensory cortical lesions mastered tactile discriminations in some of our experiments is suggestive of "reorganization" in the tactile analytic system, other models of restitution cannot easily be dismissed. Glassman (1971), for example, has argued that transient physiological shock in zones surrounding small lesions of the somatosensory cortex can contribute markedly to performance deficits in cats in the first few weeks after surgery. However, one problem with the theory of diaschisis is that it requires a reasonable equivalence of preoperative and postoperative behaviors since it is postulated that the important mediating mechanisms have been suppressed only temporaily by changes following tissue damage in anatomically distant areas. Although most reorganizational theories also tend to stress similarities in preoperative and postoperative behaviors, others (e.g., Cannon and Rosenblueth 1949) hold that some anatomical substrates may be imperfect replacements for others. This may be reflected in altered strategies and modified behaviors on some tasks that are mastered after surgery. The potential for these changes would mean that sudden learning in a complex situation does not necessarily constitute evidence for recovery of some function believed to have been lost after brain damage. In this context, it is fortunate that "functional recovery" is not always differentiated from "functional substitution" (Meyer 1973) in the behavioral literature. Indeed, a distinction in terms might hasten a delineation of the tested concept.

Along these lines, although animals with somatosensory cortical lesions compared favorably to control subjects in several of our experiments, some suggestive differences did appear between the two groups when the rats were occasionally observed at the choice point in the maze. For example, in the course of periodic examination of what the animals were doing, it was seen that the rats that preened themselves at the startbox and sometimes refused to run during the first 10 days of testing usually had sham operations. Interestingly, once these rats learned to obtain food in the maze, some showed a tendency to run so rapidly that it was occasionally difficult for a subject to rectify an incorrect response by stopping and backtracking at the choice point. In addition, many rats with SSI+II damage took considerably longer than control animals to make a choice after the first two weeks of testing, and even the operated rats that met criterion often displayed unusual care and deliberation when confronting and examining the tactile discriminanda. These observations, as well as striking deficits on some neurological tests (Finger and Frommer 1968b), would suggest that our lesion and control animals may not have been "equivalent" in those studies in which the two groups were equated on the basis of a single dependent variable measurement. Additional testing and compensatory actions and strategies, such as those described by Weiskrantz (1963), Gazzaniga (1970), and Goldberger (1972), should be considered in any experiment in which animals with brain damage appear to do well on complex behavioral tasks.

A related and equally perplexing issue is that of identifying possible anatomical substrates which might be capable of underlying complex discriminative behaviors following damage to the somatosensory cortex. In particular, the motor cortex appears well-suited for these functions. The motor areas receive both specific and non-specific afferents from thalamocortical projection systems (Nakahama 1961), and they have been shown to have both ipsilateral (Nakahama 1959a, b, 1960, 1961) and contralateral (Nakahama and Saito 1956) connections with the two somatic projection zones, at least in cat and monkey.

Subcortical participation in tactile learning and memory must also be considered (Finger, Lennard, Hammer and Ehrman 1971), even if there appears to be cortical dependence, and especially on the easier discriminative tasks. Research in this direction has been limited, but Girden et al. (1936) and Bromiley (1948) have reported that surgically decorticate dogs can learn conditioned responses to tactile stimuli, and Oakley (1971) has noted that rabbits can learn lever-pressing responses of some complexity after neodecortication. More recent studies on newborn kittens and puppies (Bacon 1973; Bacon and Stanley 1970a, b) have shown that tactile discriminations and even reversal learning are possible long before the cortex is fully developed (Fox 1970, 1971), Ochs (1966), among others, has discussed the concepts of subcortical learning and memory, and a number of experiments involving cortical spreading depression are supportive of his hypotheses (e.g., Kukleta 1966; Thompson 1964; Thompson and Hjelle 1965).

Although research on axonal sprouting (Moore, Björklund and Stenevi 1971; Raisman 1969) and denervation supersensitivity (Sharpless 1964; Stavraky 1961) may shed some light on the possibility of reorganization in the somatic afferent system, that which is clear from our series of experiments is the fact that animals with extensive somatosensory cortical damage are capable of performing well on complex discriminative tasks. Although these empirical findings may raise more questions than they answer, the data do emphasize the need for more research in this field while at the same time delineating some of the many difficulties inherent in the interpretation of individual experiments on structure-function relationships in the C.N.S.

ACKNOWLEDGMENTS

The research described in this paper was supported in part by P.H.S. Grants MH-17109 and MH-21419, by N.S.F. Grant GB-12374, and by Biomedical Sciences Support Grant FR-07054. Permission to reproduce Figure 1 was kindly granted by Pergamon Press; Figure 2 by Springer-Verlag; and Figure 3 by Clinton N. Woolsey and the University of Wisconsin Press.

REFERENCES

Adametz, J.H. (1959). Rate of recovery of functioning in cats with rostral reticular lesions. *J. Neurosurgery* 16, 85-98.

Ades, H.W. (1946). Effects of extirpation of parastriate cortex on learned visual discriminations in monkeys. *J. Neuropathology and Exp. Neur.* 5, 60-66.

Ades, H.W. and Raab, D.H. (1946). Recovery of motor function after two-stage extirpation of area 4 in monkeys *(Macaca mulatta). J. Neurophysiol.* 9, 55-60.

Bacon, W.E. (1973). Aversive conditioning in neonatal kittens. *J. Comp. Physiol. Psych.* 83, 306-313.

Bacon, W.E. and Stanley, W.C. (1970). Avoidance learning in neonatal dogs. *J. Comp. Physiol. Psych.* 71, 448-452 (a).

Bacon, W.E. and Stanley, W.C. (1970). Reversal learning in neonatal dogs. *J. Comp. Physiol. Psych.* 70, 344-350 (b).

Benjamin, R.M. and Thompson, R.F. (1959). Differential effects of cortical lesions in infant and adult cats on roughness discrimination. *Exp. Neur.* 1, 305-321.

Berger, B.D., Wise, C.D. and Stein, L. (1973). Nerve growth factor: Enhanced recovery of feeding after hypothalamic damage. *Science* 180, 506-508.

Bland, B.H. and Cooper, R.M. (1969). Posterior neodecortication in the rat: Age at operation and experience. *J. Comp. Physiol. Psych.* 69, 345-354.

Bromiley, R.B. (1948). Conditioned responses in a dog after removal of neocortex. *J. Comp. Physiol. Psych.* 41, 102-110.

Cannon, W.F. and Rosenblueth, A. (1949). "The Supersensitivity of Denervated Structures", New York: Macmillan Co.

Chow, K.L. (1952). Conditions influencing the recovery of visual discriminative habits in monkeys following temporal neocortical ablations. *J. Comp. Physiol. Psych.* 45, 430-437.

Chow, K.L. (1967). Effects of ablation. *In* G.C. Quarton, T. Melnechuk and F.O. Schmitt (Eds.), "The Neurosciences", vol. 1. New York: Rockefeller University Press. pp. 705-713.

Chow, K.L. and Randall, W. (1964). Learning and retention in cats with lesions in reticular formation. *Psychonomic Science* 1, 259-260.

Chow, K.L. and Survis, J. (1958). Retention of overlearned visual habit after temporal cortical ablation in monkey. *Arch. Neur. Psychiat. (Chicago)* 79, 640-646.

Cowey, A. (1967). Perimetric studies of field defects in monkeys after cortical and retinal ablations. *Quart. J. Exp. Psych.* 19, 232-245.

Dawson, R.G. (1973). Recovery of function: Implications for theories of brain function. *Behav. Biol.* 8, 439-460.

Dobrzecka, C., Konorski, J., Stepień, L. and Sychowa, B. (1972). The effects of the removal of the somatosensory areas I and II on left-leg-right leg differentiation to tactile stimuli in dogs. *Acta Neurobiologia Experimentalis* 32, 19-33.

Douglas, R.J. and Isaacson, R.L. (1964). Hippocampal lesions and activity. *Psychonomic Science* 1, 187-188.

Downer, J. de C. and Zubek, J. (1954). Role of the cerebral cortex in temperature discrimination in the rat. *J. Comp. Physiol. Psych.* 47, 199-203.

Emmers, R. (1965). Organization of first and second somesthetic regions (S1 and S2) in the rat thalamus. *J. Comp. Neur.* 124, 215-218.

Finger, S. (1972). Lemniscal and extralemniscal thalamic lesions and tactile discrimination in the rat. *Exp. Brain Res.* 15, 532-542.

Finger, S., Cohen, M. and Alongi, R. (1972). Roles of somatosensory cortical areas 1 and 2 in tactile discrimination in the rat. *Int. J. Psychobiol.* 2, 93-102.

Finger, S. and Frommer, G.P. (1968). Effects of somatosensory thalamic and cortical lesions on roughness discrimination in the albino rat. *Physiol. Beh.* 3, 83-89 (a).

Finger, S. and Frommer, G.P. (1968). Effects of cortical lesions on tactile discriminations graded in difficulty. *Life Sciences* 7, 897-904 (b).

Finger, S. and Frommer, G.P. (1970). Effects of cortical and thalamic lesions on temperature discrimination and responsiveness to footshock in the rat. *Brain Res.* 24, 69-89.

Finger, S., Lennard, P.R., Hammer, R. and Ehrman, R. (1971). Retention of tactile discriminations following somatosensory cortical lesions in the rat. *Exp. Brain Res.* 12, 354-360.

Finger, S.; Marshak, R.A., Cohen, M., Scheff, S., Trace, R. and Niemand, D. (1971). Effects of successive and simultaneous lesions of somato-sensory cortex on tactile discrimination in the rat. *J. Comp. Physiol. Psych.* 77, 221-227.

Finger, S., Scheff, S., Warshaw, I. and Cohen, M. (1970). Retention and acquisition of fine temperature discriminations following somato-sensory cortical lesions in the rat. *Exp. Brain Res.* 10, 340-346.

Finger, S., Walbran, B. and Stein, D.G. (in press). Brain damage and behavioral recovery: Serial lesion phenomena. *Brain Res.*

Fox, M.W. (1970). Reflex development and behavioral organization. *In* W.A. Himwich (Ed.), "Develop-mental Neurobiology", Springfield, Ill.: Charles C. Thomas, pp. 553-580.

Fox, M.W. (1971). "Integrative Development of Brain and Behavior in the Dog", Chicago: The Univer-sity of Chicago Press.

Gazzaniga, M.S. (1970). "The Bisected Brain", New York: Appleton-Century-Crofts.

Girden, E., Mettler, F.A., Finch, G. and Culler, E. (1936). Conditioned responses in a decorticate dog to acoustic, thermal and tactile stimuli. *J. Comp. Psych.* 21, 367-385.

Glassman, R.B. (1970). Cutaneous discrimination and motor control following somatosensory cortical ablations. *Physiol. Beh.* 5, 1009-1019.

Glassman, R.B. (1971). Recovery following sensori-motor cortical damage: Evoked potentials, brain stimulation and motor control. *Exp. Neur.* 33, 16-29.

Glassman, R.B. (in press). Similar effects of infant and adult sensorimotor cortical lesions in cats' posture. *Brain Res.*

Glick, S.D. and Greenstein, S. (1972) Facilitation of recovery by α-methyl-p-tyrosine after lateral hypothalamic damage. *Science* 177, 534-535.

Glick, S.D. and Zimmerberg, B. (1972). Comparative recovery following simultaneous- and successive-stage frontal brain damage in mice. *J. Comp. Physiol. Psych.* 79, 481-487.

Goldberger, M.E. (1972). Restitution of function in the CNS: The pathologic grasp of *Macaca mulatta*. *Exp. Brain Res.* 15, 79-96.

Goldman, P.S. (1971). Functional development of the prefrontal cortex early in life and the problem of neuronal plasticity. *Exp. Neur.* 32, 366-387.

Hall, J.F. (1966). "The Psychology of Learning", Philadelphia: Lippincott Co.

Harlow, H.F. (1939). Recovery of pattern discrimination in monkeys following unilateral occipital lobectomy. *J. Comp. Neur.* 27, 467-487.

Hughes, K.R. (1965). Dorsal and ventral hippocampus lesions and maze learning: Influence of preoperative environment. *Canadian J. Psych.* 325-332.

Isaacson, R.L. (Ed.) (1968). "The Neuropsychology of Development: A Symposium", New York: John Wiley & Sons.

Jackson, J.H. (1879). On affections of speech from disease of the brain. *Brain* 2, 323-356.

Joynt, R.J. (1970). Language disturbances in cerebrovascular disease, Presentation 5. *In* A.L. Benton (Ed.), "Behavioral Changes in Cerebrovascular Disease", New York: Harper & Row. pp. 37-39.

Joynt, R.J. and Benton, A.L. (1964). The memoir of Marc Dax on aphasia. *Neurology (Minn.)* 14, 851-854.

Kennard, M.A. (1936). Age and other factors in motor recovery from precentral lesions in monkeys. *Amer. J. Physiol.* 115, 138-146.

Kennard, M.A. (1938). Reorganization of motor function in the cerebral cortex of monkeys deprived of motor and premotor areas in infancy. *J. Neurophysiol.* 1, 477-496.

Kennard, M.A. (1940). Relation of age to motor impairment in man and in subhuman primates. *Arch. Neur. Psychiat.* 44, 377-397.

Kennard, M.A. (1942). Cortical reorganization of motor function. *Arch. Neur. Psychiat.* 48, 227-240.

König, J.F.R. and Klippel, R.A. (1963). "The Rat Brain", Baltimore: Williams and Wilkins.

Kukleta, M. (1966). Learning in functionally decorticate state and its transfer to normal state. *J. Comp. Physiol. Psych.*62, 498-500.

Lukaszewska, I. and Thompson, R. (1967). Retention of an overtrained pattern discrimination following pretectal lesions in rats. *Psychonomic Science* 8, 121-122.

McIntyre, M.M. and Stein, D.G. (1973). Differential effects of one versus two-stage amygdaloid lesions on activity, exploratory and avoidance behavior in the albino rat. *Behav. Bio.* 9, 451-465.

Meyer, P.M. (1973). Recovery from neocortical damage. *In* G.M. French (Ed.), "Cortical Functioning in Behavior", Glenview, Ill.: Scott, Foresman and Co., pp. 115-138.

Moore, B.Y., Björklund, A. and Stenevi, U. (1971). Plastic changes in the adrenergic innervation of the rat septal area in response to denervation. *Brain Res.* 33, 13-35.

Nakahama, H. (1959). Cerebral response in somatic area II of ipsilateral somatic I origin. *J. Neurophysiol.* 22, 16-22 (a).

Nakahama, H. (1959). Cerebral response of anterior sigmoid gyrus to ipsilateral posterior sigmoid stimulation in cat. *J. Neurophysiol.* 22, 573-589 (b).

Nakahama, H. (1960). Cerebral response in somatic area I of ipsilateral somatic II origin. *J. Neurophysiol.* 23, 74-86.

Nakahama, H. (1961). Functional organization of somatic areas of the cerebral cortex. *Int. Rev. Neurobio.* 3, 187-250.

Nakahama, H. and Saito, M. (1956). Interconnections of the somatic area I and II. *Japan. J. Physiol.* 6, 200-205.

Norrsell, V. (1971). A comparison of function of the first and second somatosensory areas of the dog. *Experientia* 27, 1284.

Oakley, D.A. (1971). Instrumental learning in neodecorticate rabbits. *Nat. New. Biol.* 233, 185-187.

Ochs, S. (1966). Neuronal mechanisms of the
  cerebral cortex. *In* R.W. Russell (Ed.),
  "Frontiers in Physiological Psychology",
  New York: Academic Press. pp. 21-50.
Orbach, J., and Fantz, R.L. (1958). Differential
  effects of temporal neocortical resections on
  overtrained and non-overtrained visual habits
  in monkeys. *J. Comp. Physiol. Psych.* 51, 126-
  129.
Raisman, G. (1969). Neuronal plasticity in the
  septal nuclei of the adult rat. *Brain Res.* 14,
  25-48.
Reyes, R., Finger, S. and Frye, J. (1973). Serial
  thalamic lesions and tactile discrimination in
  the rat. *Behav. Biol.* 8, 807-813.
Reynolds, R.W. (1965). An irritative hypothesis
  concerning the hypothalamic regulation of
  food intake. *Psych. Rev.* 72, 105-116.
Rosen, J., Stein, D. and Butters, N. (1971).
  Recovery of function after serial ablation of
  prefrontal cortex in the rhesus monkey. *Science*
  173, 353-356.
Rosner, B.S. (1970). Brain Functions. *Annual Rev.
  Psych.* 21, 555-594.
Russell, E.R. (1945). Transient disturbances
  following gunshot wounds of the head. *Brain*
  68, 79-97.
Schwartz, S. (1964). Effects of neonatal cortical
  lesions and early environmental factors on
  adult rat behavior. *J. Comp. Physiol. Psych.*
  57, 72-77.
Schwartzman, R.J. (1972). Somesthetic recovery
  following primary somatosensory projection
  cortex ablations. *Arch. Neur.* 27, 340-349.
Schwartzman, R.J. and Semmes, J. (1971). The
  sensory cortex and tactile sensitivity. *Exp.
  Neur.* 33, 147-158.
Semmes, I. (1969). Protopathic and epicritic
  sensation: A reappraisal. *In* A.L. Benton (Ed.),
  "Contributions to Clinical Neuropsychology",
  Chicago: Aldine Press. pp. 142-171.
Sharpless, S.K. (1964). Reorganization of function
  in the cerebral nervous system - Use and disuse.
  Annual Rev. Physiol. 26, 357-388.
Stavraky, G.W. (1961). "Supersensitivity Following
  Lesions of the Nervous System", Toronto:
  University of Toronto Press.

Stein, D.G., Rosen, J.J., Graziadei, J., Mishkin, D. and Brink, J.J. (1969). Central nervous system: Recovery of function. *Science* 166, 528-530.

Teuber, H.L. and Rudel, R.G. (1962). Behavior after cerebral lesions in children and adults. *Devel. Med. Child Neur.* 4, 3-20.

Thompson, R. and Rich, I. (1961). Transitory effects of interpeduncular nucleus damage. *Exp. Neur.* 4, 310-316.

Thompson, R.W. (1964). Transfer of avoidance learning between normal and functionally decorticate states. *J. Comp. Physiol. Psych.* 57, 321-325.

Thompson, R.W. and Hjelle, L.A. (1965). Effects of stimulus and response complexity on learning under bilateral spreading depression. *J. Comp. Physiol. Psych.* 59, 122-124.

Thompson, V.E. (1968). Neonatal orbitofrontal lobectomies and delayed response behavior in cats. *Physiol. Behav.* 3, 631-635.

Travis, A.M. and Woolsey, C.N. (1956). Motor performance of monkeys after bilateral partial and total cerebral decortications. *Amer. J. Phys. Med.* 35, 273-310.

Wall, P.D. (1970). The sensory and motor role of impulses travelling in the dorsal columns toward the cerebral cortex. *Brain* 93, 505-524.

Weese, G.D., Neimand, D. and Finger, S. (1973). Cortical lesions and somesthesis in rats: Effects of training and overtraining prior to surgery. *Exp. Brain Res.* 16, 542-550.

Weiskrantz, A.B. (1963). Contour discrimination in a young monkey with striate cortex ablation. *Neuropsychologia* 1, 145-164.

Woolsey, C.N. (1958). Organization of somatic sensory and motor areas of the cerebral cortex. *In* H.F. Harlow and C.N. Woolsey (Eds.), "Biological and Biochemical Bases of Behavior", Madison: University of Wisconsin Press. pp. 63-81.

Zubek, J.P. (1951). Recent electrophysiological studies of the cerebral cortex: Implications for localization of sensory function. *Canadian J. Psych.* 5, 110-121 (a).

Zubek, J.P. (1951). Studies on somesthesis: I. Role of somatic cortex in roughness discrimination in the rat. *J. Comp. Physiol. Psych.* 44, 339-353 (b).

Zubek, J.P. (1952). Studies in somesthesis: III. Role of somatic areas 1 and 2 in roughness discrimination in the rat. *Canadian J. Psych.* 6, 183-193 (a).

Zubek, J.P. (1952). Studies in somesthesis: IV. Role of somatic areas 1 and 2 in tactual form discrimination in the rat. *J. Comp. Physiol. Psych.* 45, 438-442 (b).

RECOVERY OF MOVEMENT AFTER CNS LESIONS IN MONKEYS

Michael E. Goldberger
The Medical College of Pennsylvania
Philadelphia, Pennsylvania

A. Introduction

To the anatomist concerned with the localization of motor functions within identifiably different neural structures, recovery of movement following destruction of one or more of these structures represents a chronic contradiction. For the belief that different components of the motor systems make unique, specified contributions to the control of movement is difficult to reconcile with the "recovery" of a function after the neural structure which mediated it has been destroyed. Historically, however, it was in the study of the motor system that recovery, as a phenomenon, was discovered and there that the early attempts at theoretical explanations of it were constructed (Jackson 1873; Franck 1887; Leyton and Sherrington 1917). It is possible to follow four major themes which have characterized the models constructed over the last century, in attempts to resolve the contradiction between localization and recovery.

B. Some Mechanisms

1). Equipotentiality, or mass action as expressed most clearly by Lashley (1938) rejected localization, at least for learned movements, and suggested that the mass of tissue removed, not its location, was the critical factor in determining the permanence of deficits due to central nervous system lesions. Recovery would follow naturally from such a model; in fact, one might expect it to be complete in many cases.

2). Vicarious function requires that an intact system can so alter its mode of operation as to replace the functions usually mediated by another system i.e., the one destroyed. This theory has appeared in several forms (Franz 1923; Brodal 1965; Lawrence and Kuypers

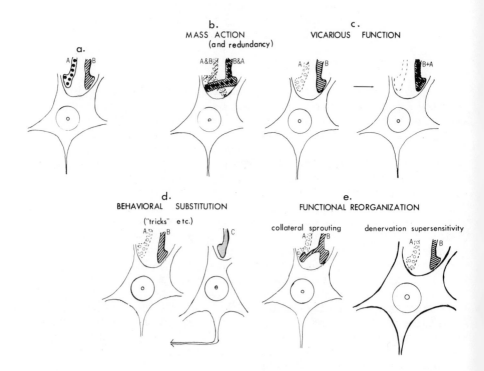

*Figure 1. (a). A unit of motor behavior is symbol-
ized by a large neuron. Two central systems, "A"
and "B" mediate control of the behavior in
question. Localization of function is indicated
by presumed different physiological properties in
"A" and in "B" shown by large dots and diagonal
stripes respectively and by the fact that they
control different parts of the post-synaptic
element. The subsequent cartoons (b-e) show several
possible responses of intact systems ("B") to the
destruction and degeneration of "A" (signified by
"A's" dotted outline). Each of these represents a
different conceptualization of the mechanisms
underlying recovery.*

     *(b). The equipotentiality of A and B is
shown by each containing the symbols (dots and
stripes) of the other and by each making similar,
synaptic contacts. Thus when "A+B" degenerates,
the function would adequately be subserved by*

"B+A". A period of deficit might be observed prior to recovery, and may be ascribed to "shock" or diaschesis.

(c). The first of the pair of drawings simply shows degeneration of A while B remains. In the second drawing, B is shown containing not only stripes but also dots signifying that, during recovery, B takes on new physiological properties, previously mediated by A, thereby functioning vicariously for the lost system. The assumption underlying Vicarious Function and Mass Action is that the returned movements are executed in the same way as they were pre-operatively and thus that true recovery of the lost function has taken place.

(d). A different assumption underlies the mechanisms of Behavioral Substitution in which apparent recovery of function is attained by return of the lost behavior. The behavior is achieved by the use of substituted functions mediated by undamaged structures indicated as "C". The restored behavior appears to be the same as that initially lost but may actually be made up of different physiological components.

(e). Two prominent mechanisms underlying Functional Reorganization are contrasted here. Collateral sprouting requires that B increases its terminal field although no change in its physiological characteristics is required. This change in the remaining pre-synaptic systems might be expected to mediate recovery of certain patterned responses which can be utilized for the return of movements, similar but not necessarily identical to those initially lost. Denervation supersensitivity in which the changes mediating recovery occur post- rather than pre-synaptically (symbolized by the increased size of the post-synaptic cell) might overcome a decreased central excitation, due to the lesion, by an increased responsiveness of the cell to all remaining inputs. One might expect certain generalized aspects of recovery to be subserved by this mechanism.

1968a, b). It often implies that a system
can possess a latent capacity to mediate
certain functions not usually attributed to
it and that this latent function is exposed
only after systems which are primary in
respect to these functions have been
abolished. This theory is closely related to
others proposing that redundancy of function
underlies recovery. The latter differs from
vicarious function in that it does not
require primary and secondary systems, but,
rather, suggests that several systems so
overlap in their properties as to be inter-
changeable or, at least indistinguishable by
the methods employed.

3). Substitution employs a behavioral rather than
strictly neural model. It was beautifully
described and documented by Sperry (1947) who
called such substituted maneuvers "tricks".
Behavioral substitution is consistent with
localization both of the initially impaired
and also of the substituted behavior
(Goldberger 1972), but implies relatively
little recovery in the usual sense, i.e.,
of the function rather than of its end-
product, behavior, which was lost.

4). Functional reorganization was formulated
(Kennard 1938) as a take-over mechanism not
unlike vicarious function. It implies,
however, a permanent change in function of
the undamaged, responsible parts of the
nervous system, rather than the expression of
a latent function. The nature of this change
was unknown at the time but the theme has
been developed over the years and may
currently be found in two quite different
variations: denervation supersensitivity and
collateral sprouting.

a. Denervation supersensitivity describes
the increased responsiveness of partially
denervated neurons to stimulation of their
remaining afferent supply (see Sharpless 1964).
The model is based on observations made on denervated peripheral nervous system structures, e.g.
striated muscle and autonomic ganglia. These
observations include: after an initial depression,
an increased reactivity to application of trans-

mitters; a loss of specificity of receptor site; and even a loss of receptor specificity, such that the denervated structure responds to stimulation by several transmitters. Demonstration of super-sensitivity in the central nervous system has been more difficult. Although increased rates of inter-neuronal firing were observed 2 weeks after lesions of the cat spinal cord (Loeser and Ward 1967) the underlying mechanism was uncertain. Partial denervation of one side of the spinal cord by dorsal rhizotomy or hemisection was found to result in an increased reactivity of the affected limb to stimulation of any of the remaining systems (Stavraki 1961). These results have not been substantiated by recent investigations (Goldberger 1973a, b; Murray 1973) in which hyperexcitability was restricted to certain reflexes. The contribution of supersensitivity to recovery of movement is not well delimited. According to that model, the burden of recovery is placed upon the denervated post-synaptic elements rather than upon adjustment on the part of remaining pre-synaptic systems. One might expect that hyper-responsiveness due to supersensitivity could contribute to recovery of movement by raising the so-called central excitatory state and mediating certain generalized, but not patterned aspects of motor performance. When, in the CNS, re-innervation takes place by regeneration or collateral sprouting, denervation supersensitivity recedes (cf Edds 1953). The chemical changes underlying supersensitivity may act as a stimulus to intact axons in the vicinity of the denervated cells, and may therefore play a role in eliciting collateral sprouting.

b. <u>Collateral Sprouting</u>. The ability of central axons to generate collateral sprouts when systems sharing with them a common post-synaptic destination have been destroyed, is a relatively recent discovery (Liu and Chambers 1958). It has been shown to occur in some parts of the adult nervous system (Rose *et al*. 1960; Goodman and Horel 1966; Goldberger and Murray 1972; Raisman 1969; Bernstein and Bernstein 1973; Lund and Lund 1971) but not in others (Kerr 1972) and to form morphologically (Raisman 1969) and functionally (Lynch 1973) competent synapses in some regions

269

but not in others (Mathers and Chow 1973). The
factors related to stimulation and prevention of
the growth of axonal sprouts are relatively
unknown as are the determinants of their ultimate
physiological success. Unusual collateral growth
can also be induced in the infant nervous system.
If certain lesions are made, undamaged systems of
growing axons can be stimulated to form larger
than normal and even aberrant terminal fields
(Schneider 1970). Such animals are spared a number
of the deficits found when similar lesions are
made in the adult (Schneider 1973). The similarity
between sparing and continued growth in infants on
one hand, and the anatomical and functional
changes which occur in the recovering adult CNS on
the other is unclear, as is the contribution of
sprouting to recovery in the adult. A relationship
between collateral sprouting and functional
recovery in the adult has in fact had some experimental support (McCouch *et al*. 1958; McCouch 1961;
Goldberger 1973a, b; Murray 1973), but the evidence
is circumstantial. In contrast to the generalized
aspects of recovery for which supersensitivity may
be responsible, sprouting appears to be quite
selective and might be expected to act as a
mechanism underlying recovery of some patterned
responses.

C.   Factors Influencing the Degree of Recovery

1.   Age: The observation that certain CNS lesions
     when made in infancy do not provoke symptoms
     nearly so severe as comparable lesions made in
     adults is by now commonplace. The relationship
     between sparing in the infant and recovery in
     the adult is unclear, however. An infant
     cannot "lose" functions which it has not yet
     developed and therefore, cannot recover
     functions it has not lost. This is not merely
     a semantic quibble; rather, it may represent
     a real distinction. In any case, there is
     little reason to assume that sparing in the
     infant and recovery in the adult are similar.
     The 'plasticity' of infant nervous systems is
     less impressive when strict parameters of
     examination (Goldman 1972; Lawrence and
     Hopkins 1972; Berman and Berman 1973) rather

than general observations are used. The
apparent lack of general motor impairment
seen in adult primates after infantile lesions
might be related to the early development of
behavioral maneuvers which mask the loss of
specific motor functions. The burden then
falls on the examiner to uncover these
deficits by rigorous testing procedures.
Small cortical lesions in infant rats produce
deficits in placing and hopping reactions
which are identical to those seen after
similar lesions in the adult (Brooks and Peck
1940). Furthermore the deficits do not appear
until the normal age of onset of the reflex
in question. Similarly, pyramidal section in
infant monkeys results in specific deficits
identical to those which follow pyramidotomy
in the adult madaque (Tower 1949) whereas the
effects on general motor behavior and on
muscle tone are far less grave. This difference in the effect of age on the ultimate
fate of general and of specific motor deficits
respectively depends for its recognition on
the use of test parameters which distinguish
between these two categories of movement.
Further, it implies that, at least in some
systems, the potential of residual motor
functions to compensate for those abolished by
lesions is greater in the infant than in the
adult, but that the degree of actual return
of function may be similar at any age.

2. Differences Among Different Components of the
Motor Systems: Even the precisely organized
corticospinal tract of the monkey exhibits a
dual anatomical organization partly topographical, partly diffuse (Liu and Chambers 1964).
The former type is reflected in the somatotopic projection of hand motor cortex to motor
neurons (and those of the nucleus proprius) in
cervical but not lumbar cord; the latter is
exhibited in the projection from the same
cortical region to the interneurons of the
zone intermedia of all segmental levels. The
former projection is overlapped only by
afferents from the dorsal roots, while the
latter projection is shared by multiple inputs
(Petras 1967). The diffuseness of the cortico-

interneuronal projection can be demonstrated
physiologically by the facilitation of stretch
reflexes at many different spinal segments
elicited by stimulation of a somatopic area
in the monkey's motor cortex (Bernhard and
Bohm 1954). It is perhaps this organization
and the presence of a generalized component
of the cortical efferent system that underlies
the recovery of movement in the limb paralyzed
by subtotal motor cortex lesion, for the
recovery in that limb is far greater than that
seen after complete motor cortex ablations
even though the cortical remnant spared is not
somatotopically related to the recovering limb
(Hines 1937). The behavior mediated by topographically organized pathways is somewhat
different from that subserved by systems
referred to as diffuse and it is therefore
difficult to compare the two. Nevertheless,
there are a number of reasons to believe that
recovery from lesions of non-topographical
("loosely coupled") systems is greater than
that seen after destruction of those whose
point-to-point organization can be demonstrated. For example, lesions involving
reticulospinal systems in the monkey have
persistently failed to reveal any trace of
topical arrangement (Mettler 1944; Wagley
1945; Goldberger 1965; 1969). The severity of
resultant deficits appears to be a function of
the size of the lesion and, unless the amount
of destruction is devastating, recovery of
movement is both rapid and extensive. In
contrast, ablation of only the hand area of
the monkey's motor cortex provokes a loss of
reflex tactile placing (hair bend) which is
localized to the contralateral hand, and that
loss is permanent (Bord 1938). The point-to-
point nature and exquisite specificity of the
motor cortex may preclude the possibility of
recovery due to any sort of substitution by
remaining tissue. Alternatively, this apparent
inflexibility may be a property of the post-
synaptic neurons which, in normal life, were
innervated by the destroyed tissue.
It is common experience that the view of
recovery in general revealed by lesion

experiments will reflect, in large part, the nature of the particular system under investigation. Most workers studying "association cortex" have been impressed by recovery, as a phenomenon and especially by the degree of recovery which follows subtotal and serial lesions (Rosen *et al.* 1971; Butters *et al.* 1972). In contrast, investigators of the functions of primary somato-sensory (Glassman 1971), or primary visual cortex (Teuber 1973), or motor cortex-pyramidal tract (Tower 1940; Hines 1960) have been struck by the functional specificity or uniqueness of these regions, lesions of which produced some impairments for which there was no recovery. Since there are such clear differences in recovery from lesions of different parts of the cortex alone, it may be premature to attempt to characterize recovery as a process in general. Rather, it must be determined what the degree and mechanism of recovery is for different systems. Provisionally, it would appear that the capacity for recovery in a particular system is related to the diffuseness and overlap of its afferent and efferent projections which can be determined by analysis of its anatomical organization.

3. The Most Variable Variable. It is the investigator who must not only determine the extent and mode of recovery of function but also, as a first step, define the function initially lost. Both are accomplished by the use of tests which, for the motor systems range from elicitation of the simplest reflexes and casual inspection of spontaneous movement to sophisticated conditioned tasks and recording of muscles or nerve cells suspected of contributing to the recovery process. The definition of the function of a particular component of the motor systems is no less problematical than defining the recovery which follows its destruction. Usually transient deficits are not used as criteria for function. It is the permanent deficit which cannot be corrected by coaxing or formal conditioning that is generally used to designate the function, in mirror image, of

the neural region destroyed. But since the
irretrievable function shows us what the
undamaged parts of the nervous system cannot
do, we are defining not only the lost function
but also the limits of recovery. This is
perhaps an unavoidable difficulty stemming
from the lesion method rather than from the
testing procedures used.

There are some systems in which the tests
used to elicit movement (and therefore motor
deficits) have been crucial to the interpretation of function. For example, it is commonly
held that one major function of the pyramidal
tract is the control of movements of distal
musculature whereas proximal muscle usage is
mediated by brainstem-spinal systems. This
view has been supported and strengthened by
the use of testing and conditioning procedures
which have demonstrated the persistent difficulty in making isolated finger movements
which follows corticospinal lesions (Growden *et
al*. 1967; Wiesendanger 1969; Hepp-Raymond *et
al*. 1972; Kuypers 1973). Whether the pyramidal
tract plays an equally important role in
mediating isolated movements of proximal
muscles is unknown, for discrete movements of
proximal muscles have not been examined by
these conditioning procedures. The categories
of movement relevant to the study of pyramidal
function may be quite different. For example,
following pyramidal lesions, group (rather
than discrete) movements can be performed both
by distal and by proximal muscles. Yet the
retractors of the hip, (clearly proximal
musculature) which normally lead in backward
stepping never do so in the pyramidal monkey
(Hines 1943; Tower 1940). In fact, backward
hopping is not performed at all (Goldberger
1969; 1972)! Thus the interpretation of
pyramidal function as mediator of distal
movements may reflect the difficulty in
testing discrete movements of proximal
muscles.

To illustrate and re-emphasize the methodological problems involved in defining motor
functions, it will be useful to examine some
recent history of cerebellar function in

monkeys. Lesions of the dentate-interpositus
nuclei provoke a characteristic ataxia-tremor
upon "goal-directed" movements of the limbs.
Secondary lesions made anywhere along the
corticospinal pathway appeared to abolish
cerebellar tremor (Aring and Fulton 1936;
Carrea and Mettler 1955; Carpenter and
Correll 1961). This suggested that the defect
was primarily an expression of corticospinal
mismanagement due to loss of cerebellar
modulation of the thalamocortical-(VL-motor
cortex)-pyramidal system. Thus it was not
inconsistent to find that thalamic lesions
including the VL nucleus (Carpenter and Hanna
1962) corrected the tremor and ataxia. These
conclusions were based on the results of
lesions made in untrained monkeys. If,
however, the animals are pre-operatively
trained to perform certain motor tasks
(Growden et al. 1967) the ataxia and tremor
provoked by the initial cerebellar damage
persists after the addition of pyramidal and
corticospinal tract lesions at least in the
conditioned tasks. Apparently, the untrained
monkey shows so little "goal-directed"
movement after corticospinal lesions that its
cerebellar tremor is submerged and masked by
general paresis and poverty of movement. The
general problem brought out by this example
is one of asking the appropriate questions
of a particular system under investigation.
If the expression of cerebellar disorder
depends upon the experimenter's ability to
evoke a specific category of movement (e.g.
"goal-directed") which is suppressed by
pyramidotomy then cerebellar symptoms will
disappear following the pyramidal lesion.
It is likely then that cerebellar function
will mistakenly be assumed to be mediated by
the pyramidal tract. Our interpretations not
only of the pathways involved in the mediation of certain types of movement and
therefore, in mediation of disordered
movements as well but also of motor
mechanisms, depends on the most thorough
exploration of all categories of movement
before and after lesions. Our ability to

275

define the capacities and limitations of the
intact CNS for recovery after destruction of
one part is constrained precisely by our
ability to describe the results of that
destruction.

4. Stimulation, Specific and Non-Specific
    Variables in this category include "motiva-
    tion", excitation (drug induced or other),
    practice, and formal training and conditioning
    procedures. As suspected by Lashley (1938) and
    documented by Tower (1940) part of the
    impairment which follows corticospinal lesions
    in the Macaque results from the discouragement
    experienced by the animal at the initial
    post-operative failure of its affected limbs
    to execute movement in a rewarding manner.
    This may be especially critical during the
    first two weeks when spinal shock (from
    corticospinal loss) is maximal (Liu *et al*.
    1966). Thereafter, a disuse atrophy of move-
    ment may set in; the animal gives up.
    According to this view, increased motivation
    could counteract some of the effects of
    spinal shock. Later patterned movement could
    recover based on this non-patterned general
    stimulation. The role of motivation has been
    questioned by Schwartz (1969) who showed that
    reinforcements of opposite valence did not
    alter the time-course of recovery from motor
    cortex lesions. The possibility that graded
    intensities of reinforcement do effect
    recovery has not been studied in the motor
    systems.
    The action of excitant drugs on the undamaged
    motor systems might be equivalent to that
    of motivation. Contact placing is reported to
    be temporarily restored by amphetamine in
    pyramidal monkeys (Beck and Chambers 1970).
    The restored movement in monkeys was thought
    to differ however from a true placing response
    in that 1) it was not elicited by tactile
    (hair bend) stimulation 2) it lacked
    spatiality and specific orientation and 3)
    appeared to be related to the animal's
    general agitation and increased generalized
    movements in response to the drug. Such non-
    specific increases in the central excitatory

state as can be provided by motivation or
drugs seem far removed from the highly
patterned movements which are known to result
from recovery. Yet generalized excitation
might provide a matrix from which patterned
movements could be molded by more specific
influences during recovery.

Formal conditioning and training serve a dual
purpose in the study of recovery of motor
function. First of all, it serves to establish
a base-line of reproducible movements for pre-
and post-operative comparison and is thus
essential for the proper analysis of certain
motor deficits (Knapp et al. 1963; Growden et
al. 1967; Beck and Chambers 1970; Liu and
Chambers 1971; Goldberger 1972; Goldberger and
Growden 1973). Secondly, conditioning pre- or
post-operatively, or both, clearly enhances
the recovery itself (Franz and Oden 1917;
Glees and Cole 1950; Taub and Berman 1968; Liu
and Chambers 1962) providing rigorous practice, the opportunity for shaping and
relearning, and incorporating motivation
through positive reinforcement. This dual
function of the conditioning procedure, i.e.
forcing the expression of motor deficits and
enhancement of recovery, represents a clear
advance in the analytic tools available for
investigation of motor disorders but, at the
same time, creates a problem in interpretation. For example, the loss of tactile
placing well-known to follow corticospinal
damage (Bard 1958) in otherwise normal
monkeys, persists as a conditioned response
in monkeys pre-operatively trained (Chambers
and Kozart 1965). These findings put us in a
quandry over the question of the role played
by the pyramid in the management of not only
tactile placing, but of a whole category of
tactually guided postural adjustments (Denny-
Brown 1966) and refined movements, each of
which, individually, can be conditioned to
survive pyramidotomy (Chambers, personal
communication). And for those motor acts
which cannot be trained so as to survive
pyramidotomy, one wonders whether it is
correct to interpret pyramidal function in

277

terms of only those few movements which cannot survive its absence (Kuypers 1973). It is
clear that conditioning alters the motor
systems which have survived destruction of
one part in such a way that we can no longer
determine what their 'natural' function might
have been. The nature of this alteration is,
as yet, unknown. If, however, the excitability
changes which have been demonstrated in the
analysis of reflex habituation and dishabituation (Kandel *et al.* 1970) can be shown to be
permanent in the mammalian CNS, then the
effects of conditioning upon recovery might
become less mysterious.

In order to consider the usefulness of the
preceding considerations several exemplary systems
will be discussed. Their destruction provokes
familiar motor disorders followed by well-
documented recovery. Four categories of hypothetical mechanisms have been mentioned and their
applicability to specific systems should be kept
in mind:

1. Equipotentiality (or mass action)
2. Vicarious function (and redundancy)
3. Behavioral substitution
4. Functional reorganization (including
   denervation supersensitivity and collateral sprouting).

In addition several parameters were described
because they appeared to be most important in
promoting or limiting the degree of recovery. They
will be related when possible to recovery following
the specific lesions to be discussed. They are:

1. Age (of animal or of the tissue)
2. Type of organization (topographic vs.
   diffuse) of lesioned and/or spared tissue.
3. Specific and non-specific stimulation
   (motivation, excitant drugs, practice,
   formal conditioning)
4. Methods used in evaluation of the motor
   deficit and of recovery.

The motor deficits and recovery which follow
lesions of four exemplary neural structures will
be examined in the hope of revealing the relevance
of the different proposed mechanisms underlying
recovery and the factors determining the degree of
recovery:

Cerebellum (dentate and interpositus
              nuclei)
Pyramid
Premotor cortex (area 6 of Brodmann)
Dorsal roots (spinal deafferentation)

Before turning to the results of specific
lesions, it may be worthwhile to point out the
kinds of movement which are usually studied. A
convenient schema adopted by others (DeLong 1971)
has been useful in describing different classes
of movement. The definitions to be used
operationally in the foregoing discussion are:
Reflex movements e.g. tendon reflexes, are closely
bound to quantitative aspects of the stimulus as
well as to modality and local sign. Triggered
movements, e.g. placing, do not vary with intensity
of stimulation once threshold has been reached,
have a somewhat wider range of adequate stimuli and
may be somewhat less stereotyped than reflexes from
the point of view of delicacy and modifiability in
execution.
Centrally patterned e.g. 'voluntary' or
'spontaneous' movements are presumed to be initiated by command neurons within the CNS and are thus
somewhat less immediately dependent upon modality-
specific peripheral stimuli. Although central
patterning modifies and is modified by reflex and
triggered movement, the classification may be
useful in describing both the motor deficits
characteristic of the lesions to be considered
and the recovery which alters those deficits.
To these three, conditioned movements must be
added. In recent years, operant and respondant
conditioning methods have contributed greatly to
the analysis of motor deficits, and to the extent
of recovery possible after neural lesions. For
example, a triggered movement, routinely abolished
after certain lesions can, by substitution of a
pre-operatively conditioned stimulus, be elicited
in spite of the complete and permanent
ineffectiveness of the unconditioned stimulus.
Such conditioned movements may also be selected
from a repertoire of centrally patterned movements
which then become triggered conditioned responses.
This category is the most difficult to interpret,
for conditioning adds a poorly understood variable

and perhaps a permanent change to the nervous system. It increases the degree of recovery, however, as well as our ability to study it.

D. The Pyramidal Tract

The motor deficit which has received the most attention is the paralysis routinely provoked by lesions along the corticospinal pathway. It is generally conceded that since lesions of the motor cortex (Hines 1943), basis peduncle (Bury *et al.* 1966) or lateral corticospinal tract (Cannon *et al.* 1943) involve non-corticospinal systems, that a clear picture of corticospinal deficiency can only be obtained by section of the bulbar pyramid (Tower 1940; Denny-Brown 1966; Lawrence and Kuypers 1968; Goldberger 1969; Gilman and Marco 1971; Hepp-Raymond *et al.* 1970). Even this structure is complex, however. It has been pointed out (Peele 1942; Wagley 1945) that at least two cortical systems, frontal and parietal, travel in the pyramid and that they may be functionally different. Electrophysiological data obtained from the cortex during movement (Evarts 1972) showed that pyramidal tract neurons in the motor and sensory cortices exhibited different firing patterns. Furthermore, the destination of pyramidal fibers is diverse. While the major termination is on interneurons, fibers also terminate on spinal motorneurons (Chambers and Liu 1958) and on sensory relay nuclei e.g. cuneatus, gracilis and nucleus proprius (Liu and Chambers 1964). The projections to motor and sensory relay nuclei are somatotopically organized, whereas those to interneurons are overlapping. There is a further organization: although cortico-interneuronal projections stem from several cortical areas, cortico-motorneuronal fibers are derived from the motor cortex, those to sensory nuclei primarily from the sensory cortex while fibers from the pre-motor cortex end only on interneurons (Kuypers and Brinkman 1970). In spite of this rather complex anatomical organization, lesions confined to the medullary pyramid are usually thought of as "pure". Assuming that the extent and mechanism of recovery from pyramidal lesions in monkeys can be understood only to the extent that the deficit

itself is adequately described, a resumé of the
pyramidal syndrome in monkeys will precede a
discussion of recovery. Most workers (Denny-Brown
1966 is the major exception) now agree that
reflex tone judged by resistance to passive movement is decreased in most or all muscles contralateral to the lesion (Tower 1940; Goldberger 1969;
Gilman and Marco 1971; Gilman *et al*. 1971) with
some reduction in briskness and checking of the
tendon reflexes. There is a loss of the superficial, e.g. abdominal reflexes. Triggered responses
to purely tactile fore- or hind-limb stimulation,
which normally consist of placing, grasping,
evasion and orienting are permanently abolished
(Denny-Brown 1966; Goldberger 1972). Comparable
responses albeit poorly executed, can be obtained
however by other somatic stimuli e.g. heavier
contact, joint bend or nociceptive stimuli.
Visually guided placing, grasping and evasion are
intact but are slow and have a high threshold.
Thus the adequate stimulus for placing, grasping,
etc. responses are altered as is the finesse and
modifiability of their execution. The deficit in
tactually-guided movement is not sensory, for
crossed placing by the intact limb to hair stimulation of the pyramidal limb is regularly elicited.
Although the peripheral tactile input to the
monkey's motor cortex is meagre (Albe-Fessard and
Liebeskind 1966; Fetz and Barker 1969) compared
with that found in the cat (Welt *et al*. 1967;
Brooks 1969) ablation of the motor cortex in
either animal abolishes tactile placing (Bard 1933;
1938) in a manner indistinguishable from pyramidotomy. Thus the tactile input to motor cortex may
not in itself be the factor critical to tactile
placing. The change in stimulus adequate to evoke
triggered placing may be a reflection of the
"switching" of interneurons in the tactile placing
reflex pathway which can be obtained by corticospinal stimulation (Lundberg and Voorhoeve 1962;
Wall 1967). The capacity of the pyramid to switch
interneurons may be essential in determining the
stimulus modality adequate to excite the spinal
mechanism subserving the tactile placing response.
Alternatively, loss of input from motor cortex to
sensory relay nuclei may be crucial, in the change
in placing after pyramidotomy.

Among the investigators who have described centrally patterned movements following pyramidal lesions in untrained monkeys, there is little agreement as to the nature of the deficit, either with respect to its general character or with respect to the details of motor performance of the pyramidal limbs. The severity of the impairment ranges from "grave" (Tower 1940) to "no obvious deficit" (Wiesendanger 1969). The character of the impairment is most frequently described as a loss of fine control or, alternatively, force primarily in distal musculature (Wiesendanger 1969; Black *et al.* 1971) with a predominance of that deficiency in the distal flexors (Beck and Chambers 1970). It should be pointed out, however, that although the investigators describing such distal motor deficits required the monkeys to perform discrete hand or finger movements, individuated movements of proximal muscle groups were not examined. Further, distal movements were not isolated from the proximal fixation which accompanied them. When specifically tested (Tower 1949; Goldberger 1969; 1972), certain discrete movements of shoulder or hip muscles appear to be as severely impaired as those of the digits. The paralysis is nevertheless selective, affecting some muscles, both distal and proximal, more than others. An alternative view to that of disto-proximal distribution of paralysis is that the pyramidal deficit is one affecting movement of the limb projected into space in which the "multiple readjustments which are required for precise spatial orientation" (Denny-Brown 1966) are impaired. This description, appears to describe well the pyramidal deficit but in reality fails to distinguish it from the results of other CNS lesions e.g. deafferentation, nor does it localize the mechanism to any particular aspect of movement. Furthermore, the greater impairment of movements which project the limb into space compared with other types of movements has not been demonstrated convincingly. For example, the pyramidal monkey also shows a marked impairment in opening its hand to put small bits of food into its mouth, (Fig. 2) for extension of the flexed hand without an associated extensor movement of the already flexed arm is extremely difficult in these animals

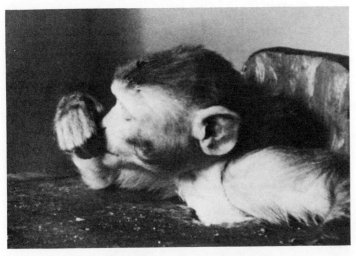

Figure 2. Monkey with left pyramidal lesion (8 weeks) showing difficulty in opening (Extending) right hand to obtain food, while arm is in a flexed position.

(Lawrence and Kuypers 1968; Goldberger 1969; denied by Beck and Chambers 1970) even after considerable training (Goldberger 1972).

What appears most striking to some workers (Tower 1940; Hines 1949) is the impaired limb fixation, which after pyramidotomy is converted into gross movement (Goldberger 1969). Equally striking is the concomittant deficit in discrete usage of muscles as prime movers. For example, monkeys trained to perform a grasp-release sequence can still open the hand, after pyramidotomy, when extension of the hand is linked to the extension of the whole arm (Fig. 3). If required to extend the hand and simulatenously flex the arm, however, the animal is faced with an apparent insurmountable difficulty (Fig. 4), even after 1 year of practice (Goldberger 1972).

The degree of recovery following pyramidal lesions ranges from "none" (Tower 1940) to "a considerable motor skill is recovered" (Wiesendanger 1969) and even "almost complete" (Bucy *et al*. 1966). Since these differences of opinion over the degree of recovery cannot be resolved here it will be preferable to try to determine what recovers (and what does not) and, if possible,

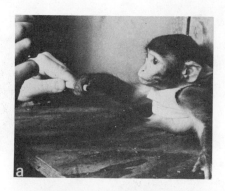

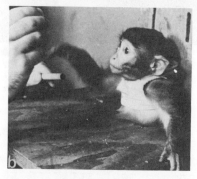

Figure 3. Monkey with left pyramidal lesion (6 months) trained to grasp and then release a stick for food reward. a. Monkey has grasped the stick with the pyramidal limb and will release the stick as b. she extends the arm to reach food which, in this case is held above the stick.

how recovery takes place. The initial post-operative picture, is dominated by diaschesis for in the monkey, the major component of post-transsection spinal shock is due to the loss of pyramidal fibers (Liu *et al.* 1966). During the subsequent weeks the 'spontaneous' reflex recovery which is seen has been explained in several ways. Denervation supersensitivity (Stavraki, 1961) and increased autochthonous firing of interneurons (Loeser and Ward 1967) may account for a generalized increase in reflex excitability; collateral sprouting from dorsal roots could sub-serve patterned reflex recovery (Goldberger 1973b; Murray 1973). Return of unconditioned movements

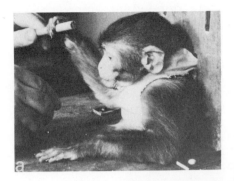
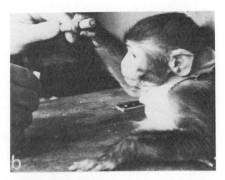
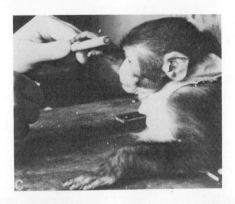
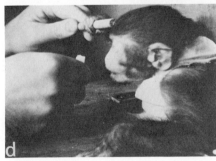
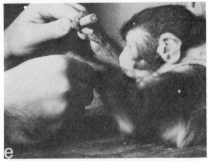

Figure 4. Same animal as in Fig. 3 but in this sequence, the food is held below the stick thus requiring synchronization of extension of the hand, to release the stick, with flexion-retraction of the arm to reach for the food. This combination of flexion and extension is very difficult for the animal to carry and Figs. 4b-4e show several ways in which the animal deals with this difficulty. 4a. The animal has lightly grasped the stick and is

appears to be related to and dependent upon the
spontaneous recovery of reflex responses which are
parallel to them in respect to form and function
(Twitchell 1951; Denny-Brown 1966). Thus the
ability to grasp an object with the paretic hand
develops as an elaboration of the emergent grasp
reflex and traction response. The pattern and
sequence of emerging spontaneous movements is
orderly and predictable from one animal to the
next, each movement appearing shortly after its
reflex counterpart. There seems to be no exception
to the sequence of reflex return, and each new
movement follows slavishly the reflex always
behind it. The "wired-in" nature of this pattern
is similar to that seen in the normal reflex
development (Hines 1942) of the infant Macaque.

   That force control is a major aspect of pyramidal function (Evarts 1968) is consistent with
the behavior of the pyramidal monkey for,
initially, the limbs show only the feeblest of
movements. The first two weeks post-pyramidotomy
are characterized by a slow improvement in the
use of whole-limb movements for feeding, reaching,
locomotion and placing (proprioceptive, visual).
The movements begin as gross, flexor or extensor,
mass limb movements which are initiated proximally
but which include the distal musculature. Although
these "synergies" (Foerster 1936) can be modified
so that proximal movements eventually become more
restrained, they are however never again converted

---

*looking at the food which is held in the examiner's
right hand. 4b. The animal has retracted the upper
arm and flexed the elbow to reach below the stick,
but this flexor movement incorporated flexion of
the digits and therefore only served to tighten the
grasp around the stick. 4c. The monkey extended the
hand by elevating the whole arm thus moving the
hand in the direction opposite to that in which she
wished it to go. She then lowered the arm to move
it toward the food and once again engaged the
stick, grasped it and, as seen in 4d. went after
the stick with her mouth. She was not rewarded for
this and is seen in 4e fighting with the examiner,
trying to get the food with the left (normal) limb
but still grasping the stick with the right
(pyramidal limb).*

into the co-contractions required for proper limb
fixation. Although some degree of impairment
fixation is permanent, it improves greatly with
time. Distal movements also improve, eventually
becoming stronger and more rapid. They are never
truly individuated however; e.g. thumb and
forefinger movements are never independent of
movements of the other three digits. In one sense,
therefore, although movement returns, the function
lost may not recover, for the manner of execution
is permanently altered. Thus the vicarious
functioning attributed specifically to the cortico-
rubro-spinal system (Kuypers 1964; Brodal 1965)
is probably ruled out; the returned function has
not been demonstrated to be the same. Recovery of
general motor behavior was shown to be dependent
not only upon the rubrospinal tract, but also
upon the extrapyramidal systems of the cortex
(Denny-Brown 1966) spinal cord (Goldberger 1969)
and Cerebellum (Growden et al. 1967). Thus many
systems appear to mediate the returned movements
through the mobilization of functions which may be
different from those subserved by the pyramidal
tract. There is a marked disparity between the
recovery of certain motor acts obtained by pre-
and post-operative conditioning (Chambers and
Kozart 1965; Hepp-Raymond et al. 1970; 1972) and
the utter failure of reflex activity and triggered
responses to improve after the first several
weeks. However, after an initial lesion in the
motor cortex, a crude form of contact (not
tactile) placing can immediately be restored and
hopping improved by subsequent lesions of the
opposite hemisphere (Bard 1938; Semmes and Chow
1955) or of the ventrolateral funiculus of the
spinal cord in a case in which the initial lesion
was in pyramid (Goldberger 1969). This improvement
is permanent and suggests that intact inhibitory
systems prevent recovery of some movements.
Temporary improvement can be produced by injections
of D-amphetamine in monkeys with incomplete
pyramidal lesions (Beck and Chambers 1970). These
findings imply that the deficit is due not only to
the loss of pyramidal facilitation but also to the
presence of inadequately opposed inhibition. Thus
brainstem systems can produce responses similar in
overall function to those mediated by the pyramid,

although cruder in execution. These are enhanced
1) by conditioning; 2) by making lesions which
affect predominantly inhibitory systems or 3) by
administering drugs which, presumably cause a
relative reduction in the level of inhibition. It
is, perhaps this inhibition which is accessible to
modification by conditioning procedures.

The improvement seen in conditioned movements
after pyramidotomy is difficult to analyze. These
learned movements, e.g. index finger-thumb
opposition, discrete grasp and its release are
performed by the trained pyramidal monkey but
only in the training situation. These monkeys,
giving almost normal performances in response to a
CS are, in their cages, indistinguishable from
untrained pyramidal monkeys, i.e. 'spontaneous'
movements do not benefit from the conditioning.
Thus it appears that a centrally patterned
movement cannot recover or be protected from the
effects of pyramid lesion, unless it can be transformed into a triggered movement, and thus placed
outside of its normal behavioral context.

Grasping can be observed as a spontaneous
movement, a triggered response and as a conditioned reflex in the pyramidal monkey. As it is
used in centrally patterned movements, it is
cruder than normal, having become inseparable
from flexion at all joints (Goldberger 1972) or
from traction responses (Denny-Brown 1966; Gilman
and Marco 1971). It is also cruder as an
unconditioned triggered movement since the normal
unconditioned stimulus, a light tactile stimulus
is no longer adequate but heavy contact or joint
bending is now required to elicit the grasp.
Conditioned grasping, however, can be evoked by
tactile as well as a variety of other conditioned
stimuli. Although the CS and US are apparently the
same (tactile stimulation of the palm), only the
CS is effective. This suggests different
mechanisms for the normal and for the conditioned
responses. Furthermore, unconditioned triggered
responses (e.g. proprioceptively triggered grasp)
and voluntary movements which remain after
pyramidotomy are abolished by subsequent cortical
(Denny-Brown 1966) spinal (Goldberger 1969)
brainstem (Lawrence and Kuypers 1968b) or cerebellar (Growden *et al*. 1967) lesions. Conditioned

motor habits are abolished neither by pyramidotomy
nor by subsequent, additional ablations (Hepp-
Raymond *et al*. 1972) and appear to have either
very widespread or no localization (Lashley 1924).
In the pyramidal monkey each recovered conditioned
movement is treated as an individual motor act;
it is not used spontaneously by the animal. It is
conceivable that each component of the total
pyramidal deficit might be conditioned separately,
and thus restored. Even discrete thumb-index
finger opposition was protected from the effects
of pyramid section or motor cortex ablation by
pre-operative conditioning (Hepp-Raymond *et al*.
1972). These and other conditioned movements
which persist or return after pyramidotomy may
thus be characterized as follows: 1) there is no
generalization from one conditioned movement to
the next. 2) there is no generalization of the
trained movement from the training situation to
'natural' conditions involving triggered responses
or spontaneous motor acts utilizing the same
movement 3) these movements lack variability and
the fine adjustments which orient them to changes
in external conditions. These observations suggest
that after pyramidal lesions recovery for different categories of movement might depend upon
quite different mechanisms.

E. Lesions of Area 6

The 'premotor' cortex of Fulton (1934) has had
a rather stormy history. This is related in part
to the use of different cytoarchitectural maps by
different workers. Fulton and his co-workers
defined the premotor area according to the Vogts'
map and therefore included the anterior part of
Brodmann's area 4. Hines (1937) and others used
Brodmann's map. Thus it is not surprising that the
results of premotor ablation vary from investigator
to investigator. For the purpose of this survey,
the premotor area will be identified as Brodmann's
area 6, and, for convenience, the caudal border of
Fulton's premotor region which coincides with the
rostral part of the motor cortex of most workers
will be referred to as the anterior border of 4
or 4-S.
The most commonly described defect following

bilateral premotor lesions is the inability to
resist grasping any object making contact with the
palmar surface of the hand or foot with a concomittant loss of normal tactile evasion. Once grasped,
the object cannot be released so long as tension
on the flexors of the fingers is maintained by
stretch (Fig. 5a), (Richter and Hines 1932;
Fulton and Kennard 1934; Seyfforth and Denny-Brown
1948). The closing phase is elicited by tactile
stimuli while the maintained phase (Proprioceptive
grasping) is a stretch reflex (Rushworth and
Denny-Brown 1959) related to the traction response
of the decerebrate monkey (Denny-Brown 1962).
Together, these two related phenomena make up the
forced grasp.

The immediate effects of the lesion are
remarkable for their intensity: closure of the
hand is elicited from a wide zone and flexion of
one digit recruits the flexors in the other digits
(Fig. 5b). Reinforcement of the grip of the hand
recruits all of the flexors of the arm and the
adductors of the shoulder. Regression of the disorder is seen first in lessening of response in
proximal muscles and in a narrowing of the
reflexogenous zone. The response then becomes
limited to the hand only and is elicited from a
discrete zone on the palmar surface. As the
response wanes, the opposing, normal response,
tactile evasion returns, becoming slightly
hyperactive, and after 2-3 weeks forced grasping
cannot be elicited (Goldberger 1972).

The recovery described here has also been
studied in monkeys with area 6 lesions trained to
perform a conditioned grasp and release (Goldberger 1972). If, some time after recovery from
forced grasping was 'complete', one pyramidal
tract was cut, the forced grasp returned
immediately, contralateral to the pyramidotomy.
It was evoked not by tactile but by proprioceptive
stimuli i.e. stretch, and by the conditioned
stimulus. The pyramidal tract itself does not
mediate inhibition of the grasp reflex but is
necessary for all unconditioned, tactually guided
responses of the hand and limb. Thus after pyramidotomy, tactile evasion disappeared and with it,
the recovery from the proprioceptive phase of
forced grasping. It appeared that the underlying

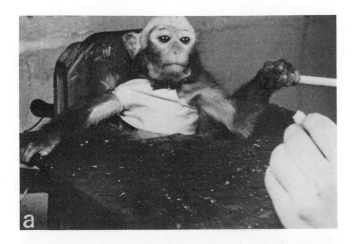

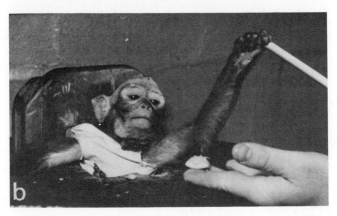

Figure 5. Monkey with bilateral area 6 ablation (9 days) trained as in Figs. 3 and 4 in a conditioned grasp-release sequence for food. In 5a. monkey has grasped the stick but is unable, because of forced grasping, to release it to obtain the food which she is obviously looking at with concentration. The examiner is pulling on the stick making it impossible for the animal to let go and the tension in the flexor muscles of the animal's left arm can be seen. In 5b., the animal's fifth finger is grasping the stick, pulling opposite to the direction in which the examiner is pulling. This is enough to elicit forced grasping and to recruit the flexors of the digits.

deficit, i.e., impaired inhibition of the grasp, remained impaired during recovery but was masked by the use of an opposing reflex, tactile evasion, normally mediated by the pyramids and (Denny-Brown 1966) parietal cortex (Denny-Brown and Chambers 1958). The mechanism of recovery proposed here is one of behavioral substitution. According to this model, the pyramid does not take over the function of the ablated premotor region (e.g. vicarious function) or change qualitatively its normal mode of operation. Rather, the readjustment is one of enhancement of a pyramidally mediated tactile response to mask a permanent proprioceptive deficit. The permanence of the original deficit is shown by the immediate return of the grasp reflex following pyramidotomy. This is also followed by a permanent loss of tactile evasion and, concomittantly, the failure to recover any behavioral manifestation of inhibition of the grasp thereafter.

The functional significance of the monkey's premotor cortex has been disputed widely since the initial experiments demonstrated that inhibition of the infantile grasp reflex depended upon its presence. To a number of workers (Woolsey *et al.* 1952; Kuypers 1958; Kuypers and Brinkman 1970) this region was simply the rostral extent of the motor cortex in which the axial musculature controlling posture is represented. This is consistent with the interpretation of the pathologic grasp reflex as a release of brainstem postural mechanisms after cortical control of proximal musculature is removed (Bieber and Fulton 1938; Fulton and Dow 1938). This view is difficult to reconcile with the fact that after area 6 lesions distal muscles (hand and fingers) are the most affected by the grasp reflex, and that proximal muscle involvement recovers first even though the cortical representation of proximal musculature is supposedly removed. An alternate view suggests that area 6 functions as an association area for the motor cortex (Hines 1949) since complex rather than discrete movement are elicited by area 6 stimulation (Foerster 1936; Hines 1947). The proposed associative function serves distal as well as proximal musculature. The forced grasp would then represent only one aspect of the total

functional impairment attributed to area 6 which
has been described as a perseveration or "abnormal persistence" of posture, or apraxia (Denny-
Brown 1958). This is consistent with the finding
of other apraxic disorders of the limbs
(Jacobsen 1936; Delacour *et al.* 1972) and face
(Watson 1973) following lesions in area 6 or of
that and adjacent cortex of area 8 (Deuel 1969).
    Perhaps the difficulty in interpretation of the
results of area 6 ablation can be used to illustrate an important problem in the study of recovery
of function. Recovery can be determined only if the
lost function and the region upon which it depends
can reliably be defined. Area 6 can be included
with equal justification as part of several
different functionally and anatomically defined
areas. Caudally, it merges with the rostral border
of the motor cortex. When both are destroyed,
marked spasticity as well as the forced grasp
appear (Fulton and Kennard 1934). According to
Fulton, areas 6 and "4S" consituted a unit, the
premotor cortex which regulated brainstem postural
reflexes and muscle tone. Medial area 6 is the
'supplementary motor cortex' to which has been
attributed (Travis 1955b; Travis and Woolsey 1956)
all of the functions of the premotor as defined by
Fulton. Immediately rostral in the periarcuate
region, a different functional organization
suggests itself. Whereas stimulation of area 6
elicits "synergistic" movements of the limbs and
trunk, representation of eye movements (Smith 1944;
Crosby *et al.* 1952; Bizzi 1968) or coordinated eye-
head movements (Bizzi and Schiller 1970) is located
just rostrally, in area 8. Thus these areas, taken
together, may be considered as a region related to
orienting movements.
    Periarcuate ablations limited to area 8
provoke only transient symptoms (Kennard and Ectors
1938; Welch and Stuteville 1958) but if the lesion
is defined in terms of its cortical association
connections (Pandya and Kuypers 1968) to include
parts of area 6 and 8, a long-lasting syndrome
results (Deuel 1969) which includes polysensory
neglect, 'efferent' apraxia (Luria 1963), and a
strong tendency to grasp, with some forced
grasping. The rate of recovery of the grasp is
rather rapid and depends on the pyramidal tract

(Goldberger 1972); recovery from neglect is slower and may be related to posterior parietal cortex (Eidelberg 1973) but loss of some motor habits due to apraxia may be enduring, unless re-learning is instituted (Deuel, personal communication).

Since interpretation of these behavioral results must determine the extent and location of cortex to be removed, recovery following lesions in this area may also be interpreted as sparing due to incompleteness or failure to destroy completely a functional unit. For example, if area 6 is considered to be simply a rostral extension of the motor cortex, only a bilateral 4 + 6 lesion will be complete and result in a permanent grasp reflex. If on the other hand, the region is thought of as "association" cortex related to the apraxias, area 8 must be added for production of an enduring deficit. In looking for recovery, one may well be beset by doubts arising from either interpretation; the criterion for function used in defining the region in question is just that functional loss from which there is no recovery.

F. Lesions of the Dentate-Interpositus Nuclei in Macaques

Recent studies (Goldberger and Growden 1973; 1974) have been carried out in order to re-evaluate certain aspects of the sequellae of dentate-interpositus lesions in monkeys, to describe the pattern of recovery which follows and to determine the contribution of several regions of the cerebral cortex to that recovery. The traditional division of symptoms (tremor, ataxia, hypermetria, etc.) within this classical cerebellar disorder (Holmes 1922; Carrea and Mettler 1947; 1955; Carpenter and Stevens 1957) was not supported by observations of conditioned standardized movements and quantitative measures of the oscillations ("intention tremor" and "ataxia") and other motor deficits accompanying these movements. For example, it was demonstrated by serial accelerometer recordings of frequency, regularity and amplitude of the oscillations which typically follow cerebellar destruction that ataxia and tremor should properly be unified and seen as a series of wide-slow (ataxia) versus small-amplitude-fast (tremor) oscillations as previously suggested by Growden *et al.* (1967). Typical ataxia was seen with relatively insecure limb positions (extension-abduction) whereas characteristic cerebellar tremor was evoked by limb positions closer to the body (flexion-adduction) (Fig. 6). In addition, "ataxia", seen in the initial post-operative period was replaced by "tremor" in the later stages with an intermediate phase during which both were seen. Analysis of learned, standardized compound movements requiring a fixed end-point (e.g., reaching-grasping) based on filmed records matched with accelerometer tracings of the oscillations revealed an underlying deficit: an inability to stop a motor act by limb fixation at the precise moment required for the beginning of a distal or proximal phasic movement (Fig. 7). This impairment in synchronization of fixation with phasic movement produced an error in any compound movement having a fixed end-point. The error, usually expressed as hypermetria or over-reaching, was then over-corrected by a movement in the opposite direction which again bypassed the bait e.g. food or a conditioned stimulus. A series of oscillations followed, stemming from the initial error which was repeated over and over as the animal attempted to correct the misplacement of its limb. The deficit underlying the repeated error, however, was in the timing of the original movements. Continuous movements as used in locomotion, and other movements with no fixed end-point which, therefore, did not require limb-fixation to be synchronized with phasic movement, were free of oscillations.

Although cerebellar as well as extra-cerebellar structures have been suspected of playing a role in mediation of recovery after dentate-interpositus lesions, it is likely that extracerebellar structures are the more important. Vermal lesions in the Rhesus monkey do not have a marked or lasting effect upon movement, (Yu 1973) nor do those of the fastigial nucleus (Carpenter 1959). Furthermore, fastigial ablation does not have an additive effect upon the impairments in limb movement due to a prior dentate-interpositus lesion: it only adds an apparently independent axial component (Goldberger and Growden 1974).

Selective lesions of either dentate or interpositus nuclei did not provoke recognizable cerebellar symptoms such as tremor and ataxia (Sprague 1967; Zervas 1967; 1970) and it was therefore assumed that each nucleus was able to compensate for the loss of the other. The overlapping distribution of efferents from the two nuclei to thalamus and brainstem (Carpenter and Stevens 1957) was thought to provide anatomical support for a functional similarity between dentate and interpositus. Isolated lesions of dentate or interpositus do, however, produce motor deficits which can be distinguished from each other (Goldberger and Growden 1973) and under rigorous testing conditions (Brooks 1972), reversible dentate lesions alone provoke the typical errors of over- and under-shooting which underlie cerebellar tremor. A qualitatively different deficit followed reversible (Brooks *et al.* 1970) or permanent interpositus lesions. These findings

---

Figure 6. This composite of film clips and accelerometer records shows the effect of limb position on the frequency of oscillations in a monkey with bilateral dentate-interpositus lesions. The electrolytic lesions were placed stereotaxically in the cerebellum 6 weeks before these photographs were taken. The rate of oscillations (per second) is shown below the corresponding photograph. The animal was trained to grasp the stick which is cut in two halves separated by foam rubber, squeeze the two halves together and then take food with the other hand. Three different arm positions are shown, determined by the location of the stick. The arm is reaching out in a semi-extended abducted position in a., and in a mid-flexed adducted position in c. As he moves through these three positions, the accelerometer records show a decreasing amplitude and increasing frequency of the oscillations. The oscillations in a. were more ataxia-like and those in c. more tremor-like, with those in b. in between the two.

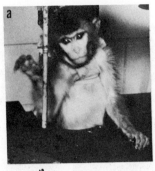

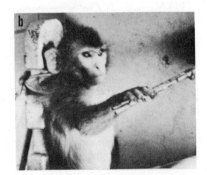

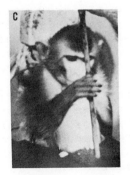

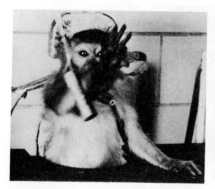
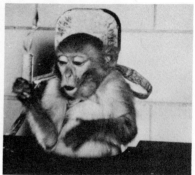

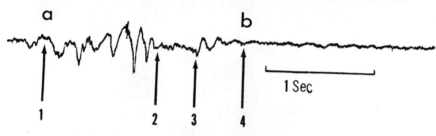

Figure 7. These photographs with corresponding accelerometer tracings below them are intended to show the differential effects of cerebellar lesions on a compound movement and on a maintained limb position, respectively. The animal is trained to take the cylinder in her hand and to hold it in a fixed position while the rubber band from which the cylinder is dangling, remains slack. She received a bilateral dentate-interpositus lesion 8 weeks before these pictures were taken. In a. the monkey is reaching for and trying to grasp the cylinder, which she misses. This compound movement elicits a series of oscillations (6 per second) shown below on the accelerometer recording, between 1 and 2. At 2 the monkey successfully grasps the cylinder and the oscillations cease until 3 when she tightens her grip setting off a new but brief series of oscillations. In b. she is maintaining the required position with no superimposed phasic movement; thus the movement is no longer compound and there is no accompanying tremor. The corresponding accelerometer tracing at 4 is flat.

suggested an alternative interpretation of the
compensatory relations between the two nuclei.
Dentate control was thought to be related primarily
to velocity or timing of phasic movements while the
interpositus was related more to the tonic and
reflex functions involved in limb fixation and
postural aspects of phasic movements. Full blown
cerebellar dyskinesia was interpreted (Goldberger
and Growden 1973; 1974) as the expression of two
underlying disorders; one related to the phasic
component of a movement, the other to fixation of
the limb at an end-point determined by the movement's goal. These two functions may be mediated
differentially by dentate and interpositus
respectively. Only the impairment in both of these
motor functions by destruction of both nuclei
provokes the oscillations, known as ataxia and
intention tremor, typical of cerebellar syndromes.
Thus the anatomical unit related to tremor includes
both nuclei; the failure of tremor to appear
following lesions of one or the other nucleus may
be viewed as a result of sparing of a part of that
unit rather than due to compensatory activity of
one nucleus after loss of the other. Indeed,
recent anatomical studies in the monkey (Flummer-
felt *et al.* 1971; Stanton 1973) have shown that
dentate and interpositus projections although
overlapping are certainly not identical.

During the year following dentate-interpositus
lesions, gradual attentuation was seen so that
oscillations during movement were eventually
difficult to elicit. The recovery period was
divided into three stages by comparison of quantitative data obtained during performance of conditioned and unrehearsed movements (Fig. 8), as well
as testing of postural responses e.g., placing,
hopping and vestibular responses, observations of
posture and locomotion and neurological examination. During recovery, the animals exhibited deft
and subtle changes in limb position which minimized
or even avoided the oscillations which had been
elicited by their movements. It seemed that the
inaccuracy in timing of movement could be compensated for by greater accuracy in position due to
unusually adept and facile use of muscles for limb
fixation. Such a complex behavioral maneuver
suggested mediation of recovery, at least in part,

Weeks Post-operative

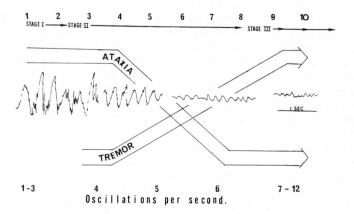

Figure 8. *This chart summarizes the changes which occur during a 10 week recovery period during which the oscillations provoked by bilateral dentate-interpositus lesions become attentuated, i.e. the amplitude becomes smaller and the frequency becomes more rapid and the rhythm more regular. This period is divided into 3 stages on the basis of the change in rate and amplitude of oscillations as well as recovery in specific and general motor performance (see text). The chart also shows the preponderance of ataxia or tremor as defined by the usual clinical criteria during the post-operative period and shows the transition from ataxia in stage I to tremor which predominates in stage III. The observations of tremor and ataxia and the serial accelerometer recordings were made with the animal's forelimb in a mid-flexed position, as in Fig. 6c.*

through the cerebral cortex. This is in contrast to the traditional view that cerebellar control (rather than recovery from loss of cerebellar control) was mediated solely or primarily by the cortex and corticospinal system. That view was based upon the demonstration that motor cortex (Aring and Fulton 1936; Carrea and Mettler 1955) or corticospinal lesions (Carpenter and Correll 1961) abolished cerebellar tremor in untrained animals. More recently, several investigations of acute (Brooks *et al.* 1972) and chronic (Growden

300

et al. 1967) animals have questioned the role of
the motor cortex in genesis of cerebellar tremor.
When monkeys were pre-operatively conditioned,
cerebellar tremor was not abolished by total pyramidal destruction; in fact, the corticospinal
tract appeared to be important not so much for the
expression of cerebellar symptoms as for recovery
from them.

It was therefore, logical to assess the relative contribution of different parts of the
cerebral cortex to recovery from the effects of
cerebellar lesions (Goldberger and Growden 1974).
In monkeys with chronic dentate-interpositus
lesions having stabilized at an apparently maximal
level of recovery ("tremor" occasional, "ataxia"
not seen) ablations were made in areas 8, 6, 4 of
Brodmann or in the post-central gyrus (Fig. 9).
Each lesion produced decompensation, and thus the
reappearance of cerebellar oscillations. The
quantitative characteristics of the oscillations
as well as the qualitative aspects of movement
revealed that in each case the animal had returned
to one of the stages which had been seen during
the post-cerebellar recovery period. From that
stage, decompensation was followed by a series of
compensatory changes identical in sequence to
those which had followed the original post-
cerebellar recovery. The stage to which each
animal ultimately returned varied with the site of
the cortical lesions (Fig. 9). Recrudescence of
cerebellar oscillations was least following area 8
or 6 lesions although after the latter a rapid
tremor returned which appeared to be permanent.
Caudal area 4 lesions provoked a retrogression to
late stage II of the recovery period, and to early
stage II if the anterior border of area 4 was
added. In the latter animals ataxia was seen
after its absence for almost one year since the
original cerebellar lesion. Recovery proceeded
slowly to early stage III and appeared to reach a
plateau. Sensory cortex ablations limited to
rostral post-central cortex had an effect similar
to that seen after ablation of caudal area 4. If,
however the caudal part of the sensory cortex was
included in the post central lesion, the wild
ataxia (3 oscillations per second) which had
occurred only in the first days after the original

301

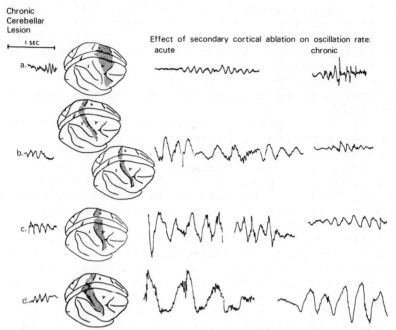

Figure 9. Cerebro-cortical lesions were made one year after cerebellar lesions. On the left of each cortical diagram is a short tremor record taken from the recovered cerebellar animal shortly before the cortical lesion was made. On the right of the cortical diagrams are accelerometer recordings taken one week and again at twelve weeks after the cortical ablations were made and shows the effect of each cortical ablation on the frequency and amplitude of the cerebellar oscillations.

a. area 6
b. rostral sensory cortex (3, 1) and caudal motor cortex (4). These were equivalent in their effects.
c. total motor cortex (4 & 4s)
d. total sensory cortex (3, 1, 2 + part of 5 and possibly infringing on 7)

These are arranged (a-d) in order of increasing decompensation judged by the increased amplitude and decreased frequency of tremor, the amount of ataxia which returned and the general impairment in reflex status and motor performance.

cerebellar lesions returned. Little recompensation was seen in the following months. That lesion was somewhat smaller in mass than the area 6 lesion which had produced only mild decompensation, thus mass of cortical tissue removed could not in itself explain the degree of decompensation which followed. The caudal part of the monkey's somato-sensory cortex may be particularly important for post-cerebellar-lesion recovery because it contains the representation of proximal and axial parts of the body (Woolsey *et al.* 1952) or because it receives the projection of joint and muscle afferents from limbs and trunk.

Structures implicated in compensation for cerebellar dyskynesia include the vestibular system for vermal-fastigial deficits (Glaser and Higgins 1966; Van der Meulen *et al.* 1966). Those shown to contribute to recovery after dentate-interpositus lesions include the dorsal roots (Liu and Chambers 1971) dorsal columns (Carpenter and Correll 1961) pre and post-central gyrus (Goldberger and Growden 1974) and pyramidal tract (Growden *et al.* 1967). These structures have in common the fact that they give rise to anatomically demonstrable projections constituting the major input to somatosensory relay nuclei of the spinal cord and brainstem (Kuypers 1960; Liu and Chambers 1964; Carpenter *et al.* 1968) which project to thalamus and then cortex. In monkeys the information projected by these structures is derived primarily from tactile and joint receptors and flower spray endings in muscle spindles (Rosen and Asanuma 1972), whereas the contribution from group I fibers from muscle is small. The major somatosensory input to cortex might therefore be expected to convey information related to position and displacement but not to the rate of change in muscle tension required for timing of movement (Glaser and Higgins 1966; Van der Meulen *et al.* 1966; Gilman 1969). Thus during recovery, the inaccuracies in timing of movement, due to loss of cerebellar circuits may be compensated for by improved use of limb position related to somatosensory feedback loops, as suggested by the behavioral observations.

If it is legitimate to parcellate the compo-nents of motor function (cf. Brooks and Stoney 1971) it appears that motor cortex is related to

changes in force (Evarts 1967; 1968) the cerebellum
to velocity (Brooks 1972) or timing and the postcentral sensory cortex, to displacement (Evarts
1972). Control of displacement by sensory cortex
may depend upon peripheral feedback resulting from
movement. In contrast, it is thought that central
feedback and feed-forward systems in addition to
peripheral information are utilized by motor
cortex and cerebellum. It may be reasonable then
to suggest that the impairment in timing of limb
movements following cerebellar lesions is permanent, but that enhanced control of force and
displacement in response to the impairment is
responsible for recovery. It is indeed possible to
observe, in monkeys recovering from dentate-
interpositus ablation, the endless series of small
limb adjustments made during movement which
appears to result in the avoidance or escape from
those positions most likely to induce tremor.
These movements are impaired or abolished after
secondary cortical ablations and thus signs of
cerebellar deficit reappear. The tremor produces
its own negative reinforcement; delay or even
failure to "zero in" on the end-point of the
movement and, therefore, its goal. Trial-and-
error shifting of limb position contains a built-
in positive reinforcement; diminution or avoidance
of tremor thereby shortening the delay in
obtaining reward. This is not recovery of
cerebellar function *per se*. It is "functional
compensation" of Luciani (1915).

G. Deafferentation:

    One of the most intriguing areas of current
investigation is that of the degree of recovery
possible after deafferentation of the limbs.
Section of the dorsal roots is not, in the strict
sense, a motor systems lesion. When performed in
monkeys however, it results in far more drastic
deterioration of movement than any other single
lesion that has been described (Mott and
Sherrington 1895; Lassek 1953; Twitchell 1954).
In addition to the loss of all intrinsic reflex
activity and of ipsilaterally triggered responses,
a loss of virtually all spontaneous or voluntary
limb movements was described.

The condition of the unilaterally deafferented forelimb in monkeys is that of a flaccid or hypotonic, almost complete paralysis; the distal muscles being the most affected (Lassek 1953). Static labyrinthine reflexes are abolished but active turning of the head evokes the expected reflex figures (Denny-Brown 1966). In fact, the mechanism underlying residual movements has been attributed to such active tonic neck reflexes (Twitchell 1954). Acceleratory vestibular responses and the scratch reflex also remain. The deafferented forelimb is excluded from quadripedal locomotion, but is able to maintain a position of tonic flexion during locomotion (Taub and Berman 1968) in spite of the absence of peripheral feedback. This is presumably the result of an active inhibitory process, since reciprocal stepping can be mediated by purely intraspinal connections (Graham-Brown 1914). In cats, the ability to maintain this flexor position and the concommitant ability to exclude the limb from reciprocal stepping takes nine days to develop after deafferentation and may be a sign of increasing descending output, including increased central feedback (Goldberger 1973b).

If the intact forelimb is restrained however, mobilization of the deafferented limb is seen (Knapp et al. 1963); under visual guidance, a variety of accurate movements emerges. In contrast, when the animal is returned to a free situation, the limb shows not a trace of improvement over its previous status. If however, intact limb immobilization is maintained for three or more days, improved use of the deafferented limb is permanent (Taub et al. 1972a). Either interlimb inhibition is not involved in the failure of the deafferented limb to express its capacity for movement, as previously suspected (Taub et al. 1966) or, this inhibition is successfully suppressed by descending systems during the period of limb-restraint. Emergence of movement could presumably be facilitated by such a descending inhibitory mechanism.

In contrast to the unilateral deafferent, the bilaterally operated animal is capable of impressive "spontaneous" recovery of movement (Knapp et al. 1963; Taub and Berman 1968; Liu and Chambers 1971). The bilaterality either "forces the issue" as in the bilateral pyramidal monkey (Tower 1940), or abolishes interlimb inhibition of some sort, or overcomes "learned non-use" (Taub et al. 1972a). Most observers (e.g. Denny-Brown 1966; Bossom 1972) have emphasized the recovery of movements of proximal muscles which precede that of distal muscles and show a greater degree of eventual improvement. Others (Liu and Chambers 1971) have found that nibbling of the fingers, which requires discrete distal control, and emptying of the cheek pouch with the dorsum of the wrist were the first movements to emerge post-operatively, thus suggesting a disto-proximal sequence of recovery. Other interpretations are possible however, since biting of the fingers and pouch-emptying involve contact between the deafferented hand and an intact part of the body i.e. the face. Most significantly perhaps, both of those movements involve the limb flexors and coordinated fixation by proximal, primarily flexor musculature. In the initial post-operative stage, the deafferented forelimbs manifest a distinct 'flexor bias' as does the hindlimb following partial denervation due to spinal transsection (Sherrington 1898). This "flexor bias" is so strong as to convert certain extensor reflexes (e.g. vestibular) and extensor movements to flexion (Denny-Brown 1966; Liu and Chambers 1971). Thus the movements which emerge during the first few days might express the unopposed bias of the intersegmental spinal mechanism as well as its relative refractoriness to most stimuli, rather than a predominant distal or proximal recovery pattern. The analysis of movement according to proximal versus distal control, although time-honored, may be limited due to its dependency upon the method of examination. The dexterity of individual finger and other distal movements is more accessible to observation than the complex coordination and fine modulation of limb fixation which accompanies such distal movements.

Projection of the limb away from the body develops later than hand-to-face movements (Bossom 1972). Visually-guided reaching begins as a ballistic circumduction of the whole arm; controlled reaching which occurs later, requires that the 'flexor bias' be inhibited. Even then,

stabilized extension of the arm with accurate
grasping of the whole hand have to be superimposed
on the original reaching act as motor status
improves. Thumb-finger opposition can be performed
later for picking up small bits of food or
grooming. Before that, dependency on visual
guidance wanes, so that after first seeing the
food, successful reaching and grasping take place
without further vision of the food or of the
limb.

Unlike most lesions affecting movement,
deafferentation in the infant or fetal monkey does
not result in a greater degree of ultimate
recovery than that found in adult deafferents
(Lassek and Moyer 1953; Taub *et al.* 1972b; Berman
and Berman 1973). In fact, the eventual motor
status attained by these animals may be somewhat
less than in their adult counterparts, although
damage of the fingers and the precautions taken
to prevent such damage (bandaging the limbs, etc.)
make this conclusion uncertain. Despite some
differences between the results of infant and
adult deafferentation, the motor development of
infant deafferented monkeys shows most of the
features of the normal developing Rhesus (Taub *et
al.* 1972b; Berman and Berman 1973), even without
visual guidance (Taub *et al.* 1973). Although the
rate of development is slower in deafferents,
the sequence of emerging movements, as defined for
the normal Macaque (Hines 1942), is remarkably
similar in normal and deafferented infants. In the
normal monkey some correlation has been found
between reflex development and synaptogenesis
(Bodian *et al.* 1968), thus it is remarkable that
fetal deafferentation alters motor development so
little. These observations do not suggest that
dorsal roots are unimportant in normal movement
and its maturation but, rather, that the development and performance of many motor patterns can
take place in the absence of segmental reflexes,
somatic sensation and peripheral feedback. Thus
these movements are "wired into" the organization
of the neuraxis at least in the deafferented
monkey.

The fact that infant deafferents do not conform
to the general rule of improved motor status of
infants compared with adults with the same lesion,

suggests the possibility that at least some central
neurons fail to recover from early lesions due,
perhaps to a greater sensitivity to partial
denervation in the infant than in adults. This
might limit the extent of recovery. Anatomical
evidence for such sensitivity is ample in the
visual system (Wiesel and Hubel 1963; Guillery and
Scott 1971).

Less is known about the morphological
sequelae of motor systems lesions. Cells of
Clarke's nucleus in cat spinal cord appear to be
affected permanently by deafferentation at birth
(Smith 1969; 1973; Loewy 1972) but not in the
mature animal. Conceivably, these alterations
might prevent the cell from being reinnervated by
collateral sprouting from intact systems. In hemi-
deafferented adult cats, the partially denervated
cells of Clarke's nucleus are reinnervated by
collateral sprouting from descending systems
(Goldberger and Murray 1972; Goldberger 1973a; b).
This provides an additional central feedback
pathway to the cerebellum which may subserve some
aspects of recovery. Whether this occurs also in
Clarke's cells made morphologically abnormal by
infant deafferentation is not known, but in the
visual system, atrophic geniculate cells fail to
be re-innervated by collateral sprouts (Guillery
1972) even though the sprouting may occur
(Ralston and Chow 1973). If this were true also
of the spinal gray matter after infantile
deafferentation, it might explain the less
developed motor status of deafferented infants
compared with adult counterparts. It would be the
morphological counterpart of a permanent
diaschisis.

As impressive as the 'spontaneous' recovery
in the deafferented monkey may seem, it is less
than that obtained through the use of classical
and operant conditioning methods (Knapp *et al.*
1958; Taub *et al.* 1966; Bossom and Ommaya 1968; Liu
and Chambers 1971). Although this fascinating area
cannot be reviewed here, certain points should be
mentioned. In the present context, it appears
noteworthy that there is a greater correspondence
between recovery of conditioned and of untrained
movements in the bilaterally deafferented monkey,
when compared with that found after other lesions,

e.g. pyramidal, cerebellar. The fact that these
deafferented animals are able to learn a maintained limb position without vision may be
important for the performance of many recovered
movements, both conditioned and unconditioned.
That the maintained position can be mis-performed,
if the starting neutral position is changed
without the animal's knowledge (Liu and Chambers
1971) suggests that they learn a displacement
rather than a fixed position. These observations
have led to the elaboration of several important
concepts which emphasize the connections of
descending motor systems with neural structures
which are not, by convention, motor. Some of
these are known; corticostriate projections (Petras
1972) must surely be important since caudate
ablations in deafferented monkeys abolished
recovered, accurate reaching movements when vision
is occluded (Bossom and Ommaya 1968). With vision,
these movements are well performed so that the
added deficit is not considered motor in the
usual sense, but is thought to be due to loss of
a corollary discharge dependent on fronto-striate
connections.

Central feedback related to "sensory"
structures has ample physiological and anatomical
basis e.g. pyramidal (Kuypers 1960) and extrapyramidal (Levitt *et al*. 1964) projections to
dorsal column nuclei and to the dorsal horn of the
spinal cord. Presumably these would reach sensory
cortex and influence motor output. But a role for
the primary and association somatosensory cortex
in recovery from deafferentation, although looked
for, has not been found (Chambers and Liu 1973).
Many central feedback systems of unknown function
e.g. cortico-thalamic, cortico-ponto-or-olivo-
cerebellar are present in normal animals and may
be important in recovery from deafferentation.
Others may be formed by collateral sprouting only
after deafferentation e.g. descending projections
to Clarke's nucleus in the cat (Goldberger 1973a;
b) and cortical projections to external cuneate
nucleus in the deafferented monkey (unpublished).
Recovery may depend not only upon feedback systems
but also upon increased efficiency of central
patterning and, related to this, enhanced motor
output which might result from increased

309

descending innervation of interneurons (Goldberger and Murray 1972). That such recovery can in fact be related to collateral sprouting is suggested by the enormous difference between a completely deafferented animal and one in which a single root is spared (Twitchell 1954). The lone dorsal root provides recovery not only for segments of the limb it normally innervates, but for most of the limb. When studied anatomically a dorsal root so isolated has been shown to have increased its extent of spinal termination over several segments by collateral sprouting (cat: Liu and Chambers 1958) during the recovery period.

H. Summary and Discussion

1. Summary of the effects of four lesions.
Each of the lesions described provokes a characteristic array of motor deficits, followed by subsequent recovery of movement. The gravity of the deficit, following any one of the lesions discussed here, is non-uniform however, in respect to the impairment and the degree of recovery seen in different categories of movement: reflex, triggered and centrally patterned.
Pyramidal lesions affect tendon reflexes by raising their thresholds (Gilman *et al.* 1971). There is evidence that the subsequent recovery of these reflexes is related to collateral sprouting of the dorsal roots (McCouch *et al.* 1958; Murray 1973) and that recovery of at least some centrally patterned movements is dependent upon recovery of the stretch reflexes (Twitchell 1951). Although dorsal root function cannot be said to replace pyramidal function, it is possible that loss of force control (Evarts 1967; 1968) which must follow pyramidotomy may be compensated for, in part, by the increase in dorsal root input. On the other hand, the loss of certain triggered responses, unless they are conditioned pre-operatively, is complete and permanent.
Deafferentation abolishes intrinsic limb reflexes, and reduces crossed reflexes arising in the intact limb whereas descending reflexes, initially depressed, eventually become exaggerated. The return of centrally patterned movements may reflect an elaboration of this exaggerated

descending reflex activity, although the centrally patterned movements are far more extensive and are also better controlled especially in bilaterally deafferented monkeys. Visual guidance is important but, for many movements, not essential. The significance both of central feedback and corollary discharge has been stressed especially in the performance of limb positions maintained without visual guidance (Bossom and Ommaya 1968; Taub and Berman 1968; Liu and Chambers 1971). These corollary systems exist in the undamaged nervous system. They may also increase in effectiveness or even develop *de novo* in response to deafferentation.

Cerebellar lesions of the dentate-interpositus nuclei have transient effects on reflexes (Gilman 1959) but a lasting effect on those movements, centrally patterned or triggered, in which a fixed end-point must be attained by limb-fixation. The oscillations, which may result from a deficit in the timing of movements, become attentuated in time. This recovery may be due to an unusually deft use of limb positions which avoid cerebellar oscillations. After recovery, such oscillations can be reinstated by lesions of the somatosensory system or of the pyramidal tracts, provided that the type of movement which brings out the cerebellar deficit can still be elicited. For after the second lesion the execution of movement with a fixed end-point is, in untrained animals, often abolished; and with it, cerebellar tremor.

Lesions of the premotor cortex affect all classes of movement. Tendon reflexes of the digits are hyperactive. Grasping, triggered by tactile stimulation and maintained by stretch, is exaggerated and apraxia, a disruption of complex sequential motor acts, is seen. Recovery from the forced grasp, mediated by the pyramidal tract, may be achieved by substitution of the opposing response, tactile evasion. The recovery from apraxia is slower and may depend upon the integrity of other parts of the frontal lobe or of the parietal association cortex. The difference in duration of the forced grasp and of apraxia as well as the difference in pathways which mediate recovery suggest that term premotor cortex may actually refer to more than one functionally

distinct cortical region. The functional diversity
of the region makes difficult the interpretation
of its contribution to movement and therefore of
the recovery which follows its destruction.
    2.   Summary of the factors which enhance or
        limit recovery.
    The factors determining the degree of
recovery seen after each of these lesions have a
relative rather than uniform importance; they
differ in the case of each lesion. For example,
the age at which an animal is deafferented has
relatively little effect on the ultimate status
of its motor performance. The infant-lesioned
animals fail to show more improvement than their
adult counterparts. This may be related to the
failure of normal development of the partially
denervated spinal cord (Smith 1969; 1973; Loewy
1972) after infant or fetal deafferentation.
Abnormal development might render certain cell
groups, e.g. Clarke's nucleus, unable to receive
collateral sprouts from descending systems as they
do in adult deafferents (Goldberger 1973a; b). In
contrast, the age at which lesions of the pyramid
or motor cortex are performed is, apparently,
critical. The general motor performance of the
adult monkey, pyramidal lesioned in infancy
greatly surpasses, that of its adult-lesioned
counterpart. Specific performance, however, at
least for certain types of responses, is severely
impaired or abolished by pyramidotomy regardless
of the age at which it is performed (Tower 1949;
Lawrence and Hopkins 1972). Why pyramidal lesions
made in infancy discriminate between different
classes of movement with respect to the differing
degree of recovery possible for each class, is
unknown. It has been shown in other systems,
however, (Goldman 1972; 1973) that the age of the
animal at the time a lesion is made, is less
important than the age of the tissue at that time,
or, at least of the differential development
within the infant's nervous system. If different
classes of movement were mediated by different
pathways with non-uniform developmental rates,
then pyramidal lesion in infancy should be
expected to affect these pathways in a non-uniform
manner.
    The type of organization within a system

("loose" vs. "tight" coupling: Brooks and Stoney 1971; Glassman 1971; 1973) also affects the degree of recovery possible after its destruction. Destruction of those regions showing least localization, are followed by the most extensive recovery. For example, the intensity of forced grasping following area 6 lesions varies with the amount of that cortex, rather than the subdivision of the area which is removed. The rate and completeness of recovery is greater than in e.g., motor-cortex lesions and varies inversely with the intensity of the original deficit. Area 6 may be diffusely organized in terms of its afferent and efferent connections. Other systems, however appear to contain more than one type of organization. For example, the dorsal roots (as well as the pyramidal tract) manifest a dual organization, specific and diffuse, and after rhizotomies, the pattern of recovery reflects both. If, for example, the brachial roots are cut but one is spared, recovery of centrally-patterned movements is seen throughout the limb (Twitchell 1954) rather than being confined to the part of the limb innervated by the spared root. These movements can be classed as 'general' since there are a number of ways in which they can be executed. On the other hand the specific, segmental deficits due to loss of dorsal roots, are permanent. A similar, dual organization was reflected in the deficits following subtotal motor cortex lesions in which a bit of residual cortex provided recovery for limbs to which it was not somatotopically related. In the pyramidal and in the dorsal root systems there are discrete, topographical projections to motorneurons and sensory relay nuclei, as well as overlapping inputs to interneurons. Specific and general deficits may reflect these two types of anatomical organization and these types of deficits appear to differ in the degree and rate of recovery possible. Thus destruction of a region with no demonstrable topographical projection might be expected to provoke generalized deficits from which behavioral recovery is relatively complete and rapid. Such is the case with cortical lesions of area 6.

The effects of conditioning and other training procedures upon recovery also differ from one type

313

of lesion to the next. For example the extent of recovery following cerebellar lesions has not been found to be greater in trained animals, although training is often essential in exposing well-hidden cerebellar symptoms. Recovery appears to take place spontaneously according to a very stereotyped pattern in which cerebellar oscillations become progressively more controlled. Ataxia is replaced by tremor which, itself, eventually becomes attenuated. These changes are paralleled by greater control over reflex activity and progressive decrease in hypotonia. In contrast to the cerebellar monkey one with a unilaterally deafferented forelimb makes very little recovery without training. The dependency of the animal on the normal limb and a hypothesized (Taub and Berman 1968) inter-limb inhibition may prevent the development of the ability to utilize central feedback mechanisms. If the normal limb is restrained for three days however, a marked and lasting improvement in the use of the deafferented limb is seen. With training, the use of such limbs is remarkable. So important is central feedback and/or corollary discharge to movement that deafferented animals can learn to distinguish movement, direction and degrees of active joint rotation with no peripheral feedback or visual guidance. Is it this central feedback which is essential for the enhancement of recovery by conditioning? If so, then the lack of significant effects of conditioning on recovery from cerebellar lesions may be related to the reliance of the cerebellar-lesioned animal on peripheral feedback systems. The latter may be less educable. The animals in which peripheral feedback is removed by deafferentation show the greatest beneficial effects of conditioning which, in this case can act only upon central feedback and feed-forward systems, such as those of the cerebellum.

3. Discussion

Of the mechanisms considered to be relevant to recovery, the evidence suggests that there is no one mechanism common to all lesions, nor is there one which accounts for all the recovery following any one lesion. Rather it would appear that the behavioral changes which we interpret as recovery result from the collective contribution made by several mechanisms acting together upon an altered nervous system. The mechanisms were grouped into four major classes: 1) Mass action (and equipotentiality) 2) Vicarious function, 3) Behavioral substitution and 4) Functional reorganization (collateral sprouting, denervation supersensitivity).

The evidence for mass action in the motor systems is slight except, perhaps, in the regulation of muscle tone. Initially, pyramidotomy, deafferentation and cerebellar lesions each reduce muscle tone rather drastically which then undergoes recovery to a variable extent. If that recovery were complete, so would be the equipotentiality of the structures mediating control of muscle tone. These three systems appear to utilize somewhat different mechanisms (Gilman 1969; Gilman et al. 1971), although, after lesions, they do appear to be able to act one for the other. Within each system, the mass action which exists may be a reflection of the degree of overlap found in the anatomical projections of its subdivisions. The functional manifestations of diffuseness appear to be overshadowed in most cases by the effects of a lesion attributable to the somatotopic and/or functional localization which is present. The theory of equipotentiality or mass action as formulated by Lashley (1938) focused on the post-lesion retention of learned movements, but ignored the question of recovery of execution or quality of motor performance per se: "I found perfect retention of manipulative habits in monkeys after destruction of the motor cortex, although the retention could not be demonstrated until the paralysis has recovered," (p. 737). How the paralysis might have recovered was not determined. His conclusions relating recovery to mass action of a system were thus based upon retention studies rather than upon the mode of execution of movement after lesions and the changes which took place during the recovery period. Had he examined the nature of the motor performance in his lesioned monkeys he undoubtedly would have described both an immediate, grave deficit, and later, a permanent one which was less marked due to recovery.

The ability of one system to change its normal

315

modus operandi and thereby to function vicariously (rather than because of mass action) for another which has been destroyed has been thought to be an innevitable consequence of the observation that recovery took place. The candidacy of vicarious function as a mechanism may be assessed by the deterioration of recovery which takes place after a sequence of lesions is made in different neural systems. There is good evidence that such deterioration takes place when destruction of one system is superimposed upon chronic lesions of another even after long recovery periods. The interpretation of this sequence of events as vicarious function however is questionable. If the term is to be used rigorously, it should imply that after a first lesion the contribution to recovery made by a secondary system is due to its ability to subserve specific motor performances by mediation of the same mechanisms which, initially, had been impaired or abolished. The results of many investigators have failed to support this proposition, for it has not been demonstrated that the recovered motor act is performed in the same way as it was prior to the lesion. For example, the somatosensory system, which is essential for recovery from cerebellar lesions has not been shown to contribute to accuracy in movement in the same way as the cerebellum does. If it did the many small compensatory adjustments during movement seen in the animal recovering from cerebellar lesions should not be necessary. The compensatory use of position for impairment in timing was suggested instead. There was a similar failure to demonstrate that the pyramidal tract functioned vicariously for the loss of the premotor cortex as the lesioned animal recovered from forced grasping. The manner in which the pyramidal tract and premotor cortex mediated control of the grasp did not appear to be the same. Thus vicarious function may not be a common mechanism underlying recovery of unconditioned movements. An argument can be made, however that the retention or post-lesion performance of certain conditioned movements may depend upon the vicarious functioning of undamaged neural tissue (see below).

There is, perhaps, better evidence for behavioral substitution as a mechanism of signifi-

cance for recovering systems. The distinction
between this and vicarious function is often overlooked. What is meant by behavioral substitution
is that, although the undamaged systems responsible
for recovery may become more efficient in
mediating the responses attributed to them, that
their normal functions may become enhanced, but
that their functions do not change in order to
replace those which were lost and, therefore, that
they do not act vicariously. It is not the function
but, rather, the behavior which is replaced in the
sense that the original ends are achieved by
different means. The results of several investigations reviewed here have suggested this possibility
which stems from Sperry's (1947) analysis of the
recovery of movement in monkeys with crossed
nerves to flexor and extensor muscles. It is
inferred from apparent take-over by the pyramid of
control of grasping following area 6 lesions and
by the control of cerebellar tremor and ataxia by
the somatosensory and pyramidal systems. In
neither case was there evidence that the undamaged
systems mediated restitution by taking on novel or
anomalous functions. Rather it was thought that
the behavior mediated normally by these systems
could be utilized by the animal to mask a permanent
underlying impairment of a specific function. The
underlying impairment in inhibition of the grasp
(area 6) or timing of movements (cerebellum)
could then be unmasked by a second lesion following
which motor performance deteriorated to such a
degree that the initial deficit could no longer be
covered up. The only requirement imposed by this
model is that the functions of the pathways
responsible for recovery become enhanced during
the recovery period as a compensatory response to
brain damage. One mechanism which has been proposed for such enhancement of function, at the
synaptic level, is dishabituation of reflex
responses by presynaptic facilitation (Kandel *et
al.* 1970). This mechanism fulfills the requirement
imposed by the model suggested for behavioral
substitution. That is, presynaptic facilitation
would be capable of producing enhancement of an
already existing reflex or centrally-patterned
movement without a qualitative change in the
pathways responsible.

There are two major lines of evidence for
mechanics underlying <u>functional</u> <u>reorganization</u>,
anatomical e.g. collateral sprouting and
biochemical e.g. denervation supersensitivity.
Either of these could be responsible for the
neuronal hyperexcitability found in some partially
denervated neurons of the spinal cord (Loeser and
Ward 1967) and brainstem (Kjerulf and Loeser 1973;
Kjerulf *et al.* 1973). The hyperactive spinal
interneurons could be recipients of reinnervation
from collateral sprouts (Liu and Chambers 1958)
but hyperactive cells in the cats external cuneate
nucleus were presumed to be supersensitive since
no electron microscopic evidence for such
sprouting could be found (O'Neal and Westrum 1973).
The functional implications of anatomically
demonstrable collateral sprouting are still
uncertain, however. Sprouting has been observed
in the spinal cord by degeneration and radioauto-
graphic techniques in animals in which reflex and
behavioral recovery were also demonstrated. There
was a correlation between the time course of recovery and that of increased dorsal root
projections determined by quantitative radioauto-
graphy. There was also a correlation between the
anatomical system which increased its spinal
projection field and the reflex system which
recovered or became hyperactive (Goldberger and
Murray 1972; Murray 1973; Goldberger 1973a; b).
For example in hemi-deafferented cats, in which
descending reflexes (e.g. vestibular) became
unilaterally hyperexcitable, it was the
descending tracts on that side which showed signs
of sprouting. It has also been possible to show a
similar correlation between reflex recovery,
increased electrophysiological response to dorsal
root stimulation and in increase in anatomically
determined dorsal root projections in transsected
cat and monkey spinal cord (McCouch 1961; McCouch
et al. 1958).

One obvious question here is the usefulness of
such reflex and anatomical changes to the animal's
general adaptation to a lesion. It has been shown
in several systems that recovery of spontaneous
movement proceeds in a manner parallel to reflex
changes (Growden *et al.* 1967; Goldberger 1969;
Beck and Chambers 1970; Goldberger and Growden

318

1973; 1974). In particular, Twitchell (1951; 1954) has shown a temporal relationship not only between post-lesion return of a reflex and the subsequent use of that reflex in the recovery of centrally patterned and triggered motor responses, but also between the exaggeration of certain reflexes and the recovery of movements related to them. For example extensor hypertonus of the hindlimbs may be the basis for the return of standing and loco-motion after motor cortex destruction. Furthermore if the exaggerated reflexes underlying recovered movements are abolished by a second lesion, the recovered movements too are destroyed (Denny-Brown 1966). It can therefore be proposed that collateral sprouting and/or denervation supersensitivity mediate recovery and exaggeration of certain reflexes which may, in turn, constitute the elements from which recovery of unconditioned, centrally-patterned and triggered movements are reconstructed during recovery.

The persistence and the recovery of conditioned movements after lesions expected to abolish them is an even more complex problem. Each of these movements can be pre-operatively shaped by the investigator as a superstructure, utilizing an apparently identical triggered response or 'spontaneous' movement as a base. Yet the condi-tioned movement may persist after the destruction by a lesion, of its unconditioned counterpart. Such is the case when lesions of the pyramid (Liu and Chambers 1962; Chambers and Kozart 1965) or, bilaterally, of the motor cortex (Goldberger, unpublished data) are made in monkeys pre-operatively trained to perform tactile placing. The conditioned placing response is retained after the lesion but tactile placing, tested in the usual manner is permanently abolished. Several interpre-tations of this data are possible. The pathways which mediate the learned and the triggered response in the normal animal may not be the same, even though the conditioning procedure makes use of the unlearned movement in shaping the condi-tioned response. It would appear that although the unconditioned response is reinforced during conditioning, the reinforcement must act upon pathways other than, or in addition to those normally mediating it. Alternatively it is possible

319

that the conditioning procedure recruits additional, or reinforces 'latent' collateral pathways for
conditioned tactile placing rather than strength-
ening those subserving the normal placing
responses. The pathways upon which unconditioned
tactile placing depend are relatively simple in
the monkey: medial lemniscus and pyramidal tract
(Bard 1938). They may also be relatively
resistant to modification by conditioning whereas
other systems which respond to tactile stimuli
may be more responsive to repeated experience and
reinforcement. Alternatively, conditioning may
serve to disinhibit other systems which then
express a previously 'latent' function. Evidence
has been presented for pathways which inhibit
tactile placing and may prevent its recovery in
untrained monkeys (Semmes and Chow 1955; Goldberger
1969). If such collateral systems subserved
performance of the learned response, there would
be no reason to expect a loss of conditioned
tactile placing following pyramidal or motor cortex
lesions. Data supporting or rejecting one of these
alternative formulations might have implications
not only for the theoretical understanding of the
effect of conditioning upon recovery of movement
following neural lesions, but also for the
rehabilitation of patients with such lesions.
        It should be emphasized that different
mechanisms are being proposed for the recovery of
unconditioned triggered, centrally-patterned or
'voluntary' movements on one hand and for recovery
of movements triggered by conditioned stimuli on
the other. The former requires certain anatomical
and/or biochemical changes which result in reflex
return and hyperactivity i.e. the "organic recovery" of Luciani (1915), and that the recovered
reflex activity be transformed into useful
movement by the undamaged motor systems. This
transformation may result from selective
enhancement of some reflexes and concomittant
suppression of others (Spencer *et al*. 1966; Kandel
et al. 1970). Or, recovery of unconditioned movements may reflect the compensatory substitution of
one mode of executing a movement when the usual
mode has been severely impaired by the lesion i.e.
the "functional compensation" of Luciani.
Vicarious function need not play a role in this

process. As for learned movements, however, when collateral systems exist or are recruited by repeated reinforcement, they may indeed function vicariously for those destroyed, at least in the environment imposed by conditioning methods. Both with the recovery of spontaneous and of conditioned movements the ultimate performance will not be as beautiful as it was before the lesion was made. Motor patterns may normally be 're-represented' in several parts of the nervous system or, this multiple representation may be a result of post-lesion adaptations which can be enhanced by training. Although the apparent re-representation of movements within a number of neural structures or functional units may provide a basis for considerable recovery "compensation, sometimes 'practically' perfect, can never be absolute since no two units represent the whole region (of the body) in quite the same way" (Jackson 1882).

ACKNOWLEDGMENTS: Supported by NSF GB 35505. The author gratefully acknowledges the expert assistance of Ms. Beverly Brown for technical work, Mr. Mel Oster and Ms. Shirley Aumiller for the photography, Ms. Terri Krupa for the secretarial work and Dr. Marion Murray for the criticism and advice.

REFERENCES

Albe-Fessard, D. et Liebeskind, J. (1966). Origine des messages somatosensitifs activant les cellules du cortex moteur chez le singe. *Exp. Brain Res.* 1, 127-146.

Aring, C.D. and Fulton, J.F. (1936). Relation of the cerebrum to the cerebellum. *Arch. Neurol. Psychiat.* 35, 439-466.

Bard, P. (1933). Studies on the cerebral cortex. I. Localized control of placing and hopping reactions in the cat and their normal management by small cortical remmants. *Arch. Neurol. Psychiat.* 30, 40-74.

Bard, P. (1938). Studies on the cortical representation of somatic sensibility. *Harvey Lectures* 33, 143-169.

Beck, C.H., Chambers, W.W. (1970). Speed, accuracy and strength of forelimb movement after unilateral pyramidotomy in rhesus monkeys. *J. Comp. Physiol. Psychol.* 70, 1-22.

Berman, A.J. and Berman, D. (1973). Fetal deafferentation: The ontogenesis of movement in the absence of peripheral sensory feedback. *Exp. Neurol.* 38, 170-176.

Berman, A.J., Taub, E., Pomina, A.D., and Knapp, H.D. (1960). Further observations on deafferentation in the monkey. *Trans. Amer. Neurol. Assoc.* 85, 198-199.

Bernhard, C.G., Bohm, E. (1954). Monosynaptic cortico-spinal activation of forelimb motorneurons in monkeys (*macaca mulatta*). *Acta Physiol. Can.* 31, 104-122.

Bernstein, M.E. and Bernstein, J.J. (1973). Regeneration of axons and synaptic complex formation rostral to the site of hemisection in the spinal cord of the monkey. *Intern. J. Neuroscience* 5, 15-26.

Bieber, I. and Fulton, J.F. (1938). The relation of the cerebral cortex to the grasp reflex and to the postural and righting reflexes. *Arch. Neurol. Psychiat.* 39, 435-454.

Bizzi, E. (1968). Discharge of frontal eye field neurons during saccadic and following eye movement in unanesthetized monkeys. *Exp. Brain Res.* 6, 69-80.

Bizzi, E. and Schiller, P.H. (1970). Single unit activity in the frontal eye fields of unanesthetized monkeys during eye and head movement. *Exp. Brain Res.* 10, 151-158.

Black, P., Cianci, S.N. and Markowitz, R.S. (1971). Differential recovery of proximal and distal motor power after cortical lesions. *Trans. Am. Neurol. Assoc.* 96, 173-177.

Bodian, D., Melby, E.C. and Taylor, N. (1968). Development of fine structure of spinal cord in monkey fetuses: II. Pre-reflex period to period of long intersegmental reflexes. *J. Comp. Neur.*, vol. 133, no. 2. 113-166.

Bossom, J. (1972). Time of recovery of voluntary movement following dorsal rhizotomy. *Brain Res.* 45, 247-250.

Bossom, J. and Ommaya, A.K. (1968). Visuo-motor adaptation (to prismatic transformation of the retinal image) in monkeys with bilateral dorsal rhizotomy. *Brain* 91, 161-172.

Brodal, A. (1965). Experimental anatomical studies of the corticospinal and cortico-rubro-spinal connections in the cat. *Sump. Biol. Hung.* 5, 207-217.

Brooks, C. Mc. and Peck, M.E. (1940). Effect of various cortical lesions on development of placing and hopping reactions in rats. *J. Neurophysiol.* 3, 66-73.

Brooks, V.B. (1969). Information processing motor-sensory cortex. *In* K.N. Leibovic (Ed.) "Information Processing in the Nervous System." New York: Springer-verlag. pp. 231-243.

Brooks, V.B. (1972). Some new experiments on cerebellar motor control. *EEG Clin. Neurophysiol. Suppl.* 31.

Brooks, V.B. and Stoney, S.D. (1971). Motor mechanisms: The role of the pyramidal system in motor control. *Ann. Rev. Physiol.* 33, 337-393.

Brooks, V.B., Atkin, A., Kozlovskaya, I. and Uno, M. (1970). Motor effects from interposed nuclei. *The Physiologist* 13, 157.

Brooks, V.B., Horvath, F., Atkin, A., Kozlovskaya, I. and Uno, M. (1969). Reversible changes in voluntary movements during cooling of a sub-cerebellar nucleus. *Fed. Proc.* 28, 396.

Brooks, V.B., Adrien, J. and Dykes, R.W. (1972).
Task-related discharge of neurons in motor
cortex and effects of dentate cooling. *Brain Res.*
40, 85-89.

Bucy, P.C., Ladpli, R. and Ehrlich, A. (1966).
Destruction of the pyramidal tract in the monkey.
The effects of bilateral section of the cerebral
peduncles. *J. Neurosurg.* 25, 1-23.

Butters, N., Pandya, D., Stein, D. and Rosen, J.
(1972). A search for the spatial engram within
the frontal lobes of monkeys. *Acta Neurobiol.*
Exp. 32, 305-329.

Cannon, B.W., Beaton, L.E. and Ranson, S.W. Jr.
(1943). Nature of paresis following lateral
cortico-spinal section in monkeys. *J. Neuro-*
physiol. 6, 425-429.

Carpenter, M.B. (1959). Lesions of the fastigial
nuclei in the rhesus monkey. *Amer. J. Anat.* 104,
1-34.

Carpenter, M.B. and Correll, J.W. (1961). Spinal
pathways mediating cerebellar dyskinesia in
rhesus monkey. *J. Neurophysiol.* 24, 534-551.

Carpenter, M.B. and Hanna, G.R. (1962). Effects of
thalamic lesions upon cerebellar dyskinesia in
the rhesus monkey. *J. Comp. Neur.* v. 119, 2, 127-
148.

Carpenter, M.B., Stein, B.M. and Shriver, J.E.
(1968). Central projections of spinal dorsal
roots in the monkey. II. Lower thoracic, lumbo-
sacral and coccygeal dorsal roots. *Am. J. Anato.*
v. 123, 1, 75-118.

Carpenter, M.B. and Stevens, G.H. (1957).
Structural and functional relationships between
the deep cerebellar nuclei and the brachium
conjunctivum in the rhesus monkey. *J. Comp.*
Neur. 107, 109-163.

Carrea, R.M.E. and Mettler, F.A. (1947).
Physiologic consequences following extensive
removals of the cerebellar cortex and deep
cerebellar nuclei and effect of secondary
cerebral ablations in the primate. *J. Comp.*
Neurol. 87, 169-228.

Carrea, R.M.E. and Mettler, F.A. (1955). Function
of the primate brachium conjunctivum and related
structures. *J. Comp. Neurol.* 102, 151-322.

Chambers, W.W. (1973). (Personal Communication).

Chambers, W.W. and Liu, C.N. (1958). Cortico-spinal tract in the monkey. *Fed. Proc.* 17, 24.

Chambers, W.W. and Kozart, D. (1965). Conditioned tactile discrimination of monkey with cortico-spinal or pyramidal tract lesions. *Anat. Rec.* 151, 499.

Chambers, W.W. and Liu, J.C. (1973). Effects of somatosensory (SI and SII) cortical ablations on movements of the deafferented arms of *macaca speciosa*. *Anat. Rec.* 175, 287-288.

Crosby, E.C., Yoss, R.E. and Henderson, J.W. (1952). The mammalian midbrain and isthmus regions. Part II. The fiber connections. D. The pattern for eye movements on the frontal eye field and the discharge of specific portions of this field to and through midbrain levels. *J. Comp. Neurol.* 97, 357-384.

Delacour, J., Libouban, S. and McNeil, M. (1972). Premotor cortex and instrumental behavior in monkeys. *Physio. and Behav.* 8, 299-305.

DeLong, M. (1971). Central patterning of movement. *Neurosciences Res. Prog. Bull.* 9, 10-31.

Denny-Brown, D. (1958). The nature of apraxia. *J. Nerv. and Ment. Dis.* 126, 9-33.

Denny-Brown, D. (1962). The midbrain and motor integration. *Royal Society of Medicine* 55, 527-538.

Denny-Brown, D. (1966). The cerebral control of movement. University of Liverpool.

Denny-Brown, D. and Chambers, R.A. (1958). The parietal lobe and behavior. *Proc. ARNMD.* 36, 35-117.

Deuel, R.K. (1969). Loss of motor habits after non-sensorimotor cortical lesions in monkeys. *Neurology* 19, 294.

Edds, M.V. (1953). Collateral nerve regeneration. *Q. Rev. Biol.* 28, 260-276.

Eidelberg, E. (1973). Redundancy as a compensatory mechanism. In Neuroscience research program bulletin "Functional Recovery after Lesions of the Nervous System." In Press.

Evarts, E.V. (1967). Representation of movements and muscles by pyramidal tract neurons of the precentral motor cortex. *In* M.D. Yahr and D.P. Purpura (Eds.) "Neurophysiological Basis of Normal and Abnormal Motor Activities." New York: Raven Press. pp. 215-251.

Evarts, E.V. (1968). Relation of pyramidal tract activity to force exerted during voluntary movement. *J. Neurophysiol*. 31, 14-27.

Evarts, E.V. (1972). Contrasts between activity of precentral and postcentral neurons of cerebral cortex during movement in the monkey. *Brain Res*. 40, 25-33.

Fetz, E.E. and Baker, M.A. (1969). Response properties of precentral neurons in awake monkeys. *Physiologist* 12, 223.

Flumerfelt, B.A., Courville, J. and Otabe, S. (1971). Cerebello-rubral projection in the monkey. *Anat. Rec*. 169, 318.

Foerster, O. (1936). The motor cortex in the light of Hughlings Jackson's doctrines. *Brain* 59, 135-159.

Franck, F. (1887). Fonctions motrices du cerveau. Paris.

Franz, S.I. (1923). Nervous and mental reeducation. New York.

Franz, S.I. and Oden, R. (1917). On cerebral motor control: The recovery from experimentally produced hemiplegia. *Psychobiol*. 1, 3-18.

Fulton, J.F. (1934). Forced grasping and groping in relation to the syndrome of premotor area: A physiological analysis. *Arch. Neurol. Psychiat*. 31, 221-235.

Fulton, J.F. and Dow, R.S. (1938). Postural neck reflexes in the labyrinthectomized monkey and their effect on the grasp reflex. *J. Neurophysiol*. 1, 455-462.

Fulton, J.F. and Kennard, M.A. (1934). A study of flaccid and spastic paralyses produced by lesions of the cerebral cortex in primates. *A.R.N.M.D.* 13, 158-210.

Gilman, S. (1969). The mechanism of cerebellar hypotonia. *Brain* 92, 621-638.

Gilman, S. and Marco, L.A. (1971). Effects of medullary pyramidotomy in the monkey. I. Clinical and electromyographic abnormalities. *Brain* 94, 495-514.

Gilman, S., Marco, L.A. and Ebel, H.C. (1971). Effects of medullary pyramidotomy in the monkey. II. Abnormalities of spindle afferent responses. *Brain* 94, 515-530.

Glaser, G.H. and Higgins, D.C. (1966). Motor stability stretch responses and the cerebellum. *In* "Muscular Afferents and Motor Control. Nobel Symposium I." New York: Wiley. pp. 121-139.

Glassman, R.B. (1971). Recovery following sensori-motor cortical damage: evoked potentials, brain stimulation and motor control. *Exp. Neurol.* 33, 16-29.

Glassman, R.B. (1973). Equipotentiality and sensorimotor function in cats. In Neuroscience Research Program Bulletin "Functional Recovery after Lesions of the Nervous System." In Press.

Glees, P. and Cole, J. (1950). Recovery of skilled motor functions after small repeated lesions of motor cortex in macaque. *J. Neurophysiol.* 13, 137-148.

Goldberger, M.E. (1965). The extrapyramidal systems of the spinal cord: results of combined spinal and cortical lesions in the macaque. *J. Comp. Neurol.* 124, 161-174.

Goldberger, M.E. (1969). The extrapyramidal systems of the spinal cord: II. results of combined pyramidal and extrapyramidal lesions in the macaque. *J. Comp. Neurol.* 135, 1.

Goldberger, M.E. (1972). Restitution of function in the CNS: the pathologic grasp reflex. *Exp. Brain Res.* 15, 79-96.

Goldberger, M.E. (1973a). Restitution of function and collateral sprouting in the cat spinal cord: The deafferented animal. *Anat. Rec.* 175, 329.

Goldberger, M.E. (1973b). Recovery of function and collateral sprouting in cat spinal cord. In Neuroscience Research Program Bulletin "Functional Recovery after Lesions of the Nervous System." In Press.

Goldberger, M.E. and Growden, J.H. (1973). Pattern of recovery following cerebellar deep nuclear lesions in monkeys. *Exp. Neurol.* 39, 307-322.

Goldberger, M.E. and Growden, J.H. (1974). Cerebro-
cortical contribution to recovery from cerebellar
lesions in *Macaca mulatta*. In preparation.

Goldberger, M.E. and Murray, M. (1972). Recovery
of function after partial denervation of the
spinal cord: A behavioral and anatomical study.
Soc. for Neurosciences 2, 157.

Goldberger, M.E. and Taub, E. (Unpublished data).

Goldman, P.S. (1972). Developmental determinants
of cortical plasticity. *Acta Neurobiol. Exp.* 32,
495-511.

Goldman, P.S. (1973). Recovery of function after
CNS lesions in infant monkeys. In Neuroscience
Research Program Bulletin "Functional Recovery
after Lesions of the Nervous System." In Press.

Goodman, D.C., Horel, J.A. (1966). Sprouting of
optic tract projections in the brain stem of the
rat. *J. Comp. Neurol.* 27, 71-88.

Graham-Brown, T. (1914). On the nature of the
fundamental activity of the nervous centres:
together with an analysis of the conditioning of
rhythmic activity in progression, and a theory
of the evolution of function in the nervous
system. *J. Physiol.* 48, 18-46.

Growden, J.H., Chambers, W.W. and Liu, C.N. (1967).
An experimental study of cerebellar dyskinesia
in the Rhesus monkey. *Brain* 90, 603-632.

Guillery, R.W. and Scott, G.L. (1971). Observations
on synaptic patterns in the dorsal lateral
geniculate nucleus of the cat: The C laminae and
the perikaryal synapses. *Exp. Brain Res.* 12, 184-
203.

Guillery, R.W. (1972). Experiments to determine
whether retino geniculate axons can form translaminar collateral sprouts in the dorsal lateral
geniculate nucleus of the cat. *J. Comp. Neurol.*
146, 407-420.

Hepp-Raymond, M.C., Wiesendanger, M., Brumert, M.,
Mackel, A., Unger, R. and Wespi, J. (1970).
Effects of unilateral pyramidotomy on conditioned
finger movement in monkey. *Brain Res.* 24, 544.

Hepp-Raymond, M.C., Mackel, R., Trouche, E. and
Wiesendanger, M. (1972). Effects of pyramidotomy,
motor cortical ablation and deafferentation on a
conditioned finger movement in monkeys.
Experientia 28, 728.

Hines, M. (1937). The "motor" cortex. *Bull. Johns Hopkins Hosp.* 60, 313-336.

Hines, M. (1942). The development and regression of reflexes, postures and progression in the young macaque. *Contrib. Embryol. Carnegie Inst.* 30, 154-217.

Hines, M. (1943). Control of movements by the cerebral cortex in primates. *Biol. Rev.* 18, 1-31.

Hines, M. (1947). The motor areas. *Fed. Proc.* 6, 441-447.

Hines, M. (1949). The precentral motor cortex. Ed. by P.C. Bucy, Univ. of Ill. Press, Urbana. 18, 461-499.

Hines, M. (1960). The control of muscular activity by the central nervous system. *In* G.H. Bourne (Ed.) "The Structure and Function of Muscle. II. Biochemistry and Physiology." New York: Academic Press. ch. 11, pp. 467-516.

Holmes, G. (1922). The Croonian lectures on the clinical symptoms of cerebellar disease and their interpretation. Lancet 100 (1): 1177-1182, 1231-1237: (2): 59-65, 111-115.

Jackson, J.H. (1873). On the anatomical and physiological localization of movements in the brain. Lancet, 1: 84-85, 162-164, 232-234.

Jackson, J.H. (1882). On some implications of dissolution of the nervous system. *Med. Press and Circ.* 2, 411-432.

Jacobsen, C.F., Taylor, F.B., Haslerud, G.M. (1936). Restitution of function after cortical injury in monkeys. *Amer. J. Physiol.* 116, 85-86.

Jacobsen, C.F. (1936). Studies of cerebral function in primates. *Comp. Psychol. Monogr.* 13(3), 1-68.

Kandel, E., Castelucci, V., Pinsker, H. and Kupferman, I. (1970). The role of synaptic plasticity. *In* G. Horn and R.A. Hindle (Eds.) "The Short-term Modification of Behavior in Short-term Changes in Neural Activity and Behavior." C.U.P. 281-322.

Kennard, M.A. (1938). Reorganization of motor function in the cerebral cortex of monkeys deprived of motor and premotor areas in infancy. *J. Neurophysiol.* 1, 477-496.

Kennard, M.A. and Ectors, L. (1938). Forced circling in monkeys following lesions of the frontal lobes. *J. Neurophysiol.* 1, 45-56.

Kennard, M.A. and Fulton, J.F. (1933). The localizing significance of spasticity, reflex grasping and the signs of Babinski and Rossolimo. *Brain* 56, 213-225.

Kerr, F.W.L. (1972). The potential of cervical primary afferents to sprout in the spinal nucleus of V following long term trigeminal denervation. *Brain Res.* 43, 547-560.

Kirk, E.J. and Denny-Brown, D. (1970). Functional variation in dermatomes in the macaque monkey following dorsal root lesions. *J. Comp. Neurol.* 139, 307-320.

Kjcrulf, T.D. and Loeser, J.D. (1973). Neuronal hyperactivity following deafferentation of the lateral cuneate nucleus. *Exper. Neurol.* 39, 70-85.

Kjerulf, T.D., O'Neal, J.T., Calvin, W.H., Loeser, J.D. and Westrum, L.E. (1973). Deafferentation effects in lateral cuneate nucleus of the cat. *Exper. Neurol.* 39, 86-102.

Knapp, H.D., Taub, E. and Berman, A.J. (1958). Effect of deafferentation on a conditioned avoidance response. *Science* 128, 842-843.

Knapp, H.D., Taub, E. and Berman, A.J. (1963). Movements in monkeys with deafferented limbs. *Exp. Neurol.* 7, 305-315.

Kuypers, H.G.J.M. (1958). Some projections from the pericentral cortex to the pons and lower brain stem in monkey and chimpanzee. *J. Comp. Neur.* 110, 221-256.

Kuypers, H.G.J.M. (1960). Central cortical projections to motor and somato-sensory cell groups. *Brain* 83, 161-184.

Kuypers, H.G.J.M. (1964). The descending pathways to the spinal cord, their anatomy and function. In Organization of the Spinal Cord. *Prog. in Brain Res.* 11, 178-203.

Kuypers, H.G.J.M. (1973). Recovery of motor
function in monkeys. Neuroscience research
bulletin "Functional Recovery after Lesions of
the Nervous System." In Press.

Kuypers, H.G.J.M. and Brinkman, J. (1970).
Precentral projections to different parts of the
spinal intermediate zone in the rhesus monkey.
Brain Res. 24, 29-48.

Lashley, K.S. (1924). Studies of cerebral function
in learning. V. The retention of motor habits
after the destruction of the so-called motor
areas in primates. *Arch. Neurol. Psychiat.* 12,
249-276.

Lashley, K.S. (1938). Factors limiting recovery
after central nervous system lesions. *J. Nerv.
Ment. Dis.* 88, 733-755.

Lassek, A.M. (1953). Inactivation of voluntary
motor function following rhizotomy. *J. Neuropath.
Exp. Neurol.* 12, 83-87.

Lassek, A.M. and Moyer, E.K. (1953). An ontogenetic study of motor deficits following dorsal
brachial rhizotomy. *J. Neurophysiol.* 16, 247-251.

Laursen, A.M. (1972). Static and phasic muscle
activity of monkeys with pyramidal lesions.
Brain Res. 40, 125-127.

Lawrence, D.G. and Hopkins, D.A. (1972).
Developmental aspects of pyramidal motor
control in the rhesus monkey. *Brain Res.* 40,
117-119.

Lawrence, D.G. and Kuypers, H.G.J.M. (1968). The
functional organization of the motor system in
the monkey. I. The effects of bilateral
pyramidal lesions. *Brain* 91, 1-14.

Lawrence, D.G. and Kuypers, H.G.J.M. (1968). The
functional organization of the motor system in
the monkey. II. The effects of lesions of the
descending brain-stem pathways. *Brain* 91, 15-36.

Levitt, M., Carreras, M., Liu, C.N. and Chambers,
W.W. (1964). Pyramidal and extrapyramidal
modulation of somatosensory activity in gracile
and cuneate nuclei. *Arch. Ital. Biol.* 102,
197-229.

Leyton, A.S.F. and Sherrington, C.S. (1917). Observations on the excitable cortex of the chimpanzee, orangutan and gorilla. *Quart. J. Exp.
Physiol.* 11, 135-222.

Liu, C.N. and Chambers, W.W. (1958). Intraspinal sprouting of dorsal root axons. *Arch. Neurol. Psychiat.* 79, 46-61.
Liu, C.N. and Chambers, W.W. (1964). An experimental study of the corticospinal tract of the monkey. *J. Comp. Neurol.* 123, 257-284.
Liu, C.N. and Chambers, W.W. (1971). A study of cerebellar dyskinesia in the bilaterally deafferented forelimbs of the monkey *(Macaca mulatta and Macaca speciosa). Acta Neurobiol. Exp.* 31, 263-289.
Liu, C.N. and Chambers, W.W. (1962). Conditioned tactual responses and discrete movements in monkeys with pyramidal lesions. *Fed. Proc.* 21, 367.
Liu, C.N., Chambers, W.W. and McCouch, G.P. (1966). Reflexes in the spinal monkey. *Brain* 89, 349-358.
Loeser, J.D. and Ward, A.A. Jr. (1967). Some effects of deafferentation on neurons of the cat spinal cord. *Arch. Neurol.* 17, 629-636.
Loewy, A.D. (1972). The effects of dorsal root lesions on Clarke neurons in cats of different ages. *J. Comp. Neurol.* 145 (2), 141-164.
Luiciani, L. (1915). "The Hind-brain in Human Physiology." Vol. 3, Chap. 8.
Lund, R.D. and Lund, J.S. (1971). Synaptic adjustment after deafferentation of the superior colliculus of the rat. *Science* 171, 804-807.
Lundberg, A., Voorhoeve, P. (1962). Effects from the pyramidal tract on spinal reflex arcs. *Acta Physiol. Scand.* 56, 201-219.
Luria, A.R. (1963). "Restoration of function after brain injury." New York: The MacMillan Co.
Lynch, G. (1973). The formation of new synaptic connections after brain damage and their possible role in recovery of function. In Neuroscience Research Program Bulletin "Functional Recovery after Lesions of the Nervous System." In Press.
Mathers, L.H. and Chow, K.L. (1973). Anatomical and electrophysiological studies of axonal sprouting in the rabbit visual system. *Anat. Rec.* 175(2), 385.

McCouch, G.P. (1961). Factors in the transition to spasticity. *In* G. Austin (Ed.) "The Spinal Cord." Springfield, Ill.: Thomas. pp. 256-261.

McCouch, G.P., Austin, G.M., Liu, C.N. and Liu, C.Y. (1958). Sprouting as a cause of spasticity. *J. Neurophysiol.* 21, 205-216.

Mettler, F.A. (1944). Physiological consequences and anatomic degenerations following lesions in the primate brain stem. *J. Comp. Neur.* 80, 69-148.

Moore, R.Y., Björklund, A. and Stenevi, U. (1971). Plastic changes in the adrenergic innervation of the rat septal area in responses to denervation. *Brain Res.* 33, 13-35.

Monakow, C. Von., (1914). "Die lokalisation im grosshirm und der abbau der funktion durch kortikale herde." Wiesbaden: J.F. Bergmann.

Mott, F.W. and Sherrington, C.S. (1895). Experiments on the influence of sensory nerves upon movement and nutrition of the limbs. *Proc. Roy. Soc. Lond.* 57, 481-488.

Murray, M. (1973). Restitution of function and collateral sprouting in the cat spinal cord: the hemisected animal. *Anat. Rec.* 175, 395.

O'Neal, J.T. and Westrum, L.E. (1973). The fine structural synaptic organization of the lateral cuneate nucleus. A study of sequential alterations in degeneration. *Brain Res.* 51, 97-125.

Pandya, D.N. and Kuypers, H.G.J.M. (1969). Corticocortical connections in the rhesus monkey. *Brain Res.* 13, 13-36.

Peele, T.L. (1942). Cytoarchitecture of individual parietal area in the monkey and the distribution of the efferent fibers. *J. Comp. Neur.* 77, 693-737.

Patras, J.M. (1967). Cortical, tectal and tegmental fiber connections in the spinal cord of the cat. *Brain Res.* 6, 275-324.

Petras, J.M. (1972). Corticostriate and corticothalamic connections in the chimpanzee. *In* T. Frigyesi, E. Rinvik and M.D. Yahr (Eds.) "Corticothalamic Project and Sensorimotor Activities." New York: Raven Press. pp. 201-216.

Raisman, G. (1969). Neuronal plasticity in the septal nuclei of the adult rat. *Brain Res.* 14, 25-48.

Ralston, H.J. and Chow, K.L. (1973). Synaptic reorganization in the degenerating lateral geniculate nucleus of the rabbit. *J. Comp. Neurol.* 147, 321-350.

Richter, C.P. and Hines, M. (1932). Experimental production of the grasp reflex in adult monkeys by lesions of the frontal lobes. *Am. J. Physiol.* 101, 87-88.

Richter, C.P. and Hines, M. (1934). The production of the grasp reflex in adult macaques by experimental frontal lobe lesions. *Res. Publ. Assoc., Nerv. and Ment. Dis.* 13, 211-224.

Rose, J.E., Malis, L.I., Kruger, L. and Baker, C.P. (1960). Effects of heavy, ionizing mono-energetic particles on the cerebral cortex. *J. Comp. Neurol.* 115, 243-296.

Rosen, I., Asanuma, H. (1972). Peripheral afferent inputs to the forelimb area of the monkey motor cortex: Input-output relations. *Exp. Brain Res.* 14, 257-273.

Rosen, J., Stein, D. and Butters, N. (1971). Recovery of function after serial ablation of prefrontal cortex in the rhesus monkey. *Science* 173, 353-356.

Rushworth, G. and Denny-Brown, D. (1959). The two components of the grasp reflex after ablation of the frontal cortex in monkeys. *J. Neurol. Neurosurg. Psychiat.* 22, 91-98.

Schneider, G.E. (1970). Mechanisms of recovery following lesions of visual cortex or superior colliculus in neonate and adult hamsters. *Brain Behav. Evol.* 3, 295-323.

Schneider, G.E. (1973). Role of sprouting and redirection in recovery. In Neuroscience Research Program Bulletin "Functional Recovery after Lesions of the Nervous System." In Press.

Schwartz, A.S. (1969). Recovery from motor deficit under different motivational conditions. *Physiology and Behavior* 4, 57-60.

Semmes, J. and Chow, K.L. (1955). Motor effects of lesions of pre-central gyrus and of lesions sparing this area in monkey. *Arch. Neurol. and Psychiat.* 73, 546-556.

Seyfforth, H. and Denny-Brown, D. (1948). The grasp reflex and the instinctive grasp reaction. *Brain* 71, 109-183.

Sharpless, S. (1964). Reorganization of function in the nervous system. *Ann. Rev. Physiol.* 26, 357-388.

Sherrington, C.S. (1898). Experiments in the examination of the peripheral distribution of the fibers of the posterior roots of some spinal nerves. *Phil. Trans. Roy. Soc.* 190B, 45-186.

Smith, D.E. (1969). The effect of deafferentation on synaptic development in Clarke's nucleus. *Anat. Rec.* 163, 267.

Smith, D.E. (1973). The location of neurofilaments and microtublules during the postnatal development of Clarke's nucleus in the kitten. *Brain Res.* 55, 41-53.

Smith, W.K. (1944). The frontal eye fields. *In* P.C. Bucy (Ed.) "The Precentral Motor Cortex." Urbana: University of Ill. Press. pp. 307-343.

Spencer, W.A., Thompson, R.F. and Nielson, D.R. (1966). Response decrement of the flexion reflex in the acute spinal cat and transient restoration by strong stimuli. *J. Neurophysiol.* 29, 221-239.

Sperry, R.W. (1947). Effect of crossing nerves to antagonistic limb muscles in the monkey. *Arch. Neurol. Psychiat.* 58, 452-473.

Sprague, J.M. (1967). Discussion of paper by N.T. Zervas. *Trans. Am. Neurol. Assoc.* 92, 29-30.

Stanton, G.B. (1973). Thalamic organization of some dentate and dentate-interpositus projections in *macaca mulatta*. *Anat. Rec.* 175, 450.

Stavraki, G.W. (1961). "Supersensitivity following Lesions of the Nervous System." Toronto, Canada: Univ. of Toronto Press. p. 205.

Taub, E. and Berman, A.J. (1968). Movement and learning in the absence of sensory feedback. *In* "Neuropsychology of Spatially Oriented Behavior." Homewood, Ill.: Dorsey Press. pp. 173-192.

Taub, E., Ellman, S.T. and Berman, A.S. (1966). Deafferentation in monkeys. Effect on conditioned grasp response. *Science* 151, 595-594.

Taub, E., Barro, G., Parker, B. and Gorska, T. (1972a). Utility of a limb following unilateral deafferentation in monkeys. *Soc. for Neuroscience Abstracts* 213.

Taub, E., Perrella, P.N. and Barro, G. (1972b). Behavioral development in monkeys following bilateral forelimb deafferentation on the first day of life. *Trans. Am. Neurol. Assoc.* 97.

Taub, E., Perrella, P. and Barro, G. (1973). Behavioral development after forelimb deafferentation on day of birth in monkeys with and without blinding. *Science* 181, 959-960.

Teuber, H.L. (1973). Historic and prospective view of recovery of function. In Neuroscience Research Program Bulletin "Functional Recovery after Lesions of the Nervous System." In Press.

Tower, S.S. (1940). Pyramidal lesion in the monkey. *Brain* 63, 36-90.

Tower, S.S. (1949). The pyramidal tract. *In* P.C. Bucy (Ed.) "The Precentral Motor Cortex." 2nd edition. Urbana, Univ. of Ill. Press.

Travis, A.M. (1955a). Neurological deficiencies following supplementary motor area lesions in *Macaca mulatta. Brain* 78, 155-173.

Travis, A.M. (1955b). Neurological deficiencies following ablation of the precentral motor area in *Macaca mulatta. Brain* 78, 155-173.

Travis, A.M. and Woolsey, C.N. (1956). Motor performance of monkeys after bilateral partial and total cerebral decortications. *Am. J. Phys. Med.* 35, 273-310.

Twitchell, T.E. (1951). The restoration of motor function following hemiplegia in man. *Brain* 74, 443-480.

Twitchell, T.E. (1954). Sensory factors in purposive movement. *J. Neurophysiol.* 17, 239-252.

Van der Meulen, J.P., Gilman, S. and Denny-Brown, D. (1966). Muscle spindle activity in animals with chronic lesions of the central nervous system. *In* R. Granit (Ed.) "Muscular Afferents and Motor Control." New York: Wiley. pp. 139-151.

Wagley, P.F. (1945). A study of spasticity and paralysis. *Bull. Johns Hopkins Hosp.* 77, 218-273.

Wall, P.D. (1967). The laminar organization of dorsal horn and effects of descending impulses. *J. Physiol. (Lond.)* 188, 403-423.

Ward, A.A. and Kennard, M.A. (1942). Effect of cholinergic drugs on recovery of function following lesions of the central nervous system in monkeys. *Yale J. Biol. Med.* 15, 189-230.

Watson, C.D. (1973). Functional deficits and the pattern of degeneration following lesions of the face motor cortex in *Macaca mulatta*. *Anat. Rec.* 175, 465.

Welch, K. and Stuteville, P. (1958). Experimental production of unilateral neglect in monkeys. *Brain* 81, 341-347.

Welt, C., Aschoff, J.C., Kameda, K. and Brooks, V.B. (1967). Intracortical organization of cat's motorsensory neurons. *In* M.D. Yahr and D.P. Purpura (Eds.) "Neurophysiological Basis of Normal and Abnormal Motor Activities." New York: Raven Press. pp. 255-288.

Wiesel, T.N. and Hubel, D.H. (1963). Effects of visual deprivation on morphology and physiology of cells in the cat's lateral geniculate body. *J. Neurophysiol.* 26, 978-993.

Wiesendanger, M. (1969). The pyramidal tract: recent investigations on its morphology and function. *Ergeb. Physiol.* 61, 72-137.

Woolsey, C.N., Settlage, H., Moyer, D.P., Spencer, W., Hamuy, T.P. and Travis, A.M. (1952). Patterns of localization in precentral and supplementary motor areas and their relation to the concept of a premotor area. *Res. Publ. Assoc. Nerv. and Ment. Dis.* 30, 238-264.

Woolsey, C.N., Gorska, T., Wetzel, A., Erickson, T.C., Earls, F.J. and Allman, J.M. (1972). Complete unilateral section of the pyramidal tract at the medullary level in *Macaca mulatta*. *Brain Res.* 40, 119-125.

Yu, M.G. (1973). Postural effects of cerebellar vermal zone lesions in the Rhesus monkey. *Anat. Rec.* 175, 476.

Zervas, N.T. (1970). Paramedial cerebellar nuclear lesions. *Confinia Neurologica* 32, 114-117.

Zervas, N.T. (1967). Cerebellar dentatectomy in primates and humans. *Trans. Am. Neurol. Assoc.* 92, 27-29.

CHANGES IN DRUG SENSITIVITY AND MECHANISMS OF FUNCTIONAL RECOVERY FOLLOWING BRAIN DAMAGE

Stanley D. Glick
Department of Pharmacology
Mount Sinai School of Medicine

There are generally three reasons why investigators study the effects of drugs and brain damage in the same experimental context. The most common reason is to determine the neuroanatomical "site of action" of the drug. The underlying assumption in such studies is that if one removes (i.e. damages selectively) part of the brain essential for the actions of a particular drug, then that drug will have no effect (i.e. decreased sensitivity) in the appropriately brain-damaged animal. The primary emphasis is to understand the drug; techniques of experimental brain damage are used only as a tool for this purpose.

In a second approach, the effects of brain damage and drugs are frequently compared. If a particular drug mimics the effects of damage to a specific brain structure, then it is usually surmised that the drug normally inhibits the activity of that structure. Moreover, if the drug is known to have fairly specific neuropharmacological actions, it may also be surmised what neurochemical systems mediate the normal functioning of that structure. The strength of such arguments obviously depends upon the extent to which the drug and the lesion can be shown to "mimic" each other as well as on the specificity of the drug and the selectivity of the lesion. Finally, as the major concern of this paper, changes in drug sensitivity after brain damage may be studied as a function of time and/or experience after surgery. Because the extent of recovery following brain damage generally depends upon time and experience variables, it is appropriate that interactions of these variables with drug effects be examined. The primary aim of this approach is to use drugs as a tool to understand physiological mechanisms of recovery which allow the animal to compensate functionally for an initial behavioral deficit. Secondarily, changes in drug sensitivity may reveal residual deficits in the brain-damaged animal otherwise apparent only with very subtle behavioral testing procedures. Lastly, based on recovery mechanisms inferred to occur, an attempt can be made to understand rational ways of using drugs to facilitate recovery. It must be emphasized, however, that the specificity of a drug's neuropharmacological action largely determines its usefulness in studying recovery phenomena. Furthermore, the selectivity with which a lesion interferes with particular neurochemical systems largely determines how readily post-operative drug effects may be interpreted. It is with these considerations and reservations that the following series of experiments were conducted.

A Model of Recovery

Since time after surgery is inherent to many recovery phenomena and since it appeared *a priori* important to study drug effects as a function of time, a time-dependent model of recovery of function was adopted as a heuristic scheme within which to design experiments. The model is based on findings in the peripheral nervous system usually described as evidence for "denervation supersensitivity" (Trendelenburg 1963). A review of denervation supersensitivity is not within the scope of this paper; however, several excellent reviews have been published (e.g. Sharpless 1964; Jasper, Ward and Pope 1969). Briefly, this term refers to the observation that when a post-synaptic membrane is deprived of input, usually by destruction of pre-synaptic neurons (i.e. denervation), post-synaptic sensitivity to chemical stimulation either by the neurochemical normally mediating synaptic transmission or by others, increases (i.e. supersensitivity) as a function of time after denervation. The term "disuse supersensitivity" is occasionally preferred to indicate more generally a reduction of impulse input *per se* whether this be produced by actual neuronal damage or by reversible procedures such as drugs. Sharpless (1969) has discussed these semantic problems in more detail. Because of its wider useage, "denervation" will be employed here

340

to indicate any form of disuse.

As noted, there is ample evidence for denervation supersensitivity in the peripheral nervous system. In the central nervous system, however, where it is more difficult to isolate and investigate specific neuronal pathways, evidence for denervation supersensitivity has been meager and indirectly obtained. For this reason, I refer to denervation supersensitivity as a model when applied to the central nervous system. Findings previously reported by others as well as data to be presented here are either consistent or inconsistent with the model. So far, there has been insufficient direct data to indicate that the model is a phenomenon. For purposes of the present approach, however, the model is heuristically useful in designing experiments and interpreting data.

Acute and Chronic Post-operative Changes in Drug Sensitivity

Before proceeding with the description of data, some preparatory comments concerning what kinds of post-operative drug sensitivity changes might be anticipated are warranted. To simplify matters, drugs will be considered as either agonists or antagonists. Agonists in the present context may include drugs which have direct post-synaptic actions or which act pre-synaptically to release transmitter substances, inhibit re-uptake of transmitter or increase synthesis of transmitter; all such actions would presumably enhance synaptic transmission. Conversely, antagonists may include drugs which directly block post-synaptic receptors or which act pre-synaptically to inhibit release or synthesis of transmitter. Also for conceptual reasons, two general types of brain damage will be considered: (a) damage to a site of drug action or to another site which sends facilitatory input to the site of action and (b) damage to a site which sends inhibitory input to the site of action.

Acute changes: If a site of action of an agonist is removed, partially or totally, it would be expected that an agonist would have a reduced pharmacological effect with the decrease in sensi-

tivity varying directly with the extent of
damage. If an inhibitory input to a site of
action is removed, increased sensitivity to an
agonist would be expected. In the case of an antagonist, acute changes might be more difficult to
interpret. If a site of action is partially
removed, increased sensitivity to an antagonist
might be expected because there would be less
neurons to antagonize. Following total or near-
total removal of such a site, decreased sensitivity to an antagonist might occur because the drug
could produce no further effect than the lesion
itself produced (i.e. if the lesion produces a
maximal or ceiling effect by itself). Removal of
an inhibitory input should result in decreased
sensitivity to an antagonist.

Chronic Changes: In this section reference is
made to changes occurring as a function of
increasing time after surgery. Only such changes
that would be expected on the basis of denervation
supersensitivity will be mentioned. If the drug is
an agonist and its site of action (or facilitatory
input) is partially damaged, sensitivity to the
drug should gradually return to normal and then
possibly increase above normal as the post-
operative interval increases. This would be
expected to the extent that supersensitivity of
remaining, but partially denervated, neurons
developed. Furthermore, the time-course of such
effects would be expected to parallel the time-
course of behavioral recovery after the lesion; to
the extent that recovery occurs, increasing
sensitivity to an agonist should also occur. If,
however, a site of action is totally removed, the
acutely decreased sensitivity to an agonist should
persist chronically and behavioral recovery should
be minimal. The underlying assumption in this
interpretation is that the same neuronal changes
specified by denervation supersensitivity mediate
both recovery of function and changes in drug
sensitivity. If inhibitory input to a site of
action is removed, exactly opposite chronic
changes in sensitivity to an agonist would be
expected, i.e. gradual return to normal and then
decrease below normal to the extent that behavioral
recovery occurs.

If the drug is an antagonist and its site of

action is partially damaged, sensitivity to the drug should return to normal and then possibly decrease below normal at longer post-operative intervals. This again presupposes that recovery occurs and that a supersensitive synapse is less sensitive to being blocked (Friedman *et al.* 1969). If the lesion is large but some recovery does occur, acutely decreased sensitivity to an antagonist might be expected to decrease further. Again, if behavioral recovery does not occur, acute changes would be expected to persist chronically. Opposite chronic changes should follow removal of inhibitory input, i.e. gradual return to normal and then possibly increase above normal.

An interpretative example: At this point I would like to mention one example of how the supersensitivity model may be applicable to apparently discrepant data. Several studies (Cole 1973) have attempted to determine the site of action of amphetamine's anorexic effect. Brobeck *et al.* (1956) suggested that the anorexic effect of amphetamine might be due to direct stimulation of the hypothalamic satiety center, since they recorded increased electrical activity from the ventromedial hypothalamus following amphetamine administration. This hypothesis was supported by Sharp *et al.* (1962) who reported that ventromedial lesions made cats less sensitive to the anorexic effect of amphetamine but refuted by the findings of Stowe and Miller (1957), Epstein (1959) and Reynolds (1959) who all reported that ventromedial hypothalamic lesions made rats hypersensitive to amphetamine anorexia. Kennedy and Mitra (1963) reported that rats with ventromedial hypothalamic lesions were less sensitive to the anorexic action of amphetamine during the early period of hypothalamic hyperphagia, whereas these same rats were more sensitive to the anorexic effect of amphetamine during the later static phase of hypothalamic obesity and also concluded that the ventromedial hypothalamus was not a site mediating amphetamine anorexia. Subsequently Carlisle (1964) reported that rats which had recovered from the aphagia and adipsia following lateral hypothalamic lesions were less sensitive to the anorexic effect of amphetamine and suggested that the lateral

343

hypothalamus was amphetamine's site of anorexic action. Consistent with Carlisle's view were the findings that electrical stimulation of the lateral hypothalamus can antagonize amphetamine-induced anorexia (Thode and Carlisle 1968) and that amphetamine can antagonize "forced eating" by lateral hypothalamic stimulation (Stark and Totty 1967). To maintain that the lateral hypothalamus is the site of amphetamine anorexia it must also be supposed that amphetamine inhibits this area. However, amphetamine is usually presumed to act agonistically by release of catecholamines (norepinephrine and dopamine) and/or by inhibition of catecholamine reuptake (Stein 1964; Taylor and Snyder 1970) and in most studies (Grossman 1962; Leibowitz 1971; Margules 1972) direct application of norepinephrine to the lateral hypothalamus elicits feeding. The latter findings suggest that amphetamine should induce feeding. On the basis of neurochemical postulations, several attempts have been made to reconcile these discrepancies. I should now like to make a renewed attempt based on time factors involved in the lesion studies. If it is assumed that amphetamine primarily acts on the ventromedial hypothalamus, as Brobeck et al. (1956) suggested, then all of the changes in anorexic sensitivity following lesions may be consistent with denervation supersensitivity. It would be expected that early after ventromedial hypothalamic lesions, sensitivity to amphetamine would decrease but that sensitivity would increase later -- this is exactly what Kennedy and Mitra (1963) reported; and such time-dependent changes along with variations in lesion size could readily account for the differences between the studies of Sharp et al. (1962) and Stowe and Miller (1957), Epstein (1959) and Reynolds (1959). Furthermore, if the ventromedial and lateral hypothalamus have reciprocally inhibitory connections, as several studies (Arees and Mayer 1967; Albert and Storlien 1969; Gold 1970) indicate, then recovered (i.e. chronic) lateral hypothalamic rats should be either normally sensitive or less sensitive to amphetamine and the latter was reported by Carlisle (1964). An agonistic action of amphetamine in the ventromedial hypothalamus would also be consistent with the findings of Thode and Carlisle

344

(1968) and Stark and Totty (1967). Although this interpretation is entirely hypothetical, it does tend to make intelligible a fair amount of discrepant data and indicate the importance of time factors when analyzing lesion-drug interactions.

Chronic Drug Sensitivity Changes in Frontal Monkeys

Numerous investigators have observed that monkeys with bilateral ablations of dorsolateral frontal cortex show deficits in various kinds of delayed response tests (Warren and Akert 1964). Some controversy still prevails with respect to the nature of such deficits, what areas of cortex are most critical and the extent to which recovery occurs. No attempt is made here to address these points of contention. In an initial series of studies (Glick and Jarvik 1970), this syndrome was only used to demonstrate selective changes in drug sensitivity when the brain-damaged rhesus monkey had resumed apparently "normal" function.

The particular version of delayed-response used was an automated matching-to-sample test (Glick and Jarvik 1970). Monkeys were first required to touch a center "dummy" tube after a visual-display unit above the tube projected a green or red color (sample stimulus). After a delay, two other visual-display units, situated at either side of the first unit, projected the comparison stimuli (one red, the other green). The monkey was required to match one of the side comparison stimuli with the color of the sample stimulus by touching a tube under the correct stimulus in order to receive a water reward. On each trial one of five delay conditions was used: simultaneous, 0, 2, 8 and 32 seconds. For the simultaneous condition, the sample and comparison stimuli were presented together. All monkeys were tested at the same time 7 days per week for 16 hr. per day, during which each animal received 1920 trials.

Although initially impaired following surgery, the delayed matching performance of a group (N=4) of frontal monkeys gradually recovered to preoperative levels during five weeks of postoperative testing. Various doses of d-amphetamine and scopolamine were then administered to the frontal

monkeys and to a group of unoperated control
monkeys. Both drugs impaired the matching performance of the control monkeys. However, only
scopolamine impaired the matching performance of
the frontal monkeys (Figure 1). This decreased
amphetamine sensitivity in the frontal monkeys
was somewhat task-specific: depression of rates of
responding by both drugs occurred similarly in
frontal and normal monkeys. Further drug studies
indicated the extent of pharmacological specificity (Glick and Jarvik 1970). Frontal monkeys were
less sensitive to the effect of chlorpromazine and
alpha-methyl-dopa but as sensitive as normal
monkeys to the effects of LSD, physostigmine,
mecamylamine and pentobarbital. The mechanisms of
actions of chlorpromazine and alpha-methyl-dopa
are usually presumed to involve catecholamines
whereas LSD is usually associated with serotonin,
physostigmine and mecamylamine with acetylcholine
and pentobarbital is probably nonspecific. These
data then suggested that frontal cortical lesions
have a selective influence on neuroanatomical
pathways containing catecholamines.

Studies in Frontal Rats

At the time we observed decreased amphetamine
sensitivity in frontal monkeys, other studies had
showed increased amphetamine sensitivity in
frontal rats (Adler 1961; Lynch, Ballantine and
Campbell 1969). Because the monkey experiments
involved a complex behavior whereas the rat
experiments involved measurement of locomotor
activity, two experiments were conducted to determine if species was a factor. The effect of
d-amphetamine on the locomotor activity of frontal
monkeys was determined; the frontal monkeys, like
frontal rats, were hypersensitive to amphetamine's
effect on activity (Glick and Jarvik, unpublished).
Frontal rats were next trained in a spatial
discrimination task; the frontal rats learned
slower than the control rats. D-amphetamine was
administered when the performance levels of
frontal and control rats were similar (Glick
1971); the frontal rats were less sensitive to
impairment of spatial discrimination by amphetamine (Figure 2). Thus, both frontal monkeys and

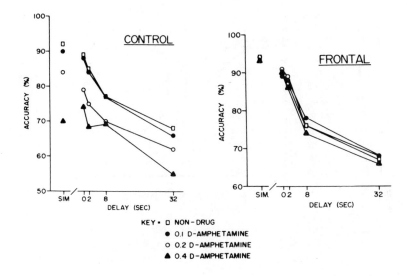

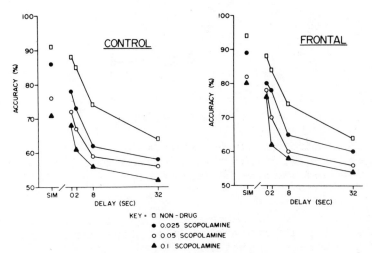

Figure 1. Effects of d-amphetamine and scopolamine on matching performance of normal (control) and recovered frontal monkeys. Results shown are for first two hours after drug administration. (From Glick and Jarvik 1970).

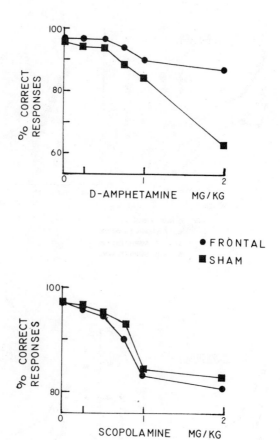

Figure 2. Effects of d-amphetamine and scopolamine on spatial discrimination performance in sham-operated and recovered frontal rats (Data derived from Glick 1971).

frontal rats could show either hyposensitivity or hypersensitivity to amphetamine depending upon the behavioral situation.

The post-operative time-course of amphetamine hypersensitivity in frontal rats was somewhat controversial. Adler (1961) showed that hypersensitivity of frontal rats to amphetamine-induced hyperactivity increased with increasing time after surgery. However, Lynch et al. (1969) found that amphetamine hypersensitivity in frontal rats gradually disappeared over a 40-day post-operative period. In an initial attempt to decide between these two trends, I (Glick 1970) reported data (Figure 3) compatible with Adler's. At about the

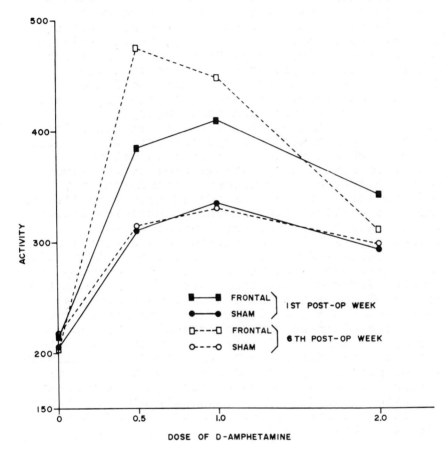

Figure 3. Effects of d-amphetamine (mg/kg) on locomotor activity (photocell counts) in sham-operated and frontal rats during the first and sixth postoperative weeks (From Glick 1970).

same time, Iversen (1971a; 1971b) reported that frontal rats were hypersensitive to amphetamine when activity testing was conducted after the third post-operative week as well as during the second and fifth post-operative months. But Lynch *et al.* (1971) then confirmed their earlier findings. The most consistent difference between

studies showing decreasing versus increasing
amphetamine hypersensitivity was the use of rats
well-habituated to their test cages prior to drug
administration versus rats with no prior habituation period, respectively. In a subsequent
experiment, I (1972) found that the habituation
variable was, in all probability, responsible for
the apparent controversy. When tested one month
after surgery, amphetamine hypersensitivity in
frontal rats was minimal if a long period of
habituation preceded testing with the drug (Table
1). This interaction with habituation was
partially attributed to a testing artifact. That
is, the apparatuses used for the activity studies
record both and do not discriminate between
normal locomotor and abnormal stereotyped movements. Different neurochemical mechanisms may
mediate these different kinds of movements (Taylor
and Snyder 1970). Since normal locomotion occurs
in response to a novel environment whereas
stereotypy is solely a drug-induced phenomenon
and probably independent of environmental stimuli,
it was reasoned that habituation, by reducing
novelty-induced locomotion, would alter the ratio
of normal locomotor and stereotyped responses
recorded as total activity after amphetamine. On
the basis of these and other results showing
directly that frontal rats are hypersensitive to
amphetamine-induced stereotypy (Iverson, Wilkinson
and Simpson 1971), it was suggested that frontal
cortical lesions denervate neurochemical systems
involved in both kinds of activity and that time-
dependent supersensitivity occurs in both cases
(Glick 1972).

Studies in Frontal Mice

Thus far, changes in sensitivity of frontal
animals to amphetamine have been cited in two
contexts: (1) The drug had been administered to
recovered frontal animals that had compensated
for an initial performance deficit with prolonged
practice (i.e. recovery as a result of use) and
(2) the drug had been administered to frontal
animals showing no postoperative deficit in
locomotor activity under particular environmental
conditions (in other situations frontal animals

Table 1

Effect of Habituation on d-Amphetamine (1.0 mg/kg)-
induced Hyperactivity[‡]

Mean Activity (photocell
counts)

		Frontal	Sham
Session 1:	d-amphetamine	4270**	3489
Session 2:	control	2649	2661
	d-amphetamine	3777***	2108
Session 3:	control	242	194
	d-amphetamine	1235*	945

*, **, *** = significantly more than sham at
$p < .05$, .01 and .001, respectively ($\underline{t}$ test).

‡ In session 1, rats were first placed in the
activity apparatus 15 min. after drug administration and activity was recorded for 30 min. In
session 2, rats were placed in the activity
apparatus for 30 min. prior to drug administration;
control value = 30 min. activity prior to drug
administration, drug value = 30 min. activity
15-45 min. after drug administration. In session
3, rats were placed in the activity apparatus for
3 hr. prior to drug administration; control
and drug values represent 30 min. pre-drug and
30 min. (15-45 min.) post-drug activity (from
Glick 1972).

---

may be hyperactive). Hyposensitivity to amphetamine
had been observed in the first paradigm and hypersensitivity in the second paradigm. Studies with
frontal mice were designed to evaluate the role
of recovery *per se* in producing this differential
sensitivity.

A model of time-dependent recovery was
established for frontal mice (Glick, Nakamura and
Jarvik 1971). Mice with frontal pole ablations

were postoperatively trained in a one-trial
passive avoidance test. Frontal mice showed a
deficit in passive avoidance learning which
recovered as a function of time within three weeks;
mice trained at 1, 4 or 10 days after surgery were
impaired in passive avoidance learning whereas
other mice trained at 19 days after surgery learned
normally. D-amphetamine was administered to frontal
and control mice prior to training at these
various postoperative intervals. The drug impaired
learning of control mice at all times; frontal
mice were found to become increasingly hyposensitive to this effect of amphetamine with increasing
time after surgery such that maximal hyposensitivity was observed when recovery was maximal. The
specificity of amphetamine's effect was again
confirmed by administering scopolamine; frontal
mice showed no change in sensitivity to
scopolamine at any time (Figure 4). D-amphetamine
was also administered to frontal mice tested on a
measure of locomotor activity at the same post-
operative intervals. As with rats and monkeys,
frontal mice were hypersensitive to enhancement
of locomotor activity by amphetamine. It therefore
appeared that when recovery of function occurred,
whether due to time alone or to use, frontal
animals became hyposensitive to amphetamine. When
recovery was not obvious or perhaps not essential
for adaptation to a particular environment,
frontal animals became hypersensitive to amphetamine. Alternatively, the results of the prior
activity studies with frontal rats, indicating
that frontal cortical lesions may affect two
different neurochemical systems, suggest that
amphetamine hyposensitivity in frontal rats may
be another artifactual consequence of interactions
between different systems. That is, amphetamine
hypersensitivity in frontal rats has been observed
when, in normal animals, amphetamine facilitates or
enhances some behavior whereas amphetamine hyposensitivity has been observed when amphetamine
normally impairs or depresses some behavior. If it
is assumed that amphetamine has two discrete
actions, perhaps via norepinephrine and dopamine
(Taylor and Snyder 1970), which respectively
facilitate and impair behavioral parameters (i.e.
producing the usual inverted U dose-response

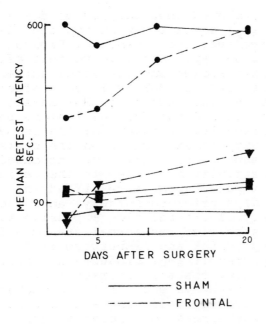

Figure 4. Effects of d-amphetamine and scopolamine on passive avoidance learning in sham-operated and frontal mice as a function of time after surgery (non-drug and d-amphetamine data derived from Glick, Nakamura and Jarvik 1971).

curve, Glick and Miller 1971) and if frontal cortical lesions result in more supersensitivity to the facilitatory action than to the depressant action, then hyposensitivity to a depressant effect of amphetamine in frontal animals might be expected. Figure 5 illustrates this possibility as a dose-response phenomenon.

Additional data consistent with the idea that recovery of function following frontal lesions in mice involves denervation supersensitivity was obtained with the use of alpha-methyl-para-tyrosine ($_a$MpT), a drug which inhibits the enzyme tyrosine hydroxlase thereby inhibiting synthesis of both norepinephrine and dopamine.

Pilot studies showed that particular doses and regimens of $_a$M$_p$T administration impaired learning of the passive avoidance response. Frontal mice were found to be hypersensitive to this effect of $_a$M$_p$T when administered one day after surgery but normally sensitive to $_a$M$_p$T by 22 days after surgery. The initial increased $_a$M$_p$T sensitivity would be expected if the frontal lesions partially denervate catecholamine pathways; the recovery of $_a$M$_p$T sensitivity is explicable on the basis of denervation supersensitivity i.e. increased post-synaptic sensitivity might negate the decrease in presynaptic input. Furthermore, if administered for several days prior to surgery, $_a$M$_p$T facili-tated recovery of frontal mice - passive avoidance learning of such mice was normal even one day after surgery (Glick and Zimmerberg 1972). This would be expected if $_a$M$_p$T produced a functional denervation (i.e. disuse) supersensitivity of catecholamine pathways such that the mechanism involved in recovery following a neuroanatomical denervation was already developed at the time of surgery.

Figure 5. Hypothetical changes in sensitivity to amphetamine following a brain lesion (indicated by arrow). The kind of change shown in (a) would occur if the lesion enhanced sensitivity to all actions of amphetamine, i.e. the entire dose-response curve is shifted to the left. The kind of change shown in (b) would occur if the lesion only enhanced sensitivity to a facilitatory action of amphetamine, i.e. the entire dose-response curve is shifted higher. The kind of change shown in (c) is a combination of (a) and (b), i.e. increased sensitivity to all actions but more so to a facilitatory action. In both (b) and (c), at particular doses on the rising and falling phases of the curve, it might be concluded that the lesion either increased sensitivity to a facilita-tory effect or decreased sensitivity to a depressant effect, respectively. At very high doses in (c), it might be concluded that the lesion produced no change in drug sensitivity. Note the resemblance of (c) to the sixth week data in Figure 3 (From Glick and Marsanico, in press).

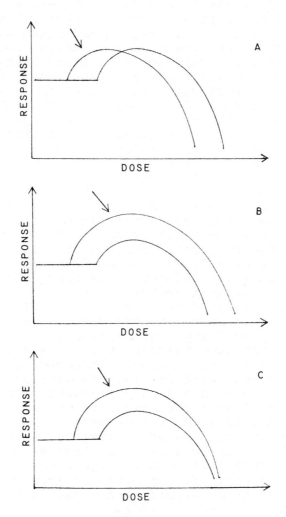

Lateral Hypothalamic Recovery

As indicated in the last experiment with frontal mice, if recovery of function involves denervation supersensitivity, it should be possible to facilitate recovery after lesion by administering treatments pre-operatively which make the system(s) responsible for recovery supersensitive at the time of surgery. It is well known that bilateral lesions of the lateral hypothalamus in the rat produce a syndrome of

aphagia and adipsia terminating in death unless
such rats are kept alive by intragastric tube
feedings. If initially maintained alive with i.g.
tube feedings, recovery of spontaneous feeding
may eventually occur (Teitelbaum and Epstein
1962). Several kinds of data have implicated an
important role of catecholamines both in feeding
behavior (Grossman 1962; Leibowitz 1971; Margules
1972) and in recovery following LH lesions (Berger,
Wise and Stein 1971; Zigmond and Stricker 1972).
According to the present denervation supersensitivity model of recovery of function, recovery
following LH lesions might be due to supersensitivity of remaining neurons involved in feeding to
remaining catecholaminergic inputs. It would also
be predicted that less severe feeding deficits
following lesions in other areas of the brain
would be due to partial removal of such catecholaminergic inputs (i.e. partial denervation of
neurons primarily related to feeding). For example,
ablation of frontal cortex in the rat results in
progressive loss of body weight for 3-4 days
followed by recovery and the changes in
sensitivity to d-amphetamine described earlier
indicate that catecholaminergic systems have been
affected by frontal lesions. It seemed possible
that if frontal cortical lesions were performed
sometime before lateral hypothalamic lesions then
recovery following the latter might be facilitated
because remaining LH neurons were already supersensitive at the time of LH surgery. Exactly this
result (Table 2) occurred when frontal cortical
ablations were performed 30 days prior to LH
lesions; no facilitation occurred when frontal
and LH lesions were performed simultaneously
(Glick and Greenstein 1972).
Another way of presumably reducing
catecholaminergic input to systems involved in
feeding would be to administer a drug which interferes with synthesis of catecholamines.
Accordingly, alpha-methyl-para-tyrosine was
administered to rats for three days prior to LH
surgery; drug administration was discontinued one
day prior to surgery. It was thought that by
administering aM_pT prior to surgery, the neurons
subserving recovery should be sufficiently
supersensitive sooner after surgery for recovery

356

Table 2

Mean Post-operative Weight Changes
(% of pre-operative weight)
Following Lateral Hypothalamic Lesions‡

Groups*

Days after LH surgery	LH	SFC-LH	10 day FC-LH	30 day FC-LH	Sham
1	87.7	87.1	89.8	89.9	99.2
2.	81.3	80.9	85.9	87.7	101.8
3	75.4	76.3	82.5**	85.7	103.8
4	70.8	72.5	78.7**	85.8	105.6
5	65.8	68.2	74.7**	86.2	108.1
6		64.8	70.5**	88.9	110.0
7			66.4	90.4	111.3
8				93.8	111.2
9				94.7	111.8
10				96.1	114.1

*LH-lateral hypothalamus, SFC=simultaneous frontal cortical; group means computed only for days on which all rats of a group still surviving.

**significantly greater than LH or SFC-LH at $p < .05$ (t test); all 30 day FC-LH rats recovered; one 10 day FC-LH rat recovered but is not included in data on table.

‡from Glick and Greenstein 1972.

357

to occur. Termination of drug treatment before surgery should allow intact inputs remaining after surgery to become functional again. Exactly this result (Table 3) occurred following doses of $aMpT$ which were effective in partially depleting the brain of catecholamines (Glick, Greenstein and Zimmerberg 1972). If $aMpT$ were administered chronically after surgery, exacerbation of the LH syndrome and perhaps an earlier death might be anticipated. Indeed, rats administered $aMpT$ (100 mg/kg twice a day) for 3 days after LH surgery lost weight at a faster rate and died sooner (5.4 vs. 7.2 days) than comparable saline-treated rats; in this case, $aMpT$ appeared to enhance catabolic changes induced by LH lesions. Some indication that the facilitatory effect of pre-operative $aMpT$ treatment on LH recovery was specific to catecholamines was obtained by administering para-chloro-phenyl-alanine (300-500 mg/kg) three days prior to LH surgery. $pCpA$, which primarily interferes with serotonin synthesis but which may also inhibit catecholamine synthesis to a lesser extent, had no effect on LH recovery suggesting that at least serotonin was not directly involved.

Thus far, when mentioning neurochemical correlates of feeding, I have purposely referred to norepinephrine and dopamine together as "catecholamines." This is because recent data have indicated considerable ambiguity with regard to which neuroanatomical structures and pathways and which neurochemicals are involved in the LH syndrome. The LH syndrome has been reported to occur following not only lesions of the lateral hypothalamus but also following bilateral sub-stantia nigra lesions or bilateral caudate lesions (Ungerstedt 1971). Since LH lesions typically encroach upon the medial internal capsule through which nigro-striatal fibers course, the possibility has been raised that the LH syndrome is really a nigro-striatal syndrome (Ungerstedt 1971). However, it has also been observed that lesions specifically avoiding nigro-striatal fibers will still produce the LH syndrome (Teitelbaum, personal communication). The neurochemical data have been just as confusing – although feeding elicited by intracerebral chemical stimulation occurs with

Table 3

Mean Post-operative Weight Changes
(% of pre-operative weight)
Following Lateral Hypothalamic Lesions‡

Days after Surgery	Groups *				
	LH-Sal	LH-aMT 10	LH-aMT 75	LH-aMT 100	Sham
1	86.8	86.2	89.3	87.5	99.2
2	80.9	80.4	87.3	85.2	101.8
3	75.0	74.6	85.9	83.6	103.8
4	70.1	69.7	83.6	84.1	105.6
5	65.2	65.0	81.8	88.7	108.1
6	61.4	61.6	79.8	90.5	110.0
7		58.6	80.1	92.2	111.3
8			82.3	95.3	111.2
9			84.4	95.6	111.8
10			85.9	96.0	114.1

*LH = lateral hypothalamus, Sal = saline,
aMT = α-methyl-p-tyrosine methyl ester
hydrochloride followed by dosage (mg/kg).
All LH-aMT 75 and LH-aMT 100 rats recovered.
Group means were computed only for days on
which all rats of a group were still
surviving.

‡ from Glick, Greenstein and Zimmerberg 1972.

norepinephrine but not with dopamine (Berger, Wise and Stein 1973), symptoms of the LH syndrome are correlated better with depletion of brain dopamine than with depletion of brain norepinephrine (Zigmond and Stricker 1973). The $_aM_pT$ results just cited are consistent with either interpretation

Cortical Modulation of Nigro-striatal Function

The facilitation of LH recovery by prior frontal cortical lesions together with the fore-going considerations implicating a role of striatal dopamine in the LH syndrome suggested that frontal cortex in the rat might be influencing the activity of the striatum more than that of the lateral hypothalamus. An attempt was therefore made to investigate a cortical-striatal relationship more directly. To do this, a behavioral phenomenon reportedly specific for nigro-striatal function was utilized (Crow 1971). Following unilateral lesions of the substantia nigra rats turn in circles or rotate towards the side of the lesion. When after a few days such rats recover from this tendency to rotate spontaneously, administration of amphetamine will re-elicit this ipsilateral rotational behavior (Ungerstedt 1971; Christie and Crow 1971). Histofluorescent data (Ungerstedt 1971) have indicated that the basis for this rotational behavior is an imbalance between the two dopamin-ergic systems ipsilateral and contralateral to the lesion, respectively. Amphetamine, by releasing dopamine from nigral input, apparently stimulates the intact nigro-striatal system and enhances the imbalance. Apomorphine, which directly stimulates dopaminergic receptors, increasingly elicits contralateral rotation with increasing time after surgery; these last data have been interpreted to indicate that time-dependent supersensitivity of the denervated striatum occurs such that apomorphine's effect is increasingly greater on the denervated striatum (Ungerstedt 1971). Although the only described dopaminergic input to the striatum of the rat ascends from the substantia nigra (Ungerstedt 1971), there has also been described a descending system of fibers originating in the rostral frontal cortex and distributing through the caudate and pallidum (Knook 1966). This latter system, though not dopaminergic, may modulate dopaminergic functions of the striatum.

Following unilateral ablation of frontal cortex, rats were tested for rotational behavior after saline or 5 mg/kg of d-amphetamine at various times after surgery. Such behavior was measured in an automated apparatus designed after one described by Ungerstedt (1971). At one day after surgery, unilateral frontal rats rotated ipsilaterally - this occurred after saline and was potentiated by amphetamine. By 3 days after surgery, frontal rats showed no significant tendency to rotate spontaneously after saline; however, amphetamine induced ipsilateral rotation at that time as well as at 7 days after surgery. At 30 days after surgery, amphetamine also induced rotation of unilateral frontal rats but the direction of rotation changed from ipsilateral to contralateral, i.e. such rats now rotated towards the side opposite the lesion (Figure 6). The spontaneous ipsilateral rotation of rats with unilateral frontal lesions at 1 day after surgery indicates a decrease in dopaminergic function of the ipsilateral striatum. Initially, amphetamine presumably potantiates the imbalance by predominantly stimulating the intact striatum. The disappearance of spontaneous rotation as well as the emergence of amphetamine-induced contralateral rotation both suggest that the ipsilateral striatum, as a result of a partial denervation, becomes supersensitive to remaining nigral input (Glick and Greenstein 1974).

Some further indication that frontal cortex influences the nigro-striatal system was obtained by making simultaneous unilateral lesions of the substantia nigra and frontal cortex. When such lesions were made contralateral to each other, there was no initial spontaneous rotational behavior one day after surgery and d-amphetamine (5 mg/kg) failed to elicit any rotation. When such lesions were made ipsilateral to each other, initial ipsilateral rotation was greater than that following either lesion alone and the potentiation of this effect by d-amphetamine was also greater.

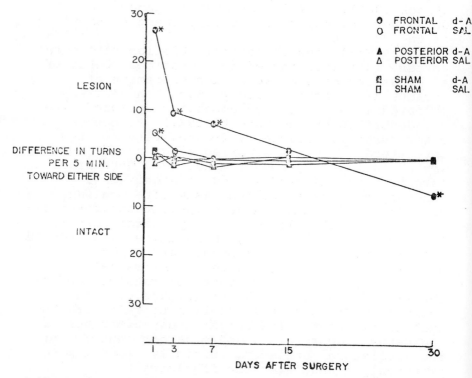

Figure 6. *Time-dependent changes in spontaneous (SALine) and d-amphetamine-induced (d-A) rotational behavior following unilateral frontal cortical, posterior cortical or sham lesions in rats; asterisks indicate significant differences between ipsilateral and contralateral turns. (From Glick and Greenstein 1973).*

Correlation of Changes in Drug Sensitivity with Recovery

In much of the preceding work, time-dependent changes in drug sensitivity after brain damage have been correlated with and/or have been used as an index of recovery of function. However, thus far no attempt had been made to see if instances of non-recovery had pharmacological correlates. Such correlates were sought in an attempt to further substantiate the rationale relating drug sensitivities to recovery. The

362

opportunity to administer drugs in a non-recovery
paradigm presented itself during a study concerned
with comparative effects of caudate, hippocampal
and septal lesions on passive avoidance learning
in mice. When trained one day after surgery and
retested a day later, mice with either of the
three lesions (bilateral) showed comparable
learning deficits. Other groups of mice with
similar lesions were trained either at 1 week or
at 1 month after surgery. Whereas mice with
caudate lesions showed time-dependent recovery
of function, mice with either hippocampal or
septal lesions had persistent and undiminished
passive avoidance deficits 1 month after surgery.
Other groups of mice were then trained at 1 day or
1 month after surgery and administered either
d-amphetamine (5 mg/kg) or scopolamine (1 mg/kg)
15 min. prior to training (Glick, Marsanico and
Greenstein 1974). In normal mice, both drugs
impair passive avoidance learning. At 1 day after
surgery, each kind of lesion decreased sensitivity
to d-amphetamine and increased sensitivity to
scopolamine (Table 4). At 1 month after surgery,
the effects of septal and hippocampal lesions on
drug sensitivities were the same as at 1 day
after surgery; in contrast, caudate lesions now
increased sensitivity to d-amphetamine and
decreased sensitivity to scopolamine. Time
dependent variations in drug sensitivity from the
initial change only occurred, therefore, in brain-
damaged mice showing time-dependent recovery of
function.

The kinds of drug sensitivity changes following
these lesions are readily explicable. If it is
assumed, as it usually is, that amphetamine's
actions are primarily agonistic (i.e. indirectly
by release of catecholamines or by inhibition of
pre-synaptic re-uptake) and that scopolamine's
action is primarily antagonistic (i.e. post-
synaptic blockade of muscarinic cholinergic
receptors) then a lesion which destroys part of
the site of action(s) of these drugs should
result in decreased sensitivity to d-amphetamine
and increased sensitivity to scopolamine.
Decreased sensitivity to d-amphetamine should
occur because there would be less neurons to
excite and consequently less action of the drug.

Table 4

Effects of Bilateral Caudate, Hippocampal or Septal
Lesions on Passive Avoidance Learning at 1 day or 1
month After Surgery (median retest latencies in
sec.) and Interaction with d-Amphetamine or
Scopolamine (% of non-drug retention)‡

1 Day After Surgery

	Lesion effect	d-Amphetamine	Scopolamine
Caudate	177.4	38.3%	12.5%
Hippocampal	158.2	34.5%	15.9%
Septal	148.4	52.2%	15.2%
Sham	584.5	21.8%	26.4%

1 Month After Surgery

	Lesion effect	d-Amphetamine	Scopolamine
Caudate	489.7*	16.7%	32.4%
Hippocampal	120.1	61.6%	17.0%
Septal	111.8	63.3%	18.3%
Sham	588.5	28.4%	24.5%

*only effect not significantly different from
sham.

‡ data derived from Glick, Marsanico and
  Greenstein, in press.

Increased sensitivity to scopolamine might be
expected because the lesion and drug should
summate, i.e. there would be less neurons to
block. These changes would all be acute. If
recovery of function occurred and if responsiveness to drugs is another correlate of such
recovery, then further changes in drug sensitivity
at later post-operative intervals would be
anticipated. The later changes in mice with
caudate lesions are consistent with a denervation
supersensitivity model of recovery; if the caudate
lesions partially denervate a system recovering
via supersensitivity, then this recovered system
should be supersensitive to an agonist,
d-amphetamine, but less sensitive to an antagonist,
scopolamine.

Mechanisms of Functional Recovery

As set forth ·in the introduction, the foregoing
data have been interpreted as consistent with a
denervation supersensitivity model. The model has
been useful in designing interesting experiments
and in predicting and interpreting complex
results. However, it might be again acknowledged
that these results provide only minimal evidence
that denervation supersensitivity is actually the
mechanism operative in recovery of function. For
example, with the exception of $_aM_pT$-facilitated
recovery, all of these results can be interpreted
as indicative of sprouting. That is, as shown in
other systems (Moore, Björklund and Stenevi 1971),
removal of one input to a specific brain area may
induce sprouting of other intact inputs to the
same area. Since sprouting is also a time-
dependent phenomenon, time-dependent recovery
results would also be explicable on this basis.
However, as sprouting appears to be a response
to degenerating terminals (Wall and Egger 1971),
this mechanism would not appear to be involved in
facilitation of recovery by drugs (i.e. $_aM_pT$). It
should be noted that in the peripheral nervous
system recovery of function following neural
lesions may involve sequentially denervation
supersensitivity, sprouting concomitant with
decreased supersensitivity and later regeneration.
It is certainly possible that at least the first

two of these sequential phenomena occur in the central nervous system. That is, denervation supersensitivity and sprouting may mediate early and later recovery of function, respectively.

In collaboration with Barbara Travis, a graduate student, and Dr. Sherwin Wilk, we have been attempting to find more direct neurochemical evidence indicative of recovery mechanisms. Because of my preceding behavioral work with frontal cortical ablations, we have assayed the hypothalamus for norepinephrine and the striatum for dopamine at several intervals after frontal lesions in rats. We have found that frontal lesions produce approximately a 20% depletion of hypothalamic norepinephrine which is maximal at 7 days after surgery; at 14 days after surgery and thereafter, hypothalamic norepinephrine levels have returned to normal. In contrast, no depletion but rather an increase in striatal dopamine levels above normal is first significant at 14 days after surgery and is larger (30%) at 28 days after surgery. The early depletion of hypothalamic norepinephrine is explicable if ablation of frontal cortex partially removes some hypothalamic input. The return to normal of hypothalamic norepinephrine and the increase in striatal dopamine are more intriguing. First, it should be noted that both of these latter phenomena occur at a time (14 days after surgery) when frontal rats have just about recovered from early feeding deficits (Glick 1971; Glick and Greenstein 1973). The major question is then what mechanism(s) underlie these increasing catecholamine levels. Sprouting would appear to be the simplest explanation. In the case of the hypothalamus, frontal lesions might partially remove noradrenergic input such that remaining noradrenergic input would sprout. In the case of the striatum, frontal lesions might remove non-dopaminergic input such remaining dopaminergic input would then sprout. However, steady state catecholamine levels may not be indicative of the number of terminals. That is, synthesis of catecholamines in remaining input may be enhanced, perhaps via feedback from neurons rendered supersensitive by a partial denervation. In other words, these steady state changes could probably occur as a consequence of either a

366

sprouting or supersensitivity mechanism. Aside from doing histochemical studies which might not be feasible because of the small magnitude of the changes, one way of deciding between these mechanisms might be to determine parameters of synthesis, i.e. enzyme levels and reuptake. The former may be increased if remaining terminals are synthesizing more transmitter whereas the latter may be increased if more terminals have sprouted. We are presently continuing our studies along these lines.

ACKNOWLEDGMENTS: This research was supported by NIMH grant MH21156 and by NIMH Research Scientist Development Award (Type 2) DA70082. I would like to thank S. Greenstein and R. G. Marsanico for indispensable technical assistance and B. Zimmerberg and J. Goldfarb for helpful comments and discussion.

REFERENCES

Adler, M.W. (1961). Changes in sensitivity to amphetamine in rats with chronic brain lesions. *J. Pharm. Exp. Ther.* 134, 204-211.

Albert, D.J. and Storlien, L.H. (1969). Hyperphagia in rats with cuts between the ventromedial and lateral hypothalamus. *Science* 165, 599-600.

Arees, E.A. and Mayer, J. (1967). Anatomical connections between medial and lateral regions of the hypothalamus concerned with food intake. *Science* 57, 1574-1575.

Berger, B.D., Wise, C.D. and Stein, L. (1971). Norepinephrine: Reversal of anorexia in rats with lateral hypothalamic damage. *Science* 172, 281-284.

Berger, B.D., Wise, C.D. and Stein, L. (1973). Nerve growth factor: Enhanced recovery of feeding after hypothalamic damage. *Science* 180, 506-508.

Brobeck, J.R., Larsson, S. and Reyes, E. (1956). A study of electrical activity of the hypothalamic feeding mechanism. *J. Physiol.* 132, 358-364.

Carlisle, H.J. (1964). Differential effects of amphetamine on food and water intake in rats with lateral hypothalamic lesions. *J. Comp. Physiol. Psych.* 58, 47-54.

Christie, J.E. and Crow, T.J. (1971). Turning behavior as an index of the action of amphetamines and ephedrines on central dopamine-containing neurons. *Br. J. Pharmacol.* 43, 658-667.

Cole, S.O. (1973). Hypothalamic feeding mechanisms and amphetamine anorexia. *Psychol. Bull.* 79, 13-20.

Crow, T.J. (1971). The relationship between lesion site, dopamine neurons and turning behavior in the rat. *Exp. Neurol.* 32, 247-255.

Epstein, A. (1959). Suppression of eating and drinking by amphetamine and other drugs in normal and hyperphagic rats. *J. Comp. Physiol. Psych.* 52, 37-45.

Friedman, M.J., Jaffe, J.H. and Sharpless, S.K. (1969). Central nervous system supersensitivity to pilocarpine after withdrawal of chronically administered scopolamine. *J. Pharm. Exp. Ther.* 167, 45-55.

Glick, S.D. (1970). Change in sensitivity to d-amphetamine in frontal rats as a function of time: Shifting of the dose-response curve. *Psychon. Sci.* 19, 57-58.

Glick, S.D. (1971). Differential sensitivity of frontal rats to d-amphetamine and scopolamine. *Comm. Behav. Biol.* 5, 341-346.

Glick, S.D. (1971). Modulation of food and water intake by frontal cortex in the rat. *Comm. Behav. Biol.* 5, 365-370.

Glick, S.D. (1972). Changes in amphetamine sensitivity following frontal cortical damage in rats and mice. *Eur. J. Pharmacol.* 20, 351-356.

Glick, S.D. and Greenstein, S. (1972). Facilitation of recovery after lateral hypothalamus damage by prior ablation of frontal cortex. *Nature New Biol.* 239, 187-188.

Glick, S.D. and Greenstein, S. (1973). Possible modulating influence of frontal cortex on nigro-striatal function. *Br. J. Pharmacol.* 49, 316-321.

Glick, S.D. and Greenstein, S. (1973). Recovery of weight regulation following ablation of frontal cortex in rats. *Physiol. & Behav.* 10, 491-496.

Glick, S.D., Greenstein, S. and Zimmerberg, B. (1972). Facilitation of recovery by α-methyl-p-tyrosine after lateral hypothalamic damage. *Science* 177, 534-535.

Glick, S.D. and Jarvik, M.E. Unpublished results.

Glick, S.D. and Jarvik, M.E. (1970). Differential impairment by drugs of delayed matching performance in frontal and normal monkeys. *Fed. Proc. Am. Soc. Exp. Biol.* 29, 279.

Glick, S.D. and Jarvik, M.E. (1970). Differential effects of amphetamine and scopolamine on matching performance of monkeys with lateral frontal lesions. *J. Comp. Physiol. Psych.* 73, 56-61.

Glick, S.D., Marsanico, R.G. and Greenstein, S. (In press). Differential recovery of function following caudate, hippocampal and septal lesions in mice. *J. Comp. Physiol. Psych.*

Glick, S.D. and Marsanico, R.G. (In press). Shifting of the d-amphetamine dose-response curve in rats with frontal cortical ablations. *Psychopharmacologia*.

Glick, S.D. and Muller, R.U. (1971). Paradoxical effects of low doses of d-amphetamine in rats. *Psychopharmacologia* 22, 396-402.

Glick, S.D., Nakamura, R.K. and Jarvik, M.E. (1971). Recovery of function following frontal brain damage in mice: Changes in sensitivity to amphetamine. *J. Comp. Physiol. Psych.* 76, 454-459.

Glick, S.D. and Zimmerberg, B. (1972). Comparative recovery following simultaneous and successive-stage frontal brain damage in mice. *J. Comp. Physiol. Psych.* 79, 481-487.

Gold, R.M. (1970). Hypothalamic hyperphagia produced by parasagittal knife cuts. *Physiol. & Behav.* 5, 23-25.

Grossman, S.P. (1962). Direct adrenergic and cholinergic stimulation of hypothalamic mechanisms. *Amer. J. Physiol.* 202, 872-882.

Iversen, S.D. (1971). The effect of surgical lesions to frontal cortex and substantia nigra on amphetamine responses in rats. *Brain Res.* 31, 295-311.

Iversen, S.D., Wilkinson, S. and Simpson, B.A. (1971). Enhanced amphetamine responses after frontal cortex lesions in the rat. *Eur. J. Pharmacol.* 13, 387-390.

Kennedy, G.C. and Mitra, J. (1963). The effect of d-amphetamine on energy balance in hypothalamic obese rats. *Br. J. Nutr.* 17, 569-573.

Knook, H.L. (1966). "The Fibre-Connections of the Forebrain", Netherlands: Royal Van Gorcum.

Leibowitz, S.F. (1971). Hypothalamic alpha- and beta-adrenergic systems regulate both thirst and hunger in the rat. *Proc. Nat. Acad. Sci. U.S.A.* 68, 332-334.

Lynch, G.S., Ballantine, P. and Campbell, B.A. (1969). Potentiation of behavioral arousal after cortical damage and subsequent recovery. *Exp. Neurol.* 23, 195-206.

Lynch, G., Ballantine, P. and Campbell, B.A. (1971). Differential rates of recovery following frontal cortical lesions in rats. *Physiol. & Behav.* 7, 737-741.

Margules, D.L., Lewis, M.J., Dragovich, J.A. and Margules, A.S. (1972). Hypothalamic norepine-phrine: Circadian rhythmns and the control of feeding behavior. *Science* 178, 640-643.

Moore, R.Y., Björklund, A. and Stenevi, U. (1971). Plastic changes in the adrenergic innervation of the rat brain septal area in response to denervation. *Brain Res.* 33, 13-35.

Reynolds, R.W. (1959). The effect of amphetamine on food intake in normal and hypothalamic hyperphagic rats. *J. Comp. Physiol. Psych.* 52, 682-684.

Sharp, J.C., Neilson, H.C. and Porter, P.B. (1962). The effect of amphetamine upon cats with lesions in the ventromedial hypothalamus. *J. Comp. Physiol. Psych.* 55, 198-200.

Sharpless, S.K. (1964). Reorganization of function in the nervous system: Use and disuse. *Ann. Rev. Physiol.* 26, 357-388.

Sharpless, S.K. (1969). Isolated and deafferented neurons: Disuse supersensitivity. *In* H.H. Jasper, A.A. Ward and A. Pope (Eds.) "Basic Mechanisms of the Epilepsies", Boston: Little, Brown and Company. pp. 329-348.

Stark, P. and Totty, C.W. (1967). Effects of amphetamine on eating elicited by hypothalamic stimulation. *J. Pharm. Exp. Ther.* 158, 272-278.

Stein, L. (1964). Self-stimulation of the brain and the central action of amphetamine. *Fed. Proc. Am. Soc. Exp. Biol.* 23, 836-849.

Stowe, F.R. and Miller, A.T. (1957). The effect of amphetamine on food intake in rats with hypo-thalamic hyperphagia. *Experientia* 13, 114-115.

Taylor, K.M. and Snyder, S.H. (1970). Amphetamine: Differentiation by d- and l- isomers of behavior involving brain norepinephrine and dopamine. *Science* 168, 1487-1489.

371

Teitelbaum, P. Personal communication.

Teitelbaum, P. and Epstein, A. (1962). The lateral hypothalamic syndrome: Recovery of feeding and drinking after lateral hypothalamic lesions. *Psychol. Rev.* 69, 74-90.

Thode, W.F. and Campbell, H.J. (1968). Effect of lateral hypothalamic stimulation on amphetamine-induced anorexia. *J. Comp. Physiol. Psych.* 66, 547-548.

Trendelenburg, U. (1963). Supersensitivity and subsensitivity to sympathomimetic amines. *Pharmac. Rev.* 15, 225-277.

Ungerstedt, U. (1971). Stereotaxic mapping of the monoamine pathways in the rat brain. *Acta Physiol. Scand. Suppl.* 367, 1-48.

Ungerstedt, U. (1971). Striatal dopamine release after amphetamine or nerve degeneration revealed by rotational behavior. *Acta Physiol. Scand. Suppl.* 367, 49-68.

Ungerstedt, U. (1971). Postsynaptic supersensitivity after 6-hydroxydopamine induced degeneration of the nigro-striatal dopamine system. *Acta Physiol. Scand. Suppl.* 367, 69-93.

Ungerstedt, U. (1971). Adipsia and aphagia after 6-hydroxydopamine induced degeneration of the nigro-striatal dopamine system. *Acta Physiol. Scand. Suppl.* 367, 95-117.

Wall, P.D. and Egger, M.D. (1971). Formation of new connexions in adult rat brains after partial deafferentation. *Nature* 232, 542-545.

Warren, J.M. and Akert, K. (1964). "The Frontal Granular Cortex and Behavior", New York: McGraw-Hill.

Zigmond, M.J. and Stricker, E.M. (1972). Deficits in feeding behavior after intraventricular injection of 6-hydroxydopamine in rats. *Science* 177, 1211-1214.

Zigmond, M.J. and Stricker, E.M. (1973). Recovery of feeding after 6-hydroxydopamine (6-HDA) or lateral hypothalamic lesions: The role of catecholamines. *Fed. Proc. Am. Soc. Exp. Biol.* 32, 754.

SOME VARIABLES INFLUENCING RECOVERY OF FUNCTION AFTER CENTRAL NERVOUS SYSTEM LESIONS IN THE RAT

Donald G. Stein
Clark University
Worcester, Massachusetts

At the present time, much neuropsychological research on the functions of the central nervous system has been concerned with delineating the role of specific areas, or anatomical structures in the control of behavior. Sometimes, underlying this approach is the assumption that structure-function relationships in the CNS are, for the most part, fixed, especially by the time the organism has reached maturity, and that damage to specific loci will result in permanent loss of function mediated by that area. In the neonate, however, brain lesions are often less debilitating and specific behavior defects sometimes disappear by the time the subject has matured (Tucker and Kling 1968). Often, the observed recovery is attributed to the possibility that the immature nervous system, being less differentiated than the adult brain, can reorganize itself so that areas not previously implicated in the behavior take over the functions of the damaged tissue (See the chapters by Goldman and Schneider for further elaboration of this point).

In general, behavioral sparing, or recovery of function in adult subjects, has been seen as an example of relearning new responses to substitute for old (e.g. Goldberger 1972). Until recently, very little serious attention was paid to the possibility that the brain could undergo some type of morphological or structural change associated with the recovery process. Rejection of the hypothesis of CNS plasticity in adult organisms is consistent with the notion that brain function is organized in a mechanistic fashion, with each defined anatomical structure or area mediating a particular aspect of behavior (see Curtis, Jacobsen and Marcus 1972 or Rosvold 1972 for examples). When behavioral recovery is observed, it is usually claimed that the tests used to measure the sparing were insensitive, and more sophisticated measurement would reveal a deficit

specifically associated with the damaged part
(Dawson 1973).

Standing in contrast to the localizationist
model of CNS function is the notion that the brain
carries out "executive activities" in a dynamic,
holistic fashion. That is, complex behavior
"depends upon an integral system of organs and
cortical areas working in close collaboration with
each other" (Luria 1963, p. xiii). In this model,
structure-function relationships in the CNS are
not necessarily considered to be fixed. Instead,
it is conceived that in a more dynamic system
under certain conditions, functional activity
could take place in such a way as to permit a
brain damaged organism to perform without demonstrating significant behavioral impairment.
Evidence of such recovery would suggest that the
structural integrity of the area(s) under study
would not be required for the behavior to occur.
Thus, if performance after brain surgery is not
disrupted, and no special training is given, the
subject could be said to have recovered "normal"
function, even though the "necessary" tissue
controlling the function has been destroyed. Many
instances of recovery after brain damage have been
carefully reviewed and discussed by Rosner (1970)
and more recently by Finger, Walbran and Stein
(1973). While there is sufficient evidence to
indicate that recovery of function occurs in adult
organisms as well as neonates, little is known
about the specific conditions under which
behavioral sparing can occur and even less can be
said about the physiological changes underlying
the process.

There are several research strategies available
for studying recovery of function and some of them
are described in this volume. One approach to the
study of CNS plasticity concerns the use of
sequential versus simultaneous lesions of an
anatomically defined locus to explore whether
temporally spaced, bilateral removals of tissue
lead to less impairment than when the same amount
of damage is inflicted in a single operation. Many
inferences about structure-function relationships
in the brain that are based on lesion experiments,
have depended primarily on results obtained from
simultaneous, bilateral damage, and it is only

within the last few years that some workers have
begun to consider the implications of the serial
phenomenon for theories of brain function (Finger,
Walbran and Stein 1973).

The seriatim technique has been employed in
many studies on recovery of function but much of
this work until very recently has been limited to
research on sensory or motor areas of the brain
(see Cole, Sullins and Isaac 1967; Kircher, Braun,
Meyer and Meyer 1970; and Meyer this volume, for
examples). In addition, these experiments often
employ either extensive preoperative behavioral
training or interlesion experience before all
surgery has been completed. For the most part,
investigators were concerned with whether sparing
or retention of a previously learned behavior
could be influenced by the type of interoperative
experience given the subjects prior to bilateral
extirpation of sensory cortex.

Instead of studying "sparing" of previously
learned behaviors after brain damage, some of us
at Clark University were interested in whether new
learning could occur in a relatively normal fashion
after all removals of tissue had been completed.
Using this strategy, we could then ask whether the
integrity of a given structure was necessary or
critical for the performance of a learned or innate
behavior pattern. In my opinion, the acquisition
paradigm deals more directly with the question of
CNS specificity than tests based upon retention of
information acquired pre-operatively. In the latter
situation, the subjects have had considerable
experience in the test situations and any obscured
sparing of function could be due to utilization of
other cues (as might be expected in a "latent
learning" situation, for example) or by shifting
to another response pattern sufficient (but perhaps
less efficient) to obtain the desired goal (e.g.
Lashley's early work in which animals were trained
to run a maze and were then given cerebellar
lesions; they still reached the goal box although
they had to tumble down the maze to do it).

In the postoperative acquisition paradigm,
testing begins after all bilateral surgery is
completed; there is no preoperative training. Here
the subject must demonstrate unimpaired performance
in the absence of the neural tissue assumed to be

375

necessary for the mediation of the behavior under study. There is no opportunity for latent learning or for developing alternative response strategies because the subjects have never before been exposed to the experimental situation.

In the studies to be reported, it will become clear that we owe much to Karl Lashley. Like him, we have tried to demonstrate that plasticity of function in adult rats may be a relatively general characteristic of the CNS. Several variables influencing recovery of function, such as age at time of surgery, sex of the experimental subjects and duration of the interoperative interval will also be discussed.

GENERAL PROCEDURES

Subjects: The subjects in all of the experiments described in this paper were albino rats (CD strain) obtained from Charles River Laboratories. Except for one study in which females of the same strain were used, and another using aged animals, the rats were random-bred males approximately 90 to 100 days of age at the beginning of the experiments and weighed approximately 275-300 gms. Prior to surgery, the rats were adapted to the laboratory and gentled by brief, daily handling for a period of 7 days to two weeks. Once operated upon, and for the duration of the experiments thereafter, the rats were maintained in individual, standard laboratory cages, under a light-dark cycle of 12 hr. on 12 hrs. off. Before surgery, and during the recovery period, the rats were allowed an *ad libitum* diet of laboratory chow and water was available at all times until behavioral testing started. The various experimental groups were all handled in the same manner during the surgical recovery period and no training or special experience was given until all surgery was completed (i.e. until bilateral removals had been affected for all groups).

Surgery:

Aspiration technic: To accomplish cortical damage to the frontal poles, the animals were mounted in a stereotaxic device under Equi-thesin anesthesia (3.33cc/kg i.p.) and atropine (.15cc standard doses i.p.) and an opening in the skull was made from bregma to the anterior tip of the frontal pole (the naves). The dura overlying the cortex was cut and retracted. A stainless steel electrode was touched to the surface of the cortex 2mm anterior to bregma and served as a reference point. Under visual guidance, the cortex between the reference pin and bregma was aspirated until white matter was exposed. All of the tissue between the reference pin and the frontal pole was aspirated down to the dorsal surface of the olfactory bulb, including the medial and lateral cortices. Figure 1 taken from a study by Teitelbaum

Maximal and Minimal Extent of Lesion

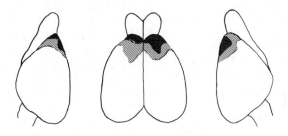

Figure 1. Maximal and minimal extent of damage after frontal cortex aspirations. Diagonal lines indicate maximal lesion; black area represents the size of the smallest lesion.

(1973) represents the typical one and two-stage lesions for this type of operation. For the subjects designated to receive a single-stage operation (1-S), both left and right frontal cortices were removed in a single operation. The animal's wounds were packed with gelfoam, their scalps sutured and the subjects returned to their home cage to recover. For those animals subjected to two-stage surgery, a unilateral lesion was made in the right or left hemisphere, their wounds were packed with gelfoam, the scalps were sutured and the animals returned to their home cage for a period of 30 days. At the end of this first

recovery period, the animals were again anesthetized and the remaining cortex contralateral to the
first operation was aspirated. Upon completion of
this surgery, the rats were allowed to recover for
two weeks prior to behavioral training. Control
operations consisted of anesthetizing the rats,
mounting them in a stereotaxic device, opening the
bone and cutting and retracting the dura overlying
the frontal cortex. Some of these sham operations
were performed in one stage, and some in two
stages.

RF Lesion technic: Except for one study to be
described below, lesions were created in subcortical structures such as the hippocampus, amygdala,
lateral hypothalamus and caudate nucleus, with a
Grass Model LM-3 or LM-4 radio frequency lesion
maker. The rats were anesthetized with Equithesin,
and mounted in a stereotaxic device for appropriate
placement of the lesion electrode. The stereotaxic
coordinates and lesion parameters for each of the
areas damaged are given in Table 1. A stainless
steel #3 insect pin (.018 inches), coated with
epoxy enamel served as the lesion electrode. The
pointed tip was slightly burnished and 0.5mm
exposed. An alligator clip attached to the fascia
usually served as the ground reference although in
some instances a rectal plug was used.

After an opening was made in the skull and the
dura incised, the electrode was lowered and removed
immediately after the burn was made. The exposed
cortical areas overlying the wounds were gently
packed with gelfoam, the animals were resutured
and returned to their home cages for the interoperative recovery period. The lesions were made in
either one or two operations as described above.
Control operations consisted of anesthetizing the
animals, mounting them in the stereotaxic device,
opening the skull, cutting the dura mater, and
lowering the electrode without passing any current.
These rats were then resutured and returned to
their home cages for the appropriate recovery
periods. These sham operations were also performed
in one or two stages in order to control for
stress, effects of anesthesia, etc.

Table 1 Summarizes the stereotaxic coordinates for the series of electrolytic lesions used to study recovery of function. Interoperative and postoperative recovery times are also given. In some cases, lesions were created at several points and these are indicated below. Coordinates for the HC, Amyg and Caudate lesions were taken from the stereotaxic atlas of deGroot; those for the LH were taken from the atlas of Pelegrino & Cushman.

	Anterior	Vertical	Lateral	Duration in Sec.	Ma	Interoperative Interval for 2-stage	Postoperative Recovery Period (after bilat. surgery, in days)
HC	3.6, 2.6	2.8, 6.0	2.2, 5.0	20	65 RF	30	14
Amyg	5.2, 4.6	8.5	4.5, 4.5	30	60–65 RF	28 – 30	14
Caud	8.0	5.0	3.4	30	70 RF	25	60
LH	1.0	8.5	2.6	15	1 DC	30	14 – 44

Histology:

Upon completion of all behavioral testing, the animals were sacrificed with Nembutal and perfused with an intracardial injection of cold, isotonic saline followed immediately by 10% formalin. The brains were mounted in albumin, frozen and sliced at 25-40u. Once the beginning of the lesion was observed, every 5th and 6th section was saved for reconstruction. The sections were stained with cresyl-echt violet and were projected upon reduced sections of the deGroot Atlas for determining the extent of damage. A polar planimeter was used to trace the perimeter of the lesion for each section and these data were subjected to t-tests to determine whether there was a significant difference in extent of damage between one and two-stage lesion groups.

The animals suffering frontal lobe removals were killed and their brains removed as described above. The brains were then photographed from dorsal, right and left lateral views. The photographic slides were then projected upon Lashley drawings of the rat brain and the perimeter of the lesion traced to determine the extent of the damage. Representative coronal sections were taken at 40u to determine the degree of insult to caudate and other subcortical structures.

Learning after simulatenous or successive lesions in the frontal cortex, limbic system and caudate nucleus: Behavioral procedures and apparutus.

In the initial series of experiments (Stein et al. 1969) we were concerned with demonstrating that recovery of function was possible in the adult organism after bilateral removals of CNS tissue thought to be critical for the mediation of learned responses. We chose hippocampus, amygdala and frontal cortex because there have been a relatively large number of studies demonstrating that bilateral removals of these areas in the adult rat causes long-standing, if not irreversible deficits, on a variety of performance variables typically associated with "learning." We wanted to show that with one stage, bilateral lesions, we could replicate the deficits obtained by others (e.g. Kimble 1963) on standard laboratory tasks.

With successive lesion groups, we hoped to demonstrate that the animals could perform as well as
normal controls even though the same amount of
tissue had been destroyed as in the rats with
simultaneous lesions. Maribeth Schultz and I later
added rats with caudate lesions to our project
because we wanted to extend the generality of the
serial lesion phenomenon to a structure that has
been implicated in motor coordination (Denny-Brown
1962), as well as "higher associative processes"
involved in learning and memory. In addition,
there have been studies showing that lesions of
the caudate nucleus result in impairments similar
to those produced by lesions of the frontal cortex
(Rosvold, Mishkin and Szwarcbart 1958; Rosvold
1972). In the rat, lesions of this area have
resulted in an inability to inhibit responses in
passive avoidance situations (Kirkby 1969) and
delayed response type tasks (Miklus and Isaacson
1965), and in deficits on tasks involving spatial
behavior (Potegal 1969; Chorover and Gross 1963).
Supposedly, caudate function is fixed early in
life; however, it has been observed that while
frontal cortex lesions in the neonatal animal
result in sparing of function as adults, neonatal
lesions of the caudate produce permanent behavioral
deficits (Goldman and Rosvold 1972). Thus, one
would expect less sparing following damage to this
structure regardless of whether surgery was performed in one or two operations. For behavioral
analysis, we chose several discriminative tasks
which have been used repeatedly by others to
demonstrate unambiguous performance deficits
following bilateral removals of the areas under
study. These tasks described in more detail below
consisted of: successive discrimination learning
and reversal, simultaneous visual pattern discrimination and reversal, delayed spatial alternation
and passive avoidance to shock.

Successive discrimination learning and reversal:
This behavioral task was employed for observing the
performance of rats with hippocampal and amygdaloid
lesions. The aparatus consisted of an enclosed
grey-painted Y-maze in which the rats were trained
to traverse the alleys in order to obtain water
reinforcement in a goal box situated at the end of
each stem. The rear walls of each goal box

381

consisted of frosted glass panels which were
illuminated by a 25w bulb just behind the glass.
An initial pretraining period was provided to
habituate the rats to a 23:45 hr. water deprivation
schedule and to their being placed in a novel
apparatus. After this period of adaptation, half of
each group was trained to run to the left for water
reward when both arms of the "Y" were illuminated,
and to the right when both arms were dark, the
other half being trained to run to the opposite
conditions, e.g. right when both arms were illuminated. The rats were given 10 trials/day under
these conditions and were trained until they
reached a performance criterion of 9/10 successively correct responses. A Gellerman schedule was
used for randomizing the sequence of right and left
reinforcements, and there was a 30 second interval
between each trial when the rats were held in the
stem of the Y behind a transparent guillotine door.
Upon reaching criterion and after a brief rest
interval of several days, the reinforcement
conditions were reversed; (e.g., if left were
correct when both arms were illuminated, and right
when both arms were dark, the conditions were now
exactly reversed). Once again, the rats were tested
until they achieved a criterion of 9/10 successively correct responses on this task.

Passive avoidance: Passive avoidance refers to
the ability of an animal to inhibit a response to
a previously reinforced stimulus or object. In our
experimental situation, the subjects were first
trained to run for water reinforcement in an
enclosed straight alley. This is a relatively
simple task which even the brain damaged rats
could acquire quickly. After they had been given
100 trials (10 trials/day) the water spout was
electrified and each time mouth contact was made,
the animals received a 1ma shock. The number of
shocks received on the test trial was the dependent
variable. If the animals refused to run the alley
after remaining there for 60 seconds or more, the
trial was terminated.

Simultaneous pattern discrimination and reversal:
This task required the rats to discriminate between
alternating black and white stripes placed in a
horizontal or vertical position on overhead swing-
ing doors. In the initial testing situation, the

animals were presented simultaneously with both
stimulus cards which blocked the entrance to the
goal boxes. The rats were required to push open
the door with the horizontal stripes to obtain the
reinforcement. The position of the correct door
could be alternated from right to left according
to a Gellerman sequence. If the animals entered
the wrong alley, they remained in the box containing a dry spout for approximately 15 seconds and
were then returned to the start box for 15 seconds
prior to being released for a subsequent trial.
The animals were obliged to achieve a criterion of
9/10 successively correct responses before the
reinforcement value of the stimulus cards was
reversed for retraining trials to the same criterion.

Delayed spatial alternation: This particular
task was chosen for use with the frontal and
caudate because previous research had shown that
spatial performance is often interrupted by
simultaneous lesions of the frontal cortex in rats
(Glick 1969; Bourke 1954) as well as higher
mammals (Rosen, Butters and Stein 1971). The
apparatus consisted of a simple, grey-painted,
enclosed T-maze in which the right or left arm
served as a goal box containing water reward,
dispensed automatically. The stem of the T served
as a start-box in which the animals were maintained
during the intertrial interval. The rats were given
16 trials/day in which the first trial represented
a free choice, i.e. the animals could go either
left or right to receive water reward. On all
subsequent trials, the animals were required to
alternate the previously correct response to
obtain water. A 30 second interval separated each
trial and responses were scored for degree of perseveration to the same side as well as latency. To
reach criterion, the rats were required to alternate 15/16 trials for two successive days.

Results and comments:

The data were subjected to an analysis of
variance followed by individual comparisons among
groups. In all cases, two-tailed levels of
significance for a priori comparisons were used.
Histological examinations revealed that there

was extensive bilateral damage to the hippocampus and amygdaloid nuclei. Most of the animals with lesions in the amygdala also had damage to the anterior portions of the ventral hippocampus and to the claustrum as well. Figure 2 shows representative photos of maximum and minimum extent of damage in rats with one or two-stage lesions of these areas. The rats with lesions in the hippo-

MAXIMUM AND MINIMUM EXTENT OF ONE AND TWO STAGE LESIONS

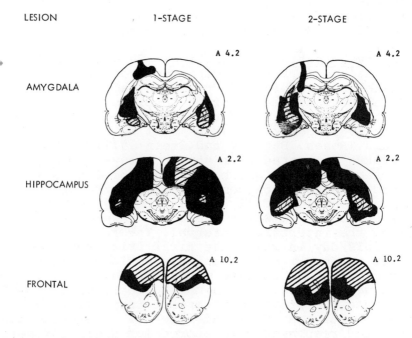

Figure 2. Representative sections of the maximum and minimum extent of damage in 3 brain structures. The hatched portions represent the minimum amount of damage indicated and the solid portions represent the maximum damage located by the coordinates shown (From Stein, et al. 1969, reprinted with permission).

campus also suffered damage to the overlying cortex, and in four cases, there was slight unilateral damage to the lateral geniculate body.

With respect to the lesions of caudate nucleus, an examination of our slides revealed that in all cases there was noticeable damage to the middle and tail of the caudate. The anterior-posterior extent of the lesion extended from A9.0 to A5.0 according to the atlas of DeGroot (1959). Most animals also showed evidence of damage to the corpus collosum and overlying neocortex. Some slight damage was noted in the areas of the lateral septum and the dorsal portions of the globus pallidus and putamen. Two animals each in the one and two-stage groups showed evidence of the lesion invading the thalamus causing damage to the n. lateralis, n. ventralis and n. reticularis. No significant differences in average size of the lesions were found for comparisons between one and two-stage lesion groups. Figure 3 shows maximum and minimum extent of damage for the anterior and posterior extent of the lesion for the one and two-stage rats with caudate lesions.

The aspiration lesions of the frontal cortex showed little variability across animals (Fig. 2). There was only one instance of slight damage to the anterodorsal caudate nucleus and this was in an animal with two-stage lesions. The planometric data from the one and two-stage groups did not reveal any significant differences in extent of lesion size.

An analysis of the behavioral data indicated that in adult rats, successive removals of approximately equal amounts of brain tissue did not produce the same deficits as single-stage removals of the same areas. Thus, while the rats with one-stage damage to the hippocampus, the amygdala or frontal cortex were impaired on all of the tests administered, animals with the same amount of tissue removed in two operations showed far less disruption of performance. In fact, the only disability observed amongst animals with two-stage lesions appeared in the group receiving damage to the amygdaloid nuclei. These animals were impaired on the initial light-dark discrimination problem but subsequently performed as well as the controls on the reversal learning tasks and on passive avoidance. The rats that received two-stage damage to hippocampus, frontal cortex or caudate nucleus performed as well as the normal controls on all of the behavioral tasks employed. In marked contrast, the rats with the same amount of tissue removed in a single operation were severely disabled on the initial tests and on all of our subsequent evaluations of their performance. Figures 4 and 5 summarize these data according to tests and lesion conditions.

One finding difficult to explain was that the rats with serial lesions of the caudate performed significantly better on the passive avoidance problem than either their one-stage or sham-operated counterparts. An analysis of the shock thresholds and motivation for water reinforcement in these animals could not account for these results. The rats with simultaneous lesions had the lowest tolerance for the shock. All three groups consumed approximately the same amount of water and did not differ significantly with respect to body weight. These data are summarized in Figure 6.

While it is clear that successive lesions in a number of CNS areas do not produce the same degree of debilitation as when the same amount of tissue is removed simultaneously, we would not be comfortable in stating that the two-stage "recovered" groups were, in fact, "just like normal controls" in all cases. The significantly better passive avoidance data obtained from animals with successive caudate lesions suggests that the actual performance of the "recovered" animal may differ from that of the normal control. Schultze and Stein (1974) suggested that statistically normal behavior on certain tasks following serial lesions does not reflect healing from the effects of the lesions but may represent the activation of an alternative neural system of the type proposed by Rosner (1970) in his recent review. Such an

Figure 3. Maximal and minimal extent of serial or simultaneous RF lesions of the caudate nucleus. The hatched portions represent the minimum amount of damage indicated and the solid portions the maximum damage. The A-P coordinates, taken from deGroot (1959) provide an indication of the extent of damage throughout the caudate nucleus.

SERIAL

SIMULTANEOUS

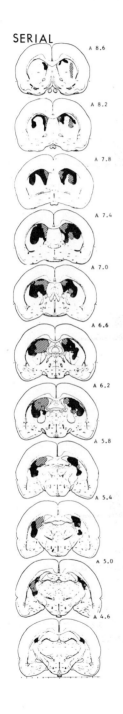

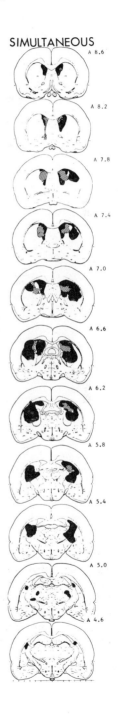

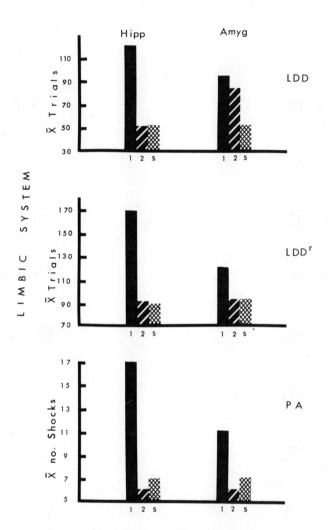

Figure 4. Postoperative performance of rats with one- or two-stage lesions of hippocampus and amygdala on light-dark discrimination (LDD); light-dark discrimination reversal (LDD^r); and passive avoidance (PA). Rats with one-stage lesions are indicated by the solid bar; those with two-stage lesions by diagonal stripes and sham controls by the hatched bar.

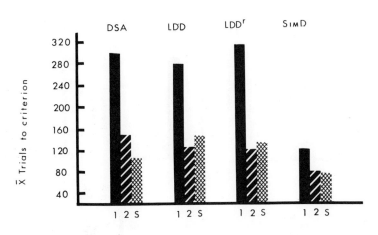

Figure 5. *Postoperative performance of rats with one or two-stage aspiration lesions of frontal cortex as compared to sham-operated controls. The tasks employed were: delayed spatial alternation (DSA); light-dark discrimination (LDD); light-dark discrimination reversal (LDDr) and simultaneous discrimination (SD). All scores are given in terms of mean trials to criterion. Rats with one-stage lesions are represented by the solid bar, those with two-stage lesions by the diagonal stripes and sham-operated controls by the hatched bar.*

alternate system could mimic behaviorally the functions of the original system along certain dimensions (i.e. no deficits on certain tasks -- performance equivalent to normals) and deviate along certain other dimensions (i.e. greater emotionality, enhanced or selective perception, etc.).

The question still remains, however, as to why one-stage removals of tissue in a number of different areas do not eventually lead to recovery of function while the same amount of tissue removed in two stages results in significantly better performance on a variety of discriminative learning tasks. One could argue that the animals with one-stage lesions eventually do learn (and recover) since,

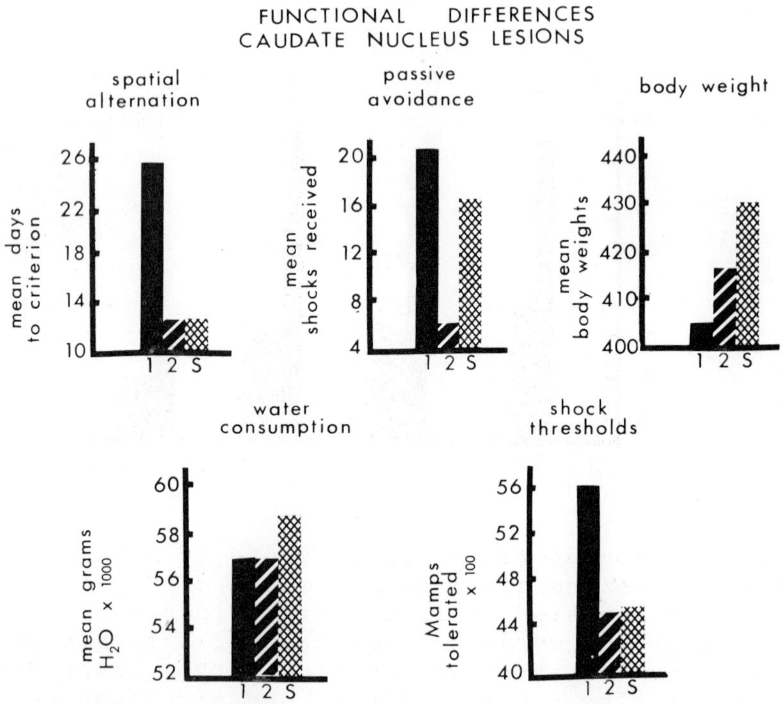

Figure 6. Effects of one or two-stage lesions of caudate nucleus on learning, body weight, water consumption and shock threshold. Rats with one-stage lesions are represented by the solid bar, those with two-stage lesions by the diagonal stripes and sham operated controls by the hatched bar.

in most cases, they achieve criterion although after many more training trials, or, in some cases, after extended post-operative recovery (see Dawson, Conrad and Lynch 1973). However, on each subsequent task, our animals were significantly impaired with respect to normal controls and to subjects with successive lesions so that eventual acquisition of task A did not necessarily produce positive transfer to task B. Thus, up to one year after all surgery had been completed, our rats (and our monkeys -- see the chapter by Butters, et al. this volume) with simultaneous removals of CNS tissue continued to show long-standing deficits in performance. This indicated that the lesion-produced impairments could not be attributed to surgical shock, diaschisis, or temporary suppression of CNS activity resulting from the operations (see also Finger, this volume).

Some temporal factors in recovery of function following frontal lobe lesions in the rat:

Since simultaneous, bilateral removals of CNS tissue can produce long standing deficits in learning and retention while sequential removals of the same locus are followed by sparing or recovery, it would appear that one of the critical variables influencing behavioral recovery is the neural change that takes place in the CNS during the time between successive operations. Although the temporal interval between surgery is important, there have only been a few systematic attempts to determine the minimum interoperative period necessary for obtaining recovery of function. Recently, Glick and Zimmerberg (1972) reported sparing of passive avoidance performance in mice subjected to serial lesions of the frontal cortex spaced 21 days apart, but not in animals with a 7 day interlesion interval. Experiments on recovery after visual system lesions in the rat showed that a 12-14 day interlesion interval was sufficient for sparing of a previously learned discrimination habit, while a 6-7 day interval resulted in subsequent disruption of the animal's performance (Meyer, Isaac and Maher 1958; Isaac 1964). In general, the above experiments were concerned with retention of materials prior to completion of all surgery. As in our previous experiments, we were interested in determining whether there was a critical period between surgical excisions which would result in sparing the acquisition of new information after all surgery had been completed. Since we had clear evidence of recovery following two-stage lesions of frontal cortex with a 30 day interoperative interval, Geoffrey Patrissi and I (1971) decided to begin our experiments with an analysis of the time factors in recovery following successive frontal cortex lesions in the rat. If the critical period was short, this would suggest perhaps a biochemical mediation of recovery. If a

relatively long period was required, one might
want to consider morphological or structural
changes (e.g. axonal sprouting as a possible
mechanism)
   The surgical, histological and behavioral
procedures for animals with frontal lesions have
been described in a previous section. In the
present experiment, 46 adult rats were randomly
assigned to the following lesion groups: sham
operates; one-stage removals; two-stage removals
(30 day interoperative interval, IOI); two-stage
removals (20 day IOI); two-stage removals (10 day
IOI). After all surgery had been completed, the
rats began training for acquisition of a spatial
alternation habit.

Results and comments:

   Figure 7 presents the mean trials to criterion
and mean errors for the different lesion groups
and sham operated controls. Briefly stated, the
sham-operated, two-stage 30 IOI and two-stage 20
IOI groups did not significantly differ from one
another. In contrast, the rats with a 10 day IOI
and the animals receiving simultaneous removals of
the frontal cortex were markedly impaired in
acquisition of this task. Although the performance
of rats with a 10 day interlesion interval was
seriously disrupted with respect to the shams, the
20- and 30-day successive lesion groups performed
significantly better than rats with one-stage
lesions and did not differ from the sham-operated
controls. These results can be interpreted to
suggest that the processes underlying sparing of
function are gradual (see Glick, this volume). For
the frontal lobes, the period for complete
behavioral recovery of spatial alternation seems
to lie somewhere between 10 and 20 days. This
temporal period seems to coincide with the time
required for the appearance of axonal sprouting
and regeneration in subcortical structures (Moore,
Bjorklund and Stenevi 1971; Raisman 1969). Similar
research for sprouting after damage to the cortex
has yet to appear. It would be tempting to suggest
that recovery of behavioral function may be
related to this sprouting of new connections from
intact neurons into the areas previously innervated

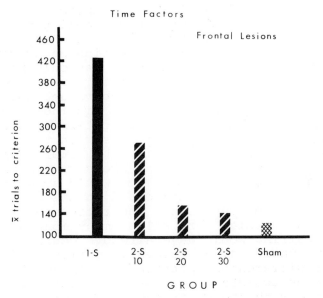

Figure 7. Temporal factors in recovery of spatial alternation performance after simultaneous or successive removals of frontal cortex in rats. The solid bar represents the performance of rats with simultaneous frontal lesions (I-S); the diagonally striped bars represent the performance of rats with successive lesions separated by a 10 day interval (2S-10); a 20 day interoperative interval (2S-20); or a 30 day interoperative interval (2S-30). The hatched bar represents the performance of the sham-operated controls.

by the damaged structures. However, there are several points to consider which tend to reduce the strength of this argument. First, in our experiments we have never observed "filling in" of the lesions even though the animals were sacrificed up to one year after all surgery had been completed. Second, except for the work of Schneider (presented at this conference) and the experiments of Lynch and his colleagues (Lynch, Deadwyler and Cotman 1973), there is little evidence to indicate that new terminals are <u>behaviorally functional</u> normally in the adult animal. Until this issue can be resolved, one could justifiably conclude that new sprouting resulting in physiological function,

could introduce "noise", or disruption, of neural
activity underlying normal behavioral patterns. In
addition, recent work by Stenevi and his colleagues
(1972) showed that neural sprouting as evidenced
by histofluorescence techniques may only be
temporary. When rats were killed several weeks
after a unilateral lesion in the visual cortex had
been created, histofluorescence did indicate
increased activity of adrenergic terminals in the
damaged areas. However, if rats with the same
lesions were killed several weeks later than the
first group, the fluorescent areas were replaced
by glial scars. This evidence would suggest that
sprouting may not be implicated in all aspects of
the recovery process since the rats used in our
behavioral studies were killed many months after
glial scarring would have already occurred.
Finally, there is, at present, no firm evidence to
suggest differential patterns of regeneration in
one versus two-stage lesioned subjects that
correlate with the clear behavioral differences we
and others have observed (see the article by
Finger in this volume).
        It is likely that some form of redundant
representation of neural patterning is involved in
the recovery process and some minimum period of
time is required for the remaining, intact brain
to regenerate the neuronal patterns associated
with specific forms of behavior. Within different
neural systems, it may be that the period required
for the development of compensatory activity will
vary as a function of the richness of afferent and
efferent connections between one area and another,
the extent to which their activities or functions
overlap (e.g. consider spatial orientation which
would involve visual, proprioceptive and sensory
motor components), and other, perhaps metabolic
factors. The fact that there does appear to be a
minimum interoperative time required to obtain
behavioral recovery of function may explain why
some workers have failed to find sparing after
sequential brain lesions. Recently, LeVere and
Weiss (1973) reported that two-stage hippocampal
lesions did not result in the recovery phenomenon
when the animals were tested on discrimination and
passive avoidance problems. In comparison to our
experiments, LeVere used a relatively short

interoperative interval (15 days). This may be one reason why he was unable to replicate our findings; his interlesion interval was half the time that we allowed between our first and second hippocampal operations. While fifteen days between surgery might be adequate for recovery from frontal lobe damage, the same period of time might not be sufficient for reorganization following hippocampal insult, or other CNS areas (Finger *et al.* 1973; Butters *et al.* 1973). Before one can claim that certain areas of the CNS fail to respond to sequential surgery, it would be important to determine if the interlesion interval is appropriate for permitting recovery of function. Thus, the degree of plasticity may vary from one area to another within the CNS; one factor in defining plasticity would be the minimum amount of time required for recovery to be observed.

Another important question needing further study involves the role of the intact, contralateral homologous structure during the interlesion interval; namely, is its integrity required for recovery of function to occur? I attempted a preliminary analysis of this question by comparing rats with large unilateral lesions of either hippocampus plus amygdala, frontal cortex plus hippocampus, or frontal cortex plus amygdala, with rats receiving bilateral lesions of hippocampus alone or amygdala alone. There were ten animals in each group and the animals were tested on the successive discrimination problem described above. The rats receiving unilateral damage, even though the extent of tissue destruction measured planometrically was the same or greater than the bilateral group, performed almost as well as the normal controls used in the previous studies. This indicated that unilateral removal of two structures results in less disruption than bilateral simultaneous removal of homologous tissue (e.g. both hippocampi). These data are only suggestive because to reach a stronger conclusion a crossed, bilateral lesion design would be required (e.g. hippocampus removed on left side, amygdala on the right, etc.) and this has not yet been accomplished. However, Finger and his students (1972) recently created two-stage, bilateral lesions of somatosensory cortex in the rat by

removing bilaterally 30-35% in the first stage and
the remaining cortex in a second operation 30 days
later. They showed that these rats performed a
tactile discrimination better than those receiving
complete extirpation in a single operation but, at
the same time, they were impaired with respect to
rats receiving two-stage removals in which the
contralateral homologue remained intact during the
interoperative interval of 35 days. The results of
Finger's experiments tend to confirm our finding
in that their rats with partial, bilateral damage
were impaired on tactile discrimination while
those with the contralateral structure intact show
considerable sparing after the second operation.
A final point in support of the notion that the
contralateral homologue may be implicated in the
recovery process can be taken from a recent study
by Zornetzer (1973). This author studied the
effects of direct, bilateral hippocampal stimulation on disruption of memory storage and found
that unless the electrode placements were
symmetrical in each hemisphere, there was no
disruption of the trace. Zornetzer argued that
this represented a high degree of functional
localization of the trace within the hippocampus.
My point is simply that for the rat, the fact that
there is such a degree of bilateral symmetry may
explain why there is considerable recovery of
function in these animals while in man, the fact
that there is considerable assymmetry (Kimura 1973)
may explain why functional reorganization after
cerebral insult occurs more slowly, if it occurs
at all.

To summarize the findings of the "critical
period" experiment, there does seem to be a minimal
interoperative interval required for recovery of
function after bilateral removals of the frontal
cortex in the rat and this seems to lie between
10 and 20 days. Second, there does appear to be
some evidence that the integrity of the contralateral homologue is required during the interoperative interval, perhaps to serve as a template
for establishing alternate neural patterns in
other areas anatomically related to the damaged
structure. Finally, at the present time, one
should be careful in ascribing recovery of
behavioral functions to axonal regenerative pro-

cesses. However, sprouting may underlie recovery
in some sensory areas and under circumscribed
conditions such as after lesions in early life
(Lynch *et al.* 1973; Schneider 1974).

Recovery of function after damage to neural systems mediating emotional and motivational behavior

Although the majority of experiments dealing
with recovery of function after successive lesions
have concentrated on the cortex, there have been
reports showing that behaviors such as eating,
sleeping and emotion remain relatively constant
after serial lesions of areas thought to be critical for the maintenance of these behaviors (Blatt
and Lyon 1968; Kesner, Fiedler and Thomas 1967).
One of the earliest experiments in which serial
lesions of brain stem structures were explored
systematically was performed by Adametz (1959).
Adametz destroyed the brain stem tegmentum of
adult cats in a series of operations and compared
their rates of survival and sleep-waking patterns
with those animals receiving similar damage in a
single operation (one-stage). He reported that
except for one case, "extensive bilateral lesions
made at a single sitting led to coma from which
the animals did not recover ... the same lesions
placed upon one side at a time with an interval of
three weeks between led to relatively quick
recovery from coma and an early return of motor
function." (page 96).
On the basis of these reports, we decided to
explore whether subcortical structures implicated
in the control of unlearned behaviors undergo
reorganization of function after serial or single
stage lesions. For this purpose, we chose to
examine disruption of ongoing behavior (drinking)
by stressful stimulation, exploration of a novel
situation, and eating in rats with one or two-
stage lesions of either the basolateral nucleus of
the amygdala or the lateral hypothalamus. In
general, we supposed that there might be considerably less recovery of function for the "more
primitive" types of behaviors such as eating and
responding to noxious stimulation since these
responses are thought to be unlearned and
controlled by highly discrete anatomical regions

of the brain.

Differential effects of one and two-stage amygdaloid lesions on emotional and exploratory behaviors

Mildred McIntyre and I (McIntyre and Stein 1973) therefore inflicted male, albino rats with one or two-stage lesions of the amygdala and compared them on a number of behavioral measures to animals receiving sham operations. We chose the amygdala because numerous studies have shown that insult to this complex often results in a variety of behavioral changes such as: alterations in eating, arousal, activity and response to aversive stimulation (e.g. Goddard 1964).

Details of the surgical and histological proce-dures have been reported elsewhere (McIntyre and Stein 1973). Before and after surgery, the rats were tested on four tasks as follows: a measure of general activity, a measure of exploratory behavior, passive avoidance to electrical shock, and passive avoidance to rotation. Passive avoidance to rotation was used because there have been reports that amygdaloid lesions produce direct, physiological alterations in response to shock and therefore any observed changes may be limited only to situations employing electrical shock (Kellicutt and Schwartzbaum 1963; Kemble and Beckman 1969). Activity was measured on a stabili-meter and movement counted automatically. Exploration was measured by attaching a runway to the animals' cages and then allowing them to leave the home cage and explore the novel environment for a ten minute period. Passive avoidance to shock utilized a simple step-down apparatus in which the subjects were placed on a small circular platform 10cm above an electrified grid floor (0.7mA). After latency of initial stepdown was recorded, the rats were given about 15 sec. of footshock, returned to the home cage for five minutes and then returned to the small platform where latencies were again recorded.

On the rotation task, the rats were required to run down a straight alley to obtain water reward. The goal box at the end of the alley was mounted on a biological shaker platform which could be oscillated or elliptically rotated, at various speeds. Initially, the rats were given 100 trials at ten trials per day to fully habituate them to the apparatus prior to surgery. As the rats approached to goal box on the 101st trial, the entire platform was rotated at a speed of 80 cpm. The time it took the subjects to reach the waterspout, the amount of time they spent in the goalbox while it rotated, and the time it took the rats to leave the goalbox were all recorded automatically. The rats were given seven trials per day with a criterion of drinking one min. in the rotating goalbox on three consecutive trials. After this point, other tests of avoidance under rotation were given and are reported in more detail in McIntyre and Stein (1973). In all cases, post-operative testing followed the same procedures described for pre-operative training.

Results and comments:

After all behavioral testing was completed, the animals were killed and their brains studied for location and extent of damage. The lesions in both the one and two-stage groups were primarily within the central and medial regions of the amygdaloid complex although there was some damage in a few cases to the basolateral nucleus, the ventral section of the nucleus caudatus putamen and the stria terminalis (Figure 8). Microscopic examination of these materials did not reveal any differences in extent or location of the lesion across the two surgical groups. Figure 8 represents one section from each of the brains of five animals in the one and two-stage groups. The blackened area at the base of each section indicates extent of damage at coordinates A3990/A4110

Figure 8. (Following pages) Representative sections of one- and two-stage amygdaloid lesions in the albino rat. The blackened area indicates extent of damage at coordinates A3990/A4110 of the König and Klippel (1963) atlas. One section from each of the brains of five animals in each group were selected for presentation (From McIntyre and Stein 1973. Reprinted with permission).

One-stage

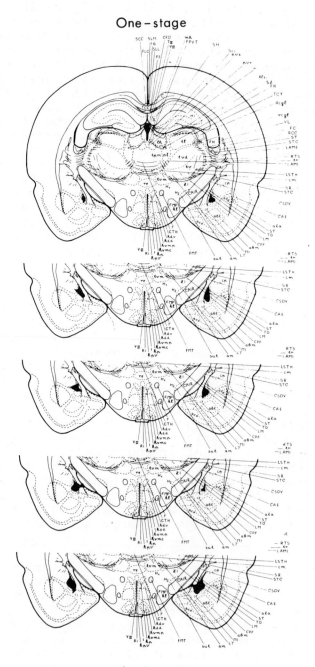

Figure 8

Two-stage

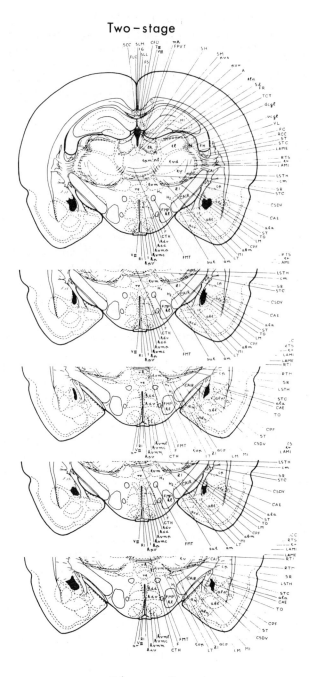

Figure 8

of the König and Klippel (1963) stereotaxic atlas.
Although there were no differences between
groups on preoperative measures of activity, a
significant change occurred after surgery had been
completed. The sham operates were relatively
constant from presurgical to postsurgical testing,
but both the rats with one and two-stage lesions
showed a marked decrease in activity scores.
However, the decrease for the one-stage group was
greater than that for the rats with two-stage
lesions.

With regard to shock avoidance behavior, there
were no differences among groups prior to surgery,
but on the postoperative measures an analysis of
the latency scores showed a significant effect.
Although the rats with one or two-stage lesions
differed significantly from each other, both groups
showed only a slight increase in step-down latency
(0.90 sec. and 4.58 sec., respectively) while sham
operates showed an increase in latency of 34.80
seconds. Thus, there was an apparent deficit in
passive avoidance to shock that was not spared,
in this case, by successive removals of amygdaloid
nuclei.

On the exploration task, no significant differences were obtained amongst the three groups of
animals for entering into the novel runway,
exploring it, or for the time the animals remained
in the alley. Apparently, this type of exploration
was not affected by damage to the amygdaloid
complex.

The rotation task (onset of 80 cpm rotation at
approach to the waterspout) yielded significant
results in the predicted direction. The rats with
one-stage lesions were the least disrupted by the
oscillation of the goalbox; i.e. they showed the
least amount of change in latency to enter the
box, and spent more time in the rotating box than
rats with two-stage lesions or sham operated
controls. Thus, their behavior is consistent with
the "sluggishness" reported after one-stage
lesions in this area of the brain. Two-stage and
sham-operated animals did not differ significantly
from each other in this phase of testing. Figure 9
summarizes the performance of the groups on
various measures of their response to 80 cpm
rotation.

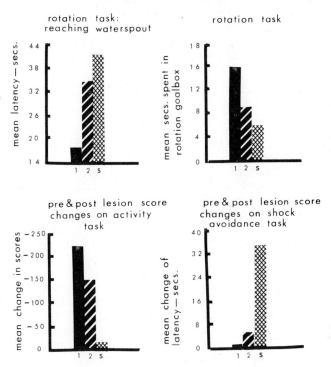

DIFFERENTIAL EFFECTS:
AMYGDALA LESIONS

Figure 9. Differential effects of one- or two-stage lesions of amygdala on passive avoidance to rotation, activity before and after lesions and passive avoidance to shock. Performance of rats with one-stage lesions is indicated by the black bar; the diagonal stripes represent performance of rats with two-stage lesions, and shams are represented by the hatched bar.

Generally, on those tasks in which a deficit was observed, the rats with two-stage lesions were less impaired than those with similar damage inflicted in a simultaneous operation. With respect to changes in activity levels and passive avoidance of shock, the rats with two-stage lesions were different from normals but they also differed significantly from the animals suffering one-stage lesions as well. This "intermediate performance"

403

indicated "some recovery of the pertinent behavioral functions" and may have been complete had we employed a longer recuperative interval. (In the study by Stein *et al.* 1969, rats with two-stage amygdaloid lesions showed a deficit on the first learning task, but performed as well as controls on all subsequent testing).

The effects of simultaneous or successive lesions of the lateral hypothalamic area (LHA) on body weight regulation[1]

This study was undertaken by my students and I in order to extend the generality of the serial lesion phenomenon to a relatively simple form of motivated behavior (eating, drinking) mediated by a specific region of the hypothalamus whose functional and anatomical connections are thought to be well understood. Typically, bilateral lesions of the lateral hypothalamic nucleus or adjacent tissue (Grossman 1972) have resulted in severe reduction of food and water intake in rats (Anand and Brobeck 1951; Teitelbaum and Epstein 1962). Often these animals will not survive the surgery unless they are force-fed or injected with glucose. However, with intensive postoperative care and special feeding, they may eventually recover sufficiently to regulate food intake and body weight in a relatively normal fashion. The rats that do survive and recover from simultaneous lesions of the lateral hypothalamus do not seem to show and increased feeding response to insulin-induced hypoglycemia. In contrast, normal rats will show increased eating and drinking under these conditions (Epstein and Teitelbaum 1967; Wayner *et al.* 1971; Booth and Brookover 1968; Steffens 1969). In the second part of this experiment, we tried to determine whether recovered rats with bilateral hypothalamic lesions inflicted in one or two-stages would respond as do normals to insulin-induced hypoglycemia.

---

[1]This research was performed in collaboration with Barry Fass, Harmon Jordan, Arna Rubman and Susan Seibel, all of Clark University.

Procedures: The subjects, male albino rats,
were approximately 120 days old and weighed 350-
450 grams at the beginning of the experiment. The
rats were handled daily for one month preoperatively. From two weeks prior to the operations and
until the animals were killed for histology, data
to the nearest tenth of a gram for body weight,
water and food consumption were collected each day.
Six rats were given one-stage LHA lesions, six
received two-stage lesions of LH area and seven
animals served as sham-operated controls. The
coordinates for the placement of the lesions are
presented in Table 1 and they were created by
passing a direct current of 1.0 mA for 15 sec.
through an anodal stainless steel electrode
covered with enamel except for 0.5mm of exposed
tip. A rectal plug served as the cathode.

Rats in the one-stage group received bilateral
damage to the LHA in a single operation. Rats in
the two-stage group first received a left
unilateral lesion and then 30 days later, a second
operation was affected in the contralateral hemisphere. For the sham operations, the electrode
was lowered to a point just above the LHA without
passing any current. Food and water intake was
measured during the inter-operative interval of
the two-stage group so that we would have an
indication of the effects of unilateral damage to
LHA on eating and drinking.

When it was determined that the rats were able
to stabilize their weight, insulin was administered
to all of the subjects in a subcutaneous injection
of Iletin U-100 (Eli Lilly & Co.). Prior to the
injections, the rats were deprived of food for 24
hours. At the time of postoperative testing, the
subjects were given at least two weeks to recover
from all phases of surgery. Each subject had to
show four or five days of weight gain or weight
maintenance and had to eat approximately 15 gms.
of dry pellets per day to be considered "recovered"
from the effects of the surgery.

As a control for the stressful effects of the
injection itself, the animals were given an
injection of saline after 24 hours of food deprivation and then measured on food and water
consumption. This procedure was carried out both
one day before and one day after injections of the

8 units of insulin.

At the end of the experiment, the rats were killed and their brains prepared for histological examination according to techniques described elsewhere in this paper. The brains were cut at 25u and every fifth and sixth section was saved for reconstruction of the lesion.

Although the lesions were not completely symmetrical in all cases, a t-test based on planometric tracing did not reveal any significant difference in lesion size between rats receiving one-stage or two-stage lesions of LHA. Figure 10 shows a representative section of each of the Ss with LHA lesions. Inspection of the slides revealed that the lesion often extended into the area beyond the LH nucleus. There was damage to the medial forebrain bundle, and several cases of unilateral encroachment into the zona incerta. The fornix, ventral portion of the internal capsule and dorsal aspect of the optic tract were also damaged. There was no substantial evidence to suggest that lesion variability was more common in one of the experimental groups than in the other.

The damage to the lateral hypothalamus was, for the most part, considered as "far lateral" and the lesion extended into fiber paths lateral and medial to the LH nucleus. There was only one case in which there appeared to be some indication of VMH involvement in the lesion zone.

Results and comments:

Three measures related to consummatory behavior served as the dependent variables in this experiment: body weight regulation, food consumption and water consumption. These measures were averaged over two-day intervals for the course of the experiment and subjected to repeated measures analyses of variance. Differences between means were tested by appropriate individual comparisons using two-tailed levels of significance.

Baseline measures taken continuously for two weeks prior to any surgical intervention revealed no significant differences amongst the three experimental groups on body weight, food or water consumption.

In order to allow for comparable recovery times

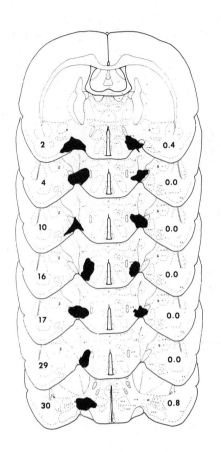 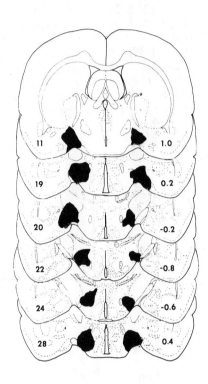

2 - STAGE   1 - STAGE

Figure 10. Representative sections of rats with lateral hypothalamic area lesions (LHA) inflicted in simultaneous or successive operations. One section from each of the animals in either the one- or two-stage lesions groups were selected for presentation. The A-P coordinates represent an approximation of the location of the lesion at its maximal extent.

and to permit assessment of the effect of unilateral damage to the hypothalamus, the rats receiving simulatenous, bilateral removals of the LH area were operated upon first and thus could be compared

to sham controls and to rats with a unilateral
(first part of the two-stage operation) lesion of
the LHA region.

   After surgery, the rats with bilateral lesions
of the LHA (i.e. 1-S lesions) showed a marked
decline in body weight in comparison to sham
operated controls. Initially, the rats with a
unilateral lesion (i.e. 2-S) were also significantly different than the sham animals and their
body weights were in a position intermediate to
that of the group with one-stage lesions (see
Figure 11). Figure 12 summarizes the results for

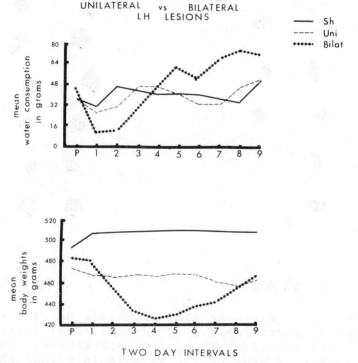

*Figure 11. Changes in water consumption and body
weight after unilateral or bilateral lesions of
the lateral hypothalamic area (LHA) in mature
rats. The solid line represents rats with sham
operations; the dotted line, those with lesions
effected in two operations; the diamonds represent
the data obtained from rats with simultaneous
bilateral LHA lesions.*

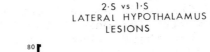

2·S vs 1·S
LATERAL HYPOTHALAMUS
LESIONS

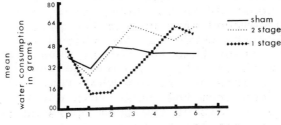

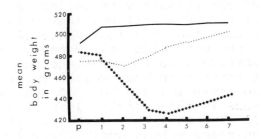

TWO DAY INTERVALS

*Figure 12. Changes in water consumption and body
weight following one- or two-stage lesions of
LHA in mature rats. Measures were taken after
all surgery had been completed.*

weight regulation and water consumption over the
entire course of the experiment. With respect to
water consumption, the 1-S rats drank significantly less than shams during the first 8 days
after surgery and the 2-S rats consumed an amount
intermediate to the one-stage and sham operated
animals. On days 9-18, there was a shift in the
pattern of water consumption. The rats with 1-S
lesions consumed significantly more than both the
rats with unilateral lesions and the sham controls.
This increased drinking is most likely due to the
fact that the 1-S animals received glucose in
their water and the sweetened flavor may have
induced more drinking in these animals. In
contrast, the difference between shams and
unilaterals disappeared for this period of

409

measurement. With respect to food consumption, there were no differences amongst any of the three groups. The rats with lesions in the LHA consumed as much food as the shams. Observation of the animal's behavior in the home cages showed that the brain-damaged rats gnawed the pellets and manipulated the powdered food they were offered to a greater extent than the shams. Thus, for example, the rats with one-stage LHA damage would grind all of their pellets and remove what remained of the powdered food from the cups. This was rarely seen in the 2-S animals or the sham operated controls. Our data are similar to those reported by Reynolds and Kim (1972) who also showed markedly increased gnawing behavior after LH lesions.

After the animals with unilateral lesions received their second operation, they were again compared with one-stage and sham operated rats. The 2-S rats, now with bilateral damage, were found to be intermediate to one-stage and sham operates with respect to body weight regulation, but the second operation did not produce any further decrease in body weight. Inspection of Figure 12 will show that rats with 1-S lesions of the LH area decrease weight over time and then begin to gain slightly after glucose treatments while the rats with 2-S lesions and the sham operated animals maintain their weights in a relatively stable manner without special diets. Thus, the second operation, inflicting damage on the remaining LH area had little effect on the animal's subsequent pattern of weight regulation. In contrast, the same tissue removed in a single stage resulted in a gradual but continuous decline in body weight during the initial period of the experiment, although the amount of food consumed did not differ significantly between the three groups.

The effects of insulin injections on the recovered animals with lesions of LH and adjacent tissue were not particularly dramatic (Figure 13). In the period of 0-3 hours after injection both the two-stage and one-stage lesioned rats tended to drink less water than sham controls receiving insulin ($p < .07$). This initial effect was not long lasting and there were no differences in water consumption among the groups 3-6 hours later. With

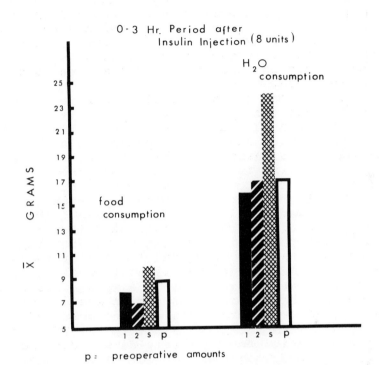

Figure 13. Effects of insulin injections on food and water consumption in rats with one- or two-stage lesions of LHA; the black bar represents rats with one-stage lesions; the diagonal stripes, those with two-stage lesions; the hatched bar represents the sham operated controls.

respect to food consumption, both lesion groups tended to eat less than the sham operated controls under insulin-induced hypoglycemia. This finding can be interpreted to suggest that there was a failure of the two-stage LH lesions to recover completely from the effects of the successive surgery. Thus, rats with two-stage lesions of the LH were able to regulate their weight more effectively than Ss with the same tissue removed in a single-stage operation, but they did not respond to insulin-induced feeding as did the sham-operated controls. This failure to recover may have been due to the surgical elimination of sensory glucoreceptors in the hypothalamus. While

411

food motivation and weight regulation may be
mediated by several systems which could compensate
for one another in case of localized destruction
of a link in the system, there is probably less
redundancy after removal of specific sensory
receptors such as those thought to monitor glucose
levels in blood.

In conclusion, our data confirm earlier studies
which indicate that the LH-area may control
several aspects of regulatory behavior since both
water consumption and weight regulation are
affected by l-S lesions in this part of the CNS.
It is interesting to note that in our experiments,
the amount of food consumed was not affected by
either single or successive LH-area lesions.
Instead, it was regulation of body weight that
seemed to be altered by LHA damage. Unilateral
lesions disrupted normal weight regulation but to
a lesser degree than bilateral lesions of the same
area. One would expect that if unilateral damage
altered body weight regulation, a second lesion in
the contralateral homologous region would disrupt
this process even more. This was not observed in
the animals with seriatum insult to the LH-zone.
The second lesion coming thirty days after the
first, appeared to have no effect on subsequent
regulation of body weight. The rats in the two-
stage group maintained their preoperative weight
levels and never required the introduction of
glucose in their drinking water, glucose injections
or the use of special diets as did their one-stage
counterparts.

This finding suggests that the LHA contralateral
to the damaged area changes its "regulatory" functions some time after the initial operation. If
this change in function did not occur, how could
one explain the finding that the second lesion,
damaging the remaining LH-area, did not alter
weight regulation in a manner similar to that produced by the initial surgery? While the integrity
of the contralateral homologous region may be
required for initiating the recovery process
during the inter-operative interval, it may not be
necessary to sustain the appropriate response
pattern once recovery has occurred.

Finally, the degree of plasticity after lesions
of the LH-area appears to be less than that

observed after two-stage cortical or limbic lesions since there is a unilateral deficit. This suggests that there is a certain degree of functional specificity associated with the lateral hypothalamic area that is not completely spared after two-stage surgery given the interoperative intervals used in this experiment.

Age and sex as factors in recovery of function after simultaneous or successive frontal lesions in rats[1]

While there is considerable evidence for recovery of function after lesions in immature and adult, but young animals, much less is known about behavioral sparing after brain damage in senescent subjects. One reason for the paucity of research on aged rats may be due to the fact that these animals are very difficult to maintain since they are quite susceptible to disease, do not respond well to anesthesia, tend to be vicious and do not perform well after even moderate food or water deprivation. Although these factors make research on aging more difficult, the question of whether aged rats show the same degree of recovery as younger conspecifics merits further investigation.

Accordingly, 27 male, albino rats approximately 2 years of age at the beginning of the experiments were subjected to either one- or two-stage lesions of frontal cortex according to procedures described earlier in this paper. The brain-damaged rats were then compared on delayed spatial alternation and discriminated shock avoidance tasks to rats of the same age subjected to sham operations. Although we started with nine animals per group, several animals in each condition died before the experiments were completed. Thus, there were 6 Ss in the one-stage group; 5 in the two-stage, and 5 rats served as sham operated controls.

---

[1]This study was performed in collaboration with Arthur Firl to whom I am indebted for much of the difficult and time-consuming testing and histology.

413

Results and comments:

Unlike their younger counterparts, aged rats with two-stage lesions of frontal cortex did not show any indication of recovery of function on spatial alternation or active avoidance when a 30 day interoperative interval was used. Indeed, on the spatial alternation task the rats with two-stage lesions performed worse than either rats with one-stage lesions or with sham operated controls. Figures 14 and 15 summarize the

SPATIAL ALTERNATION

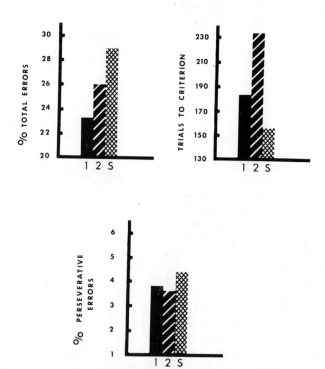

Figure 14. Spatial alternation performance in aged rats with simultaneous or successive lesions of frontal cortex. The black bars represent the performance of animals with simultaneous, bilateral damage; the bars with diagonal stripes represent the performance of rats with two-stage lesions; the hatched bars indicate performance of the sham operated controls.

ACTIVE SHOCK AVOIDANCE

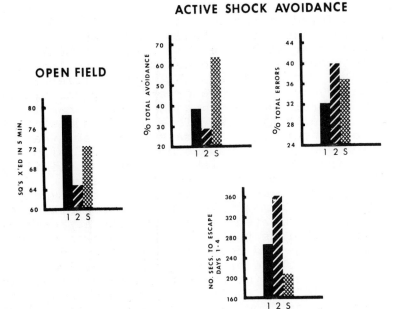

Figure 15. Active avoidance and open field performance in aged rats with one- or two-stage lesions of frontal cortex.

trials to criterion on spatial alternation, discriminated shock avoidance, and open field activity for the three groups of aged rats. On the shock avoidance task, both the rats with simultaneous and successive lesions made significantly more errors than the sham controls. However, there were no differences between the one and two-stage operated animals; both were equally impaired with respect to performance on this task. These data can be taken to suggest that recovery of function observed after lesions of the same area in younger animals does not occur as readily in rats approaching senescence. Several factors could possibly account for this failure to find recovery. First, aged rats may be more susceptible to stress than younger animals and thus the stress of repeated entry into the CNS would destroy any recovery that might be triggered by the successive operations. If true, this would suggest that a longer interoperative interval might be more effective in sparing behavioral function in aged animals; however, no data bearing on this question can be offered at the present time. Second, CNS mechanisms underlying behavior may change over time such that with advancing age, previously efficient compensatory mechanisms may no longer be available. One hypothesis that can be offered is that there may be less denervation supersensitivity following brain damage in aged animals than in younger, healthier rats. This would suggest that changes in neurochemical transmission or synaptic efficiency might be responsible for the failure to recover from serial lesions. Another possibility is that axonal sprouting, thought by some investigators to mediate CNS plasticity (Lynch, Deadwyler and Cotman 1973) may also be markedly reduced or eliminated as the subjects approach old age. It is obvious that far more research on the question of age and recovery needs to be done before any of these problems can be resolved.

One final point that should be mentioned is that the "old" rat is different in many respects from its younger conspecifics. In the first place, the old rats in our experiments did not perform well for water reward. Even the aged sham-operated controls took far longer to navigate the maze and reach criterion than younger, but mature, rats placed in the same situation. Secondly, although the animals were handled extensively, (the Ss were born in the laboratory and had been handled since birth) there were far more attempts (often success-ful) to bite and escape, suggesting different responses to stress and noise stimulation, than one finds in younger rats of the same strain. More significantly, the aged rats we used were much more sensitive to doses of the anesthetic than younger animals. In order to avoid barbituate poisoning, we were required to reduce the dose administered by more than one third to obtain the same desired level of anesthesia and avoid lethal overdose. This finding would suggest that CNS sensitivity to drugs has changed dramatically with age, and it is likely that other aspects of brain function have changed as well. In fact, Frolkis, Bezruhov and Sinitsky (1972) recently demonstrated that old rats and rabbits show significant increases in sensitivity of the brain to administration of a wide variety of neurotransmitters, stimulants and hormones.

Sex differences in recovery of function:

In general, the research described in this paper demonstrates that sparing of behavioral function after damage to the CNS is more likely to occur following sequential neural insult although there are other variables to consider such as the age of the subjects at the time of surgery, the interval of time between first and subsequent operations and the types of behavioral tasks used to evaluate recovery from brain damage. In most of the studies on recovery of function in rats, males have served as the experimental subjects and this has prevented the extrapolation of findings to females. It would be expected, however, that female animals would show the same advantages of two-stage surgical removals of CNS tissue as males although there is some evidence that females perform differently than males on a variety of learning and motivational tests (see Gray and Buffery 1971 and Broverman *et al.* 1968, for examples).

Accordingly, Bonnie Teitelbaum (1973) subjected male and female albino rats to one- or two-stage aspiration lesions of frontal cortex and then tested the subjects on the same delayed spatial alternation task described earlier in this paper. Figure 16 summarizes the results of this experiment.

Results and comments:

Briefly, she found that sham operated females learned the task significantly faster than sham-operated males. We were surprised to find, however, that no behavioral sparing followed two-stage lesions in the female group. The females with one or two-stage lesions of the frontal cortex did not significantly differ from each other; both surgical groups were markedly impaired with respect to shams and males subjected to two-stage removals. In contrast, the data from the male groups replicated results from earlier experiments; namely, animals with one-stage lesions were disrupted with

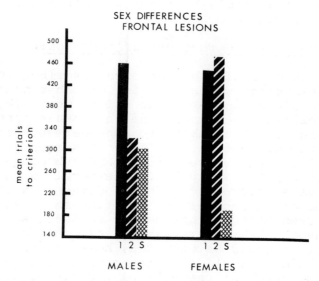

Figure 16. The effects of one- or two-stage frontal aspiration lesions on spatial alternation performance in adult, male and female rats. The black bars represent the performance of rats with one-stage lesions; the diagonal bars, those with lesions effected in two operations; the hatched bars represent the performance of non-operated animals.

respect to controls while those with two-stage ablations were not. Thus, it appears that female rats do not show recovery of function when given serial lesions under the same conditions imposed on male rats of the same age and strain.

At present, one can only speculate about the mechanisms that might underlie the differences in recovery between male and female rats. Teitelbaum suggested that the superior performance of the sham operated females on delayed alternation might be a function of the stressful nature of the experiment rather than any spatial dimensions of the task; i.e. surgical and anesthetic trauma, prolonged water deprivation, handling, non-rewarded maze trials, etc. She pointed out that there is some evidence to indicate that females are more resistant to stress than males (Swanson 1967). For example, female rats acquire an active avoidance

response faster than males (Denti and Epstein 1972)
and display greater resistance to extinction of the
response than males. These differences in performance may be due to higher levels of ACTH levels in
females according to Levine (1968) and Beatty and
Bowman (1971).

The apparent lack of behavior sparing after
frontal lesions in the females may be due to
disruption of a CNS mechanism involved in the
animal's ability to cope with stress. Teitelbaum
suggests that the surgery may disrupt rhythmic
secretion of hormones in females to a greater
extent than in males, the latter having multiple
modes of recovery less dependent upon hormonal
systems. Future research is being planned to
elucidate further the role of sex hormones in the
recovery process, but no data is presently
available on this subject. It should be pointed
out that failure to find recovery in females may
be species specific. In the subsequent chapter
dealing with recovery of function in the primate,
my colleagues and I describe a series of experiments in which both male and female animals have
been used in all phases of the research. We did
not note any major sex differences in degree of
recovery between male and female rhesus, but this
variable has not been systematically investigated.

Conclusions and comments:

The data that we have obtained as well as the
materials presented by other colleagues at this
Conference clearly indicates that recovery of
function after brain damage is not limited to
neonatal preparations nor is it limited to a
particular level in the phylogenetic scale. The
experiments carried out at Clark University have
demonstrated that behavioral recovery after CNS
lesions in the mature rat is more general and the
phenomenon more complex than we originally thought.
However, the mechanisms underlying recovery of
function are still not clearly understood, and
there are a number of important variables needing
further study.

First, there is the question of whether there
are different critical recovery periods required
for anatomically discrete areas of the brain. We,

as well as others, have shown that there is a
minimum amount of time required between operations
if the serial lesion phenomenon is to be observed.
However, it is likely that the neural processes
underlying recovery may vary from system to system
within the CNS and may also change as a function of
age or sex of the experimental subjects.

Second, we have some information which suggests
that the "recovered animal" is not the same as a
normal, unoperated control. Thus, normal
performance on certain tasks may be seen as one
symptom of a larger syndrome of behavior characteristic of the animal with successive insults to the
CNS. We have seen this difference reflected in
enhanced passive avoidance performance of rats
with two-stage lesions of the caudate nucleus, and
the alteration in body weight regulation following
unilateral lesions of lateral hypothalamus. In
addition, we have seen that behavioral sparing
after successive surgery may not occur on all
tests. For example, two-stage damage to dorsolateral amygdaloid nuclei produced sparing on some
measures of learning and emotional reactivity but
not on others, and "recovered" rats with two-stage
lesions of the lateral hypothalamus did not show
any evidence of insulin-induced hypoglycemic
feeding supposedly characteristic of intact
animals.

Third, behavioral sparing after brain damage
may be limited to certain periods of development
but not others. Our preliminary evidence obtained
from examination of senescent rats indicates that
the successive frontal lesions which result in
complete sparing in young adult animals, fail to
spare performance on spatial and discriminative
learning tasks in old rats. To date, we have also
been unable to find evidence of recovery in young,
but mature, female rats when they are tested in
the same situation as males of similar age.

These data suggest that hormonal and perhaps
non CNS mechanisms may also be implicated in
recovery of function although at the present time,
there is not sufficient evidence to indicate just
what these mechanisms might be, or what is
necessary to initiate the recovery process.

Fourth, we do not know why there should be

behavioral differences between subjects with tissue removed in a single operation, and those with the same extent and locus of damage created sequentially. Some attention should be focused on this question as well. Citing the concept of "neural shock" or diaschisis simply produces a convenient name for the observed differences in behavior but does not suggest a neural mechanism that we can manipulate experimentally.

Finally, the two-stage lesion paradigm should be considered in a broader context of exploring the organization of cognitive processes of the CNS. The evidence presented at this Conference can be taken to suggest that current concepts of localization of function may have to be reconsidered and perhaps reformulated, if we are to understand how it is that organisms can perform without the tissue thought to be critical for behavioral elicitation and control.

ACKNOWLEDGMENTS: The research described in this report has been supported by funds from NINDS (5 R01 NS08606), Clark University and by a Research Career Development Award (5 K02 MH70177) (Type II) to the author.

REFERENCES

Adametz, J. (1959). Rate of recovery of functioning in cats with rostral reticular lesions. *J. Neurosurgery* 16, 85-98.

Anand, B.K. and Brobeck, J.R. (1951). Hypothalamic control of food intake in rats and cats. *Yale J. Biol. & Med.* 24, 123-140.

Beatty, W.W., Beatty, P.A. and Bowman, R.E. (1971). A sex difference in the extinction of avoidance behavior in rats. *Psychonomic Science* 23, 213-214.

Blatt, B. and Lyon, M. (1968). The interrelationship of forebrain and midbrain structures involved in feeding behavior. *Acta. Neurol. Scand.* 44, 576-595.

Booth, D.A. and Brookover, T. (1968). Hunger elicited in the rat by a single injection of bovine crystalline insulin. *Physiol. & Behav.* 3, 439-446.

Bourke, W.T. (1954). The effects of frontal lobe damage upon habit reversal in the white rat. *J. Comp. Physiol. Psychol.* 47, 277-282.

Broverman, D.E., Klaiber, E., Kobayashi, Y. and Vogel, W. (1968). Roles of activation and inhibition in sex differences in cognitive abilities. *Psychol. Rev.* 75, 23-50.

Butters, N., Butter, C., Rosen, J. and Stein, D. (1973). Behavioral effects of sequential and one-stage ablations of orbital prefrontal cortex in the monkey. *Exper. Neurol.* 39, 204-214.

Chorover, S. and Schiller, P. (1965). Short-term retrograde amnesia in rats. *J. Comp. Physiol. Psychol.* 59, 73-78.

Cole, D.D., Sullins, W.R. and Isaac, W. (1967) Pharmacological modifications of the effects of spaced occipital ablations. *Psychopharmacologia* (Berl) 11, 311-316.

Curtis, B., Jacobsen, S. and Marcus, E.M. (1972) "An Introduction to the Neurosciences," Philadelphia: Saunders. Chapter 21.

Dawson, G. (1973). Recovery of function: implications for theories of brain function. *Behav. Biol.* 8, 439-460.

Dawson, G., Conrad, L. and Lynch, G. (1973). Single and two-stage hippocampal lesions: a similar syndrome. *Exper. Neurol.* 40, 263-277.

DeGroot, J. (1959). The rat forebrain in stereotaxic coordinates. Verhandelingen der koninklijke Nederlandse Akademie van Wetenschappen, Afd., Natuurkunder. N.V. Noord-Hollandsche Uitgevers Maatschappij, Amsterdam.

Denny-Brown, D. (1962). "The Basal Ganglia", London: Amen House. Oxford Neurological monographs, Oxford University Press.

Denti, A. and Epstein, A. (1972). Sex differences in the acquisition of two kinds of avoidance behavior in rats. *Physiol. & Behav.* 8, 611-615.

Epstein, A. and Teitelbaum, P. (1967). Specific loss of hypoglycemic control of feeding in recovered lateral rats. *Am. J. Physiol.* 213, 1159-1163.

Finger, S., Marshak, R.A., Cohen, M., Scheff, S., Trace, R. and Niemand, D. (1971). Effects of successive and simultaneous lesions of somatosensory cortex on tactile discrimination in the rat. *J. Comp. Physiol. Psychol.* 77, 221-227.

Frolkis, W., Bezrukov, V.V. and Sinitsky, V.N. (1972). Sensitivity of central nervous structures to humoral factors in aging. *Exp. Geront.* 7, 185-194.

Glick, S. (1969). Discrimination learning and reversal in frontal rats as a function of cue. *Physiol. & Behav.* 4, 389-392.

Glick, S. and Zimmerberg, B. (1972). Comparative recovery following simultaneous and successive frontal brain damage in mice. *J. Comp. Physiol. Psychol.* 79, 481-487.

Goddard, G. (1964). Functions of the amygdala. *Psychol. Bull.* 62, 89-109.

Goldberger, M. (1972). Restitution of function in the CNS: The pathologic grasp of *Macaca mulatta*. *Exp. Brain Res.* 15, 79-96.

Goldman, P.M. and Rosvold, H.E. (1972). The effects of selective caudate lesions in infant and juvenile rhesus monkeys. *Brain Res.* 43, 53-66.

Gray, J. and Buffery, A. (1971). Sex differences in emotional and cognitive behavior in mammals including man: adaptive and neural bases. *Acta Psychologica* 35, 89-111.

Grossman, S.P. (1972). Neurophysiologic aspects: Extrahypothalamic factors in the regulation of food intake. *Adv. Psychosom. Med.* 7, 49-72 (Basel).

Isaac, W. (1964). Role of stimulation and time in the effects of spaced occipital ablations. *Psychol. Rep.* 14, 151-154.

Kellicut, M.H. and Schwartzbaum, J.S. (1963). Formation of a conditioned emotional response (CER) following lesions of the amygdaloid complex in rats. *Psych. Rep.* 12, 351-358.

Kemble, E.D. and Beckman, G.J. (1969). Escape latencies at three levels of electric shock in rats. *Psychon. Sci.* 14, 205-206.

Kennard, M. (1942). Cortical reorganization of motor function. *Arch. Neurol. Psychiat. (Chic.)* 48, 377-397.

Kesner, R.P., Fiedler, P. and Thomas, G. (1967). Function of the midbrain reticular formation in regulating level of activity and learning in rats. *J. Comp. Physiol. Psychol.* 63, 452-457.

Kimble, D.P. (1963). The effects of bilateral hippocampal lesions in rats. *J. Comp. Physiol. Psychol.* 56, 273-283.

Kimura, D. (1973). The assymetry of the human brain *Sci. Amer.* 228, 70-78.

Kircher, K., Braun, J.J., Meyer, D.R. and Meyer, P.M. (1970). Equivalence of simultaneous and successive neocortical ablations in productions of impairments of retention of black-white habits in rats. *J. Comp. Physiol. Psychol.* 71, 420-425.

Kirkby, R.J. (1969). Caudate nucleus lesions and perseverative behavior. *Physiol. & Behav.* 4, 451-454.

König, J.F.R. and Klippel, R.A. (1970). "The rat brain: a stereotaxic atlas" Huntington, N.Y.: Krieger Publishing Co.

LeVere, T. and Weiss, J. (1973). Failure of seriatum dorsal hippocampal lesions to spare spatial reversal behavior in rats. *J. Comp. Physiol. Psychol.* 82, 205-210.

Levine, S. (1968). Hormones and conditioning. *In* D. Levine (Ed.) "Nebraska Symposium on Motivation," Lincoln: University of Nebraska Press. pp. 85-101.

Luria, A.R. (1963). "Restoration of Function after Brain Injury," Oxford: Pergamon Press.

Lynch, G., Deadwyler, S. and Cotman, C. (1973). Postlesion axonal growth produces permanent functional connections. *Science* 180, 1364-1366.

McIntyre, M. and Stein, D.G. (1973). Differential effects of one- vs. two-stage amygdaloid lesions on activity, exploratory and avoidance behavior in the albino rat. *Behav. Biol.* 9, 454-466.

Meyer, D.R., Isaac, W. and Maher, B. (1958). The role of stimulation in spontaneous reorganization of visual habits. *J. Comp. Physiol. Psychol.* 51, 546-548.

Miklus, W. and Isaacson, R. (1965). Impairment and perseveration in delayed tasks due to bilateral lesions of the caudate nucleus in rats. *Psychon. Sci.* 3, 485-486.

Moore, R., Björklund, A. and Stenevi, U. (1971). Plastic changes in the adrenergic innervation of the rat septal area in response to denervation. *Brain Res.* 33, 13-35.

Patrissi, G. and Stein, D.G. (1971). Time factors in recovery of function following frontal lobe lesions in the rat. Paper presented at First Annual meeting of Society for Neuroscience, Washington, D.C. October.

Potegal, M. (1969). Role of the caudate nucleus in spatial orientation of rats. *J. Comp. Physiol. Psychol.* 69, 756-764.

Raisman, G. (1969). Neuronal plasticity in the septal nuclei of the adult rat. *Brain Res.* 14, 25-48.

Reyes, R., Finger, S. and Frye, J. (1973). Serial thalamic lesions and tactile discrimination in the rat. *Behav. Biol.* 8, 807-813.

Reynolds, R.W. and Kim, J. (1972). Chronic gnawing induced by electrolytic dorsolateral and lateral to the lateral hypothalamus. *Physiol & Behav.* 8, 1179-1181.

Rosen, J., Stein, D.G. and Butters, N. (1971). Recovery of function after serial ablation of prefrontal cortex in the rhesus monkey. *Science* 173, 353-356.

Rosvold, H.E. (1972). The frontal lobe system: cortical-subcortical interrelationships. *Acta Neurobiol. Exp.* 32, 439-460.

Rosvold, H.E., Mishkin, M. and Szwarcbart, M. (1958). Effects of subcortical lesions in monkeys on visual-discrimination and single-alternation performance. *J. Comp. Physiol. Psychol.* 51, 437-44.

Rosner, B. (1970). Brain Functions. *Ann. Rev. Psychol.* 21, 555-594.

Schneider, G. (1970). Mechanisms of functional recovery following lesions of visual cortex or superior colliculus in neonate and adult hamsters. *Brain Behav., Evolution* 3, 295-323.

Schultze, M.J. and Stein, D.G. Recovery of function in the albino rat following simultaneous or seriatim lesions of the caudate nucleus. In preparation.

Steffans, A.B. (1969). The influence of insulin injection and infusions on eating and blood glucose level in the rat. *Physiol. & Behav.* 4, 823-828.

Stein, D.G., Rosen, J.J., Graziedei, J., Mishkin, D. and Brink, J. (1969). Central Nervous System: Recovery of function. *Science* 166, 528-530.

Stenevi, U., Björklund, A. and Moore, R.Y. (1972). Growth of intact central adrenergic axons in the denervated lateral geniculate body. *Exper. Neurol.* 35, 290-299.

Swanson, H.H. (1967). Alteration of sex typical behavior of hamsters in open field and emergence tests by neonatal administration of androgen or estrogen. *Animal Behav.* 15, 209-216.

Teitelbaum, B. (1973). Sex differences in delayed alternation performance following single or multiple stage frontal lesions in rats. Paper presented at 81st annual convention of American Psychological Association in Montreal, Quebec, August 29th.

Teitelbaum, P. and Epstein, A. (1962). The lateral hypothalamic syndrome: Recovery of feeding and drinking after lateral hypothalamic lesions. *Psychol. Rev.* 69, 74-90.

Tucker, T.J. and Kling, A. (1968). Sparing of function following localized brain lesions in neonatal monkeys. *In* R.L. Isaacson (Ed.) "The Neuropsychology of Development," New York: John Wiley & Sons.

Wayner, M.J., Cott, A., Millner, J. and Tartaglione, R. (1971). Loss of 2-deoxy-D-glucose induced eating in recovered lateral rats. *Physiol. & Behav.* 7, 880-884.

Zornetzer, S., Chronister, R.B. and Ross, B. (1973). The hippocampus and retrograde amnesia: localization of some positive and negative memory disruptive sites. *Behav. Biol.* 8, 508-518.

RECOVERY OF BEHAVIORAL FUNCTIONS AFTER SEQUENTIAL ABLATION OF THE FRONTAL LOBES OF MONKEYS

Nelson Butters
Boston University School of Medicine
Boston, Massachusetts

Jeffrey Rosen
Boston University
Boston, Massachusetts

Donald Stein
Clark University
Worcester, Massachusetts

Since Jacobsen's (1935) classical studies on the functions of the frontal lobes, three types of experiments have dominated the literature on this subject. In the first place there have been a large number of studies (e.g., Mishkin 1957; Gross 1963; Butters and Pandya 1969) concerned with the localization of behavioral deficits observed after large frontal lesions. These investigations have attempted to identify the smallest frontal lesion necessary and sufficient to produce the "frontal syndrome." An approach, closely associated with the first, has attempted to delineate the other cortical and/or subcortical structures that compose a frontal neural circuit (e.g., Rosvold 1972). That is, whether other structures anatomically associated with the frontal lobes, (e.g., head of the caudate nucleus) can also mediate the spatial-delay type of tasks that are impaired after frontal lobe lesions. The third problem area has focused upon specific nature of the behavioral deficits occurring after lesions rather than the anatomy of the frontal lobes (e.g., Mishkin 1964; Stamm and Rosen 1972). Thus, why do monkeys with frontal damage fail spatial delayed-alternation (DA) or delayed-response (DR)? Do these deficits reflect a problem with memory, space or motivation?

Although these three types of investigations differ in their explicit aims, they share at least one underlying neuropsychological assumption:

brain (structure)-behavior (function) relationships are innate and fixed. From this position it follows that if one ablates the critical "focus" within the frontal lobes or a sector of the frontal lobe circuit, severe deficits on DA and DR should always follow. Although exceptions are sometimes made for the few "statistically variant" adults who quickly recover behavioral functions following extensive brain damage. Once these neural circuits are destroyed it is assumed that no reorganization of behavioral functions is possible in the adult subject.

Despite the widespread acceptance of the concept of fixed structure-function relationships in the CNS there is now considerable evidence that this assumption may have limited validity. A number of studies have shown that the ablation of the monkey's prefrontal cortex during infancy is followed by normal DR performance when the monkeys are tested a year later (Harlow, Akert and Schiltz 1964; Tucker and Kling 1969; Goldman 1972). Similarly, a number of investigations have demonstrated that serial, rather than one-stage, removals of cortical structures in monkeys and rats leads to some recovery or sparing of function (e.g., Ades and Raab 1949; Meyer 1958; Stein, Rosen, Graziadei, Mishkin and Brink 1969). Ades and his collaborators (1949, 1952) found that serial removal of the monkeys' posterior associa-tion cortex did not affect perceptual abilities shown to be impaired after one-stage ablation of identical cortical regions. In rats, Meyer (1959) has reported extensive sparing of visual functions after serial striate lesions, and Stein *et al*. (1969) have shown normal spatial alternation performance after serial frontal and hippocampal lesions.

Given this demonstration of behavioral sparing after frontal lesions in infancy and the evidence suggesting that similar sparing might be evident after serial ablations in the adult, we initiated a series of studies concerned with recovery of function after serial ablation of the monkey's prefrontal association cortex. Three issues have been of major concern: (1) Does sparing of function follow serial ablation of the monkey's prefrontal association cortex? (2) If sparing or recovery does occur, is the pattern of recovery similar to that observed after lesions in infancy? (3) What neural mechanisms underlie the recovery phenomenon?

RECOVERY OF SPATIAL FUNCTIONS AFTER SERIAL ABLATION OF SULCUS PRINCIPALIS (DORSOLATERAL PREFRONTAL CORTEX)

In our initial study, monkeys with serial or one-stage lesions of sulcus principalis were assessed on three spatial tests known to be sensitive to one-stage removals of this sulcus (Mishkin 1957; Gross 1963; Butters and Pandya 1969). Ten naive adolescent rhesus monkeys (*Macaca mulatta*) ranging in weight from 3.0 to 4.0 kg served as the subjects for this experiment. All behavioral testing was conducted in a modified Wisconsin General Test Apparatus with an opaque screen (that could be raised or lowered) separating the monkey's compartment from the test tray. Raisins served as reinforcements. The animals were tested five days a week for 30 trials per day on all three tasks.

Preoperatively all monkeys learned 5-sec. spatial delayed alternation (DA). On each trial of this test the monkey was presented with two identical wooden plaques covering two recessed foodwells. One foodwell was located to the monkeys' left, one to their right. To acquire this task, the monkeys had to learn to alternate their spatial responses (right-left) on each successive trial. On the first trial of each daily test session, both foodwells were baited with raisins. On the second trial, only the foodwell not selected (i.e., responded to) on the first trial contained a reinforcement. If the monkeys made an error on any given trial, the reinforcement remained on the same side until the monkeys made a correct response on some succeeding trial (rerun correction procedure). These correction trials were counted within the 30 trial daily sessions. All monkeys continued testing until they reached a criterion of at least 90 correct responses in 100 consecutive trials.

Upon attaining DA criterion, the monkeys were assigned to one of the two surgical conditions,

the one-stage (OS) or serial-stage (SS) groups.
Surgery was performed under standard aseptic
conditions with Nembutal anesthesia (40 mg/kg).
Cortical tissue in the banks and depths of sulcus
principalis was removed by subpial aspiration. All
OS monkeys received bilateral lesions of sulcus
principalis in one operation 10 weeks after
reaching DA criterion. The SS monkeys had sulcus
principalis ablated in four operations spaced
three weeks apart, with the first operation
occurring within one week of reaching DA criterion.
Each stage of SS surgery involved the removal of
one bank of sulcus principalis. During the first
operation the inferior bank of sulcus principalis
in the left hemisphere was removed; in the second
operation, the superior bank of the sulcus in the
right hemisphere; in the third operation, the
superior bank in the left hemisphere; and finally,
in the fourth operation the inferior bank of
sulcus principalis in the right hemisphere was
ablated.

Two weeks after all surgery had been completed,
the monkeys began postoperative testing on DA
retention. The same procedures and criterion
employed preoperatively were also used for post-
operative retention. The monkeys were tested until
they met criterion or for a maximum of 1000 trials.

Following completion of DA testing, all monkeys
were trained on a 5-sec. delayed-response (DR)
task. The same testing tray (with two foodwells)
and plaques used for DA were also employed for DR.
The monkeys were initially allowed to observe the
experimenter bait and cover one of the two foodwells and then to respond immediately to either of
the two plaques. When the monkeys consistently
chose the baited foodwell (criterion was at least
27 correct responses in 30 consecutive trials) at
this nondelay interval, delay procedures were
introduced by lowering the opaque screen between
the animals and the test tray immediately after
baiting of a foodwell. At first the screen was
lowered and raised as quickly as possible (zero
delay, with screen). Upon attaining criterion at
this zero-second delay (with screen), the delay
interval between the lowering and raising of the
screen was increased by one second intervals each
day. Such increments in delay continued until the

monkeys attained criterion (at least 27 correct responses in 30 consecutive daily trials) with a five second delay. If the monkeys failed to attain criterion at any given delay (e.g., three seconds), the interval was decreased by one second on the following day (thus it would be two seconds). Testing was terminated if the monkeys failed to reach criterion at the five second delay interval within 1020 trials.

With completion of DR testing, the monkeys were trained on a series of place reversals (PR). This task required the subjects to learn and then to reverse spatial habits. The same test tray employed for DA and DR was again used. Initially the animals had to learn to respond to the right foodwell (both foodwells were covered by identical red wooden plaques) to obtain a reinforcement. Training on this spatial discrimination was continued until the monkeys reached a criterion of at least 27 correct responses in 30 consecutive daily trials. On the day following criterion attainment, the reinforcement contingencies for the two plaques were switched -- i.e., now only the foodwell on the left was baited with a reinforcement. The monkeys were tested on this reversal problem (Reversal 1) until they reached the same criterion specified for the original discrimination. This first reversal problem was followed by a second reversal (only the right foodwell was baited). In all, the monkeys learned four such reversals, each to the same criterion.

When PR training was finished the monkeys were sacrificed and their brains were prepared for histological analysis.

Table 1 shows the performance of all 10 monkeys on DA retention, DR, and PR. To evaluate overall spatial performance a total error score was derived by adding the error scores for the individual spatial tests. The SS group made significantly ($p < .05$) fewer total errors than did the OS group.

On DA, the SS group made fewer errors than did the OS group, but the difference does not approach significance. However, one monkey in each group reached DA quickly while the remaining four monkeys failed to reach criterion within 1000 trials. When the DA performances of the monkeys

Table 1

Errors compiled by OS and SS monkeys on DA
retention, DR acquisition, PR learning,
and total errors

SS Monkeys	DA	DR	PR1	PR2	PR3	PR4	Total errors
36	5	107	59	16	14	11	212
52	384	68	20	16	17	6	511
46	345	34	19	15	7	3	423
39	308	86	17	8	5	3	427
62	330	20	25	11	6	2	394
$\overline{X}$	274	63	28	13	10	5	393
OS Monkeys							
41	76	123	17	13	7	6	242
42	542	31	11	11	89	33	717
38	479	245	68	101	41	30	964
58	360	178	22	27	28	10	625
59	445	97	36	13	11	6	608
$\overline{X}$	380	135	31	33	35	17	631

that failed to relearn are compared, significant differences between the OS and SS groups emerge. Figure 1 shows the DA performance of the two groups for trials 1-500 and trials 501-1000. While the groups do not differ for trials 1-500, the SS group made significantly (p < .05) fewer errors on trials 501-1000 than did the OS group. Thus, both groups are initially (1-500) impaired on DA, but the SS group recovers the spatial alternation capacity at a faster rate than does the OS group.

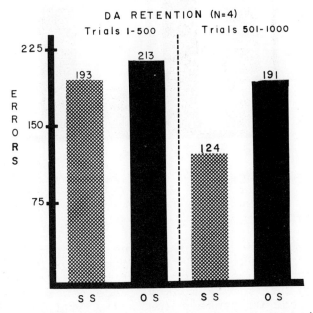

Figure 1. DA Retention: Mean errors on trials 1-500 and trials 501-1000 for OS and SS monkeys that failed to relearn within 1000 trials.

Figure 2 indicates that the improvement of the SS group during trials 501-1000 reflects the group's decreased tendency to make perseverative (repetitive errors). A perseverative error on DA is defined as every error after the first in a continuous sequence of errors. If a monkey responded erroneously to the same spatial position for seven consecutive trials, it would be credited with six perseverative errors. While the groups do not differ significantly on trials 1-500, the SS monkeys made significantly (p < .025) fewer

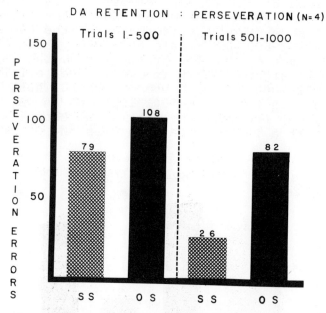

Figure 2. DA Retention: Mean perseverative errors on trials 1-500 and trials 501-1000 for OS and SS monkeys that failed to relearn within 1000 trials.

perseverative errors during the second 500 trials.
     The monkeys' performance on DR and PR also demonstrate the superiority of the serial-stage group. On DR, the SS monkeys made fewer errors than did the OS monkeys (p< .07). All five SS monkeys learned DR within 1020 trials while two of the OS monkeys failed to do so. The PR performances also indicated that the SS group was able to improve with training while the OS group failed to show such gains (Figure 3). The two groups did not differ significantly on the first two reversals, but on both the third and fourth reversals the SS group made significantly (p < .05) fewer errors than did the OS group.
     The histological findings are graphically summarized in Figure 4. For the OS monkeys, the lesions were as intended; practically all of the cortex in the banks and depths of the sulcus was ablated, and the lesion did not involve extensive amounts of surrounding dorsolateral cortex. In

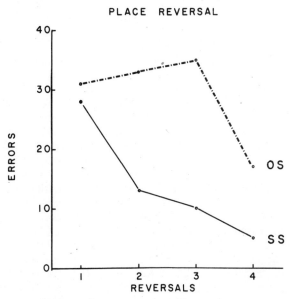

Figure 3. PR Performance: Mean errors on four place reversals for OS and SS monkeys.

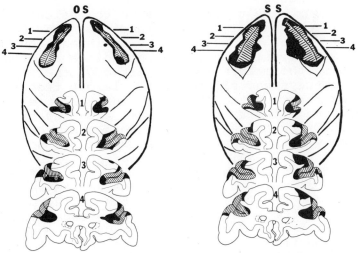

Figure 4. Dorsal views and representative coronal sections of the maximum and minimum extent of frontal damage in the one-(OS) and serial-stage (SS) surgical groups. The hatched areas represent the minimum insult observed, while the addition of the solid portions represent maximum damage.

comparison, the SS monkeys had more extensive lesions than originally intended. While the serial lesions in sulcus principalis were similar in extent to those of the OS group, they did involve extensive areas of surrounding dorsolateral cortex. This additional damage was produced by the removal of dural adhesions during the second operation on a given hemisphere (operations 3 and 4). As a consequence of this supplementary damage, the SS monkeys had significantly (p < .01) larger lesions (as judged by planimetric measurements) than did the OS animals. However, the histology did not reveal any differences between the groups in the amount of damage to the depths and banks of sulcus principalis. There was no significant (p > .10) correlation between the extent of principalis damage and the postoperative performance of either the SS or OS monkeys (P=+.24, +.21 respectively). Finally, the histology did not provide any clues as to the unusual DA performance of monkeys SS-36 and OS-41, the animals that relearned DA quickly. Neither in localization nor in extent did these animals' lesions differ from the group means.

Our results can be taken to indicate that partial recovery of spatial functions can occur not only after frontal lesions in infancy but also after serial ablation of the dorsolateral frontal cortex in the mature monkey. Although the serial-stage monkeys had significantly larger frontal lesions than did the one-stage animals, the serial animals made fewer errors on all three spatial tasks. On DR and PR the performance of the SS monkeys was essentially normal while the performance of the OS animals was impaired. On DA both the SS and OS groups were impaired (i.e., four of the five animals in each group failed to relearn within 1000 trials), but still the serial monkeys made fewer errors than did the one-stage monkeys. This serial-stage superiority on DA was most evident on trials 501-1000, a finding that underlines the gradual recovery of spatial functions for the serial-stage monkeys. It may be important to note that the present differences between DA and DR recovery closely parallel the findings of early lesion studies. Goldman, Rosvold and Mishkin (1970) have reported that frontal

lobectomies performed within the first 30 days
after birth have differing effects upon DR and DA.
When the lobectomized monkeys were tested a year
after surgery they displayed only a minimal
deficit on DR but achieved only an 80% level of
correct responses on DA after 2000 training trials.
This striking parallel between infant and serial
results suggests that these two recovery phenomena
may involve similar neural mechanisms. This
possibility was pursued in our second investigation.

A FAILURE TO FIND RECOVERY AFTER SERIAL ABLATION OF THE ORBITAL PREFRONTAL CORTEX*

While sparing of function often follows both
early and serial brain damage, it appears that
such recovery may be limited for some brain
structures and behavioral functions. Delayed-
response and delayed-alternation performance are
often considered indices of the same spatial
function (e.g., Mishkin 1964), yet the sparing of
DR is greater than for DA after early (Goldman,
Rosvold and Mishkin 1970) and sequential lesions
of the frontal cortex. Goldman (1971, 1972) has
also shown that functional recovery occurs after
lesions of the dorsolateral prefrontal cortex but
not after equally early lesions of the orbital
prefrontal region. Ablation of the orbital surface
within the first 30 days of life does not
attenuate the monkeys' learning deficits when the
animals are tested at one year of age.

In view of this functional dissociation after
early dorsolateral and orbital lesions, it seemed
appropriate to determine whether serial ablation
of the orbital cortex in the mature monkey would
result in recovery or sparing of function. If
recovery does not follow sequential lesions of
the orbital surface, this finding would provide
further evidence that sparing of function is not
characteristic of all brain structures. In
addition, although the neural mechanisms under-

---

*Dr. Charles Butter of the University of Michigan
collaborated with the authors in conducting the
following study.

lying recovery phenomena are not yet well understood, the finding of similar patterns of recovery after early and serial lesions would suggest that similar mechanisms are involved in both types of recovery.

Fifteen rhesus monkeys (weighing between 3.0-4.0 kg) were tested on three tasks, a visual go-no go discrimination (G-NG), DA, and object reversal learning (OR), on which monkeys with one-stage bilateral orbital lesions are known to be impaired (Mishkin 1964; Butter 1969). Five of the monkeys had one-stage bilateral lateral orbital ablations (OS), five had serial-stage removals of the same cortex (SS), and five served as unoperated controls (UC). Fourteen of the 15 monkeys completed all behavioral testing but one UC monkey died after DA and never attempted the OR task. All testing was performed in the same apparatus used in the previous experiment.

Preoperatively, all monkeys learned a visual G-NG problem. On each trial the monkeys were presented with a tray containing a single foodwell centered in the middle of the tray. On half the trials, the foodwell was covered by a gray cardboard plaque on which a white outlined paper square had been glued; on the remaining trials, the figure on the gray plaque was a white plus sign. If the monkeys displaced the plus plaque within five seconds, they received a reinforcement and were credited with a correct response. If the monkeys failed to displace the plus plaque within five seconds, the screen was lowered and the monkeys were credited with an error. If the monkeys displaced the square plaque within five seconds, they received no reinforcement and were credited with an error. If the monkeys refrained from displacing the square plaque for five seconds, the screen was lowered, and they received no reward but were credited with a correct response. Thus, the monkeys had to learn to respond to the plus and not to respond to the square. Thirty noncorrection trials were administered daily until the monkeys reached a criterion of at least 90 correct responses in 100 consecutive trials. After attaining criterion the monkeys were assigned to one of the surgical or control conditions.

The 10 monkeys assigned to the OS or SS groups all received bilateral removals of the lateral orbital cortex. The intended area of the lesion included all cortex on the convexity separating the dorsolateral and orbital prefrontal cortex. The intended boundary dorsally was a horizontal line five millimeters below sulcus principalis and ventrally, the lateral orbital sulcus. Anteriorly the intended lesions were supposed to extend to the frontal pole. The intended posterior extent of the lesion was the descending limb of the arcuate sulcus. The operations were performed under aseptic conditions while the animals were anaesthetized.

The five monkeys assigned to the one-stage lesion group had a single bilateral operation 10 weeks after reaching criterion. The five monkeys assigned to the sequential (i.e., serial) lesion group received four operations spaced three weeks apart. For each operation the sector of the lateral orbital cortex and/or hemisphere were switched. In the first operation the lateral orbital cortex of the left hemisphere was removed; in the second, the inferior dorsolateral surface of the right hemisphere; in the third, the inferior dorsolateral surface of the left hemisphere; and finally, the lateral orbital surface of the right hemisphere was removed in the fourth operation.

Two weeks following their last operation (or after 10 weeks of rest for the unoperated controls), the monkeys were tested for G-NG retention. The same procedures and learning criterion employed preoperatively were used again.

After completion of G-NG retention, the monkeys were trained on DA. The same procedures and criterion employed in the first experiment were followed in this study. If a monkey failed to learn DA within 1000 trials testing was terminated.

One week after completing DA training the monkeys began the OR task. On each trial the monkeys were presented with two foodwells (one to their right and one to their left) covered by wooden objects glued to wooden plaques) differing in color, shape, and size and were allowed to displace one of the plaques. If the monkey chose the correct object, it received a raisin reward;

if the monkey chose the incorrect object, it found no raisins in the foodwell. Initially, the monkeys were trained to respond to one of the two objects. When the monkeys reached criterion on the original discrimination (at least 27 correct responses on 30 consecutive daily trials), the reward value of the objects was switched (Reversal 1), and the monkeys had to learn this reversal to the same criterion as the original discrimination. Following attainment of criterion on this first reversal, the reward value of the two objects was again switched (Reversal 2) and the monkeys had to learn this reversal problem. In all, five successive reversals were learned by the monkeys.

When the monkeys completed testing on the fifth OR, they were sacrificed and their brains were prepared for histological evaluation.

Figures 5a and 5b show the histological results for the 10 operated monkeys. In general, the lesions included all of the lateral orbital cortex intended to be removed. Several animals in each operated group had lesions extending up to sulcus principalis and involving to varying degrees the lower bank of this sulcus. Assessments of total lesion size and placement (using a polar plani-meter) indicated that the two operated groups did not differ significantly.

The behavioral results for the three groups (SS, OS, UC) are shown in Figures 6, 7, and 8. All monkeys learned G-NG preoperatively and the three groups did not differ significantly in the number of errors required to attain criterion. Analyses of the monkeys' postoperative G-NG performance (Figure 6) did demonstrate major differences among the groups. Both the serial and one-stage groups made significantly ($p < .007$) more errors than did the unoperated control group, but the two operated groups did not differ significantly from each other.

The results for DA acquisition are similar to those for G-NG (Figure 7). Again there is no evidence of sparing. The control group made fewer errors than did the OS ($p < .05$) and SS ($p < .10$) groups. The difference between the OS and SS groups did not approach significance ($p > .40$).

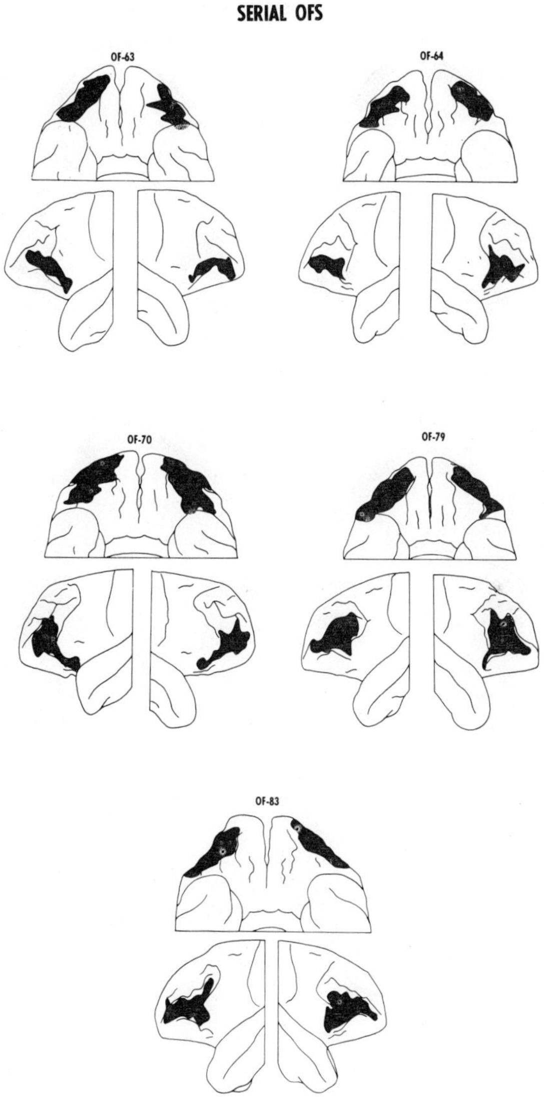

SERIAL OFS

Figure 5A. Ventral and lateral views of the serial lateral orbital frontal lesions (in black).

ONE-STAGE OFS

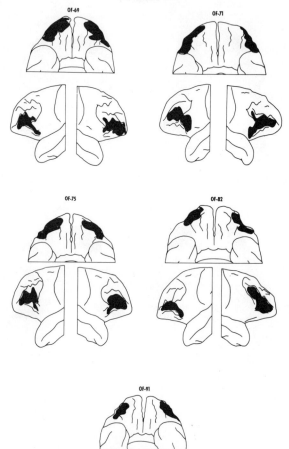

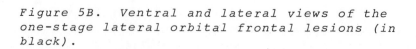

Figure 5B. Ventral and lateral views of the one-stage lateral orbital frontal lesions (in black).

GO⁻ NO GO RETENTION

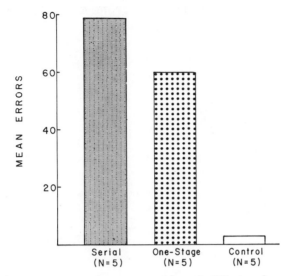

Figure 6. Mean errors on the G-NG task.

DA ACQUISITION

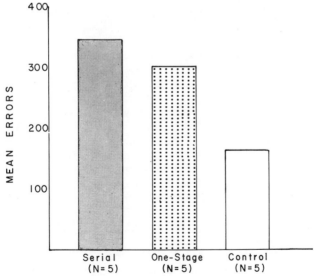

Figure 7. Mean errors in the acquisition of DA.

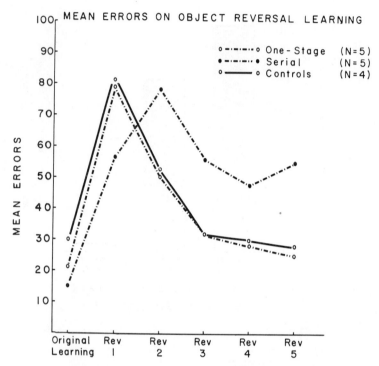

Figure 8. *Mean errors on OR learning.*

The SS vs. UC and OS vs. UC comparisons did not attain higher levels of significance because one UC monkey failed to learn DA within 1000 trials. Since this animal is the only intact monkey to fail DA acquisition in our laboratory within the last six years, its DA performance (279 errors) does not fall within the normal range. If this monkey is excluded from DA analyses, the mean error score of the UC group drops to 133 and the comparisons between the UC and the two operated groups are both highly significant (OS vs. UC, $p < .028$; SS vs. UC, $p < .034$).

The results for OR (Figure 8) also show that serial orbital removals did not lead to an attenuated behavioral deficit. Both the UC and OS monkeys made fewer errors with each successive reversal while the SS monkeys failed to show this degree of systematic improvement. When improvement

from Reversal 1-5 was computed, both the UC and
OS monkeys displayed significantly (p < .02)
greater gains than did the SS animals. The OS
and UC groups did not differ in their reversal
performance, a surprising finding in view of the
recent literature (Butter 1969; Mishkin 1967)
demonstrating the importance of orbital cortex
for OR performance.

Our present results lead us to suggest that
sequential ablation of the lateral orbital cortex
with an interoperative interval previously
successful for obtaining recovery did not reduce
the severity of the behavioral dysfunction usually
associated with lesions produced in one stage. On
all three tasks the monkeys with serial lesions
performed more poorly than did the animals with
one-stage lesions, and on one task (OR) this
difference was significant. These findings for
serial orbital lesions obviously contrast with the
previous results for serial removals of sulcus
principalis but closely parallel recent findings
for early dorsolateral and orbital lesions.
Goldman (1972) has demonstrated that recovery of
function occurs (10 months after surgery) after
removal of dorsolateral prefrontal cortex in
infancy but not after equally early ablation of
the orbital prefrontal cortex.

While these parallel findings suggest that
similar neural mechanisms may be mediating
sparing after infant and serial lesions, Goldman's
more recent results (1972) indicate that the noted
similarities in the two recovery phenomena may be
superficial. Monkeys that had their dorsolateral
cortex removed in infancy (within 30 days of
birth) and had evidenced behavioral recovery 10
months following surgery were severely impaired
when tested at two years of age. Conversely,
monkeys that had orbital lesions during infancy
and had shown little recovery 10 months after
surgery displayed considerable sparing when they
were tested at two years of age. Goldman believes
that this remarkable shift in recovery patterns
is related to the ontogenetic development of the
dorsolateral and orbital cortices (i.e., the
orbital cortex matures more quickly and assumes
its behavioral functions sooner than does the
dorsolateral region). If Goldman's interpretation

447

of her infant data is valid, it is difficult to understand how these developmental neuroanatomical factors might also be applicable to recovery after serial lesions.

This dissociation between the effects of serial ablation of dorsolateral and orbital cortices does suggest at least one hypothesis related to the limitations of the recovery phenomenon. In addition to their distinctive patterns of recovery, the dorsolateral and orbital cortices also differ in the behavioral functions they are thought to mediate and the anatomical structures with which they are associated. The dorsolateral cortex is involved with spatial and/or mnemonic functions (Mishkin 1964; Goldman and Rosvold 1970) and has major efferent connections with the basal ganglia, cingulate gyrus, and temporal neocortex (Nauta 1964; Johnson, Rosvold and Mishkin 1968). The orbital prefrontal cortex is involved with response and/or drive inhibition (Mishkin 1964; Butter and Snyder 1972) and is anatomically associated with a number of limbic structures such as the septal nuclei, amygdala, and hypothalamus (Nauta 1964; Johnson, Rosvold and Mishkin 1968). Perhaps then recovery of function after serial lesions in the adult primate is characteristic of neuroanatomical structures that are phylogenetically "new" and are concerned with sensory, motor, or associative (learning-cognitive) functions. In turn, such sparing of function may be far more restricted for structures that are phylogenetically "old" and are concerned with motivational-affective processes -- at least in the monkey.

Another possibility that cannot be overlooked at the present time is that the temporal interval between serial removals necessary to permit behavioral recovery may vary from structure to structure within the CNS. Thus 3 weeks between serial principalis lesions may have been sufficient to permit neural reorganization underlying recovery of spatial behaviors. This same interval, however, may not have been adequate for reorganization of function after orbital damage.

THE ROLE OF INTACT CORTICAL STRUCTURES IN RECOVERY
OF FUNCTION AFTER SERIAL FRONTAL LESIONS*

The first investigation demonstrated sparing
of function after sequential dorsolateral lesions,
but neither the first nor the second (orbital)
study shed much light on the neural mechanisms
underlying this recovery. If recovery after serial
lesions requires the assumption of behavioral
functions by intact neural structures, there is
some evidence to suggest that both intact cortical
and subcortical structures are involved. For
example, Glees and Cole (1950) showed in adult
monkeys that intact cortical tissue immediately
surrounding an ablated region of motor cortex may
assume the motor functions of the lesioned area.
Similarly, Doty (1961) has shown that visual
association cortex may assume the functions of
area 17 when it is ablated in infancy. In contrast
to these studies suggesting a cortical recovery
mechanism, a number of investigations have been
interpreted as supporting the role of intact
subcortical nuclei in recovery. Kling and Tucker
(1968) have suggested that the head of the caudate
nucleus mediates recovery after ablation of the
dorsolateral prefrontal cortex in infancy. Both
Meyer (1958) and Pasik and Pasik (1971) have
attributed recovery of visual functions after area
17 ablations in adulthood to subcortical
structures such as the superior colliculus and the
accessory optic system.
It is our long-range goal to examine the role
of both cortical and subcortical structures in
recovery after sequential lesions of the prefrontal
cortex. To date, however, our efforts have focused
upon cortical mechanisms. Two current studies
assess the role of intact association cortex, both
anterior and posterior, in recovery after serial
frontal lesions. The first experiment examines the

---

*Some of the monkeys reported in this section
were housed, operated, and tested at the New
England Regional Primate Center. The authors wish
to thank Drs. Trum, Jones, Garcia and their staff
for their cooperation in the use of the Center's
facilities.

possibility that intact cortex immediately surrounding the serially ablated cortex assumes the
functions of the damaged tissue. The second study
attempts to determine whether anterior and posterior association cortices, not immediately
surrounding the serially ablated region, are
involved in the sparing of frontal lobe functions.

The rationale for the first study partially
stems from earlier investigations (Butters and
Pandya 1969; Butters, Pandya, Sanders and Dye
1971) concerned with the localization of spatial-
mnemonic functions within sulcus principalis. In
these studies it was demonstrated that sulcus
principalis is not equipotential with respect to
its role in mediating spatial-mnemonic functions.
Rather, lesions limited to the middle nine
millimeters of the sulcus were necessary and
sufficient to produce severe DA and PR deficits.
In contrast, lesions limited to the anterior or
posterior nine millimeters of the sulcus had
little, if any, effect upon the spatial tasks.

When this empirical finding is considered in
conjunction with the studies by Doty (1961) and
by Glees and Cole (1950), they suggest an explanation for the partial recovery reported in our
first serial lesion study (i.e., serial vs.
one-stage ablation of sulcus principalis). After
serial ablation of the entire principal sulcus the
monkeys displayed considerable sparing in their
DR and PR performance but only limited recovery on
DA. If the intact cortex immediately surrounding
the ablated behavioral "focus" was critical in the
recovery process, the removal of the entire
principal sulcus may have included not only the
critical focus for DA performance (the middle
third of the sulcus) but also the surrounding
cortex that might normally participate in the
recovery process. To assess this possibility,
monkeys with serial and one-stage removals of the
middle third of sulcus principalis were compared
on the retention of DA.

Eight monkeys were employed in this study. All
monkeys learned DA preoperatively with the same
procedures described in the first study. After
reaching criterion, the monkeys rested for two
weeks and were then tested preoperatively for
retention of DA (Retention 1). When the monkeys

relearned DA they were assigned to one of two
operated conditions, serial (SS) or one-stage (OS)
ablations of the midprincipalis region. The four
SS monkeys had the middle nine millimeters of
sulcus principalis ablated serially. In the first
operation both banks of the middle third of the
sulcus were removed (by subpial aspiration) in the
left hemisphere. An attempt was made to ablate
both superficial tissue and all cortex in the
depths of the sulcus. Care was taken to insure
that the lesions did not involve the anterior or
posterior sectors of the sulcus. Four weeks
following the first operation, the midprincipalis
region in the right hemisphere was ablated in a
similar manner. For the four OS monkeys, the
midprincipalis region was ablated in a single
bilateral operation four to five weeks after
reaching criterion on DA Retention 1.

Two weeks following their last operation all
monkeys were retrained on DA (Retention 2), again
employing the same procedures described previously
in this paper. When DA testing was completed,
seven of the eight monkeys were sacrificed. The
eighth monkey, a SS animal, received further
testing and surgery that will be discussed later
in this section.

The results of this experiment are shown in
Figure 9. In addition to the postoperative DA
retention scores of the serial and one-stage midprincipalis monkeys, the DA performance of the 10
monkeys used in the first study (serial vs.
one-stage removals of the entire sulcus) are
shown for comparison. While the serial and
one-stage groups did not differ significantly in
the previous investigation (removals of the
entire sulcus), there is no overlap in the
performance of the SS and OS monkeys with limited
midprincipalis lesions. All four SS midprincipalis
monkeys relearned DA within 1000 trials while all
four OS midprincipalis monkeys failed to relearn
the task. It should also be noted that the two OS
groups do not differ significantly ($p > .25$), but
the SS midprincipalis monkeys perform significantly
($p < .05$) better than the SS monkeys with total
sulcus principalis lesions.

These results are taken to indicate that
limiting the serial lesions to the cortical focus

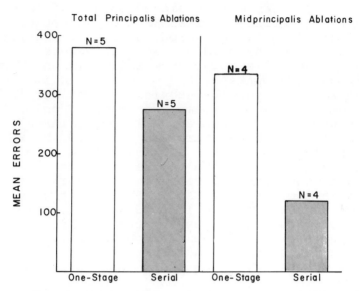

Figure 9. DA Retention: Mean errors of OS and SS monkeys with total sulcus principalis or midprincipalis lesions.

for DA, and thereby sparing the tissue immediately surrounding the focus (i.e., the anterior and posterior thirds of the sulcus), results in more extensive recovery than found in the initial experiment. This finding permits us to suggest that the posterior and/or anterior sectors of the sulcus may be important in the recovery process. Although inclusion of these anterior-posterior sectors in a one-stage lesion does not significantly increase the size of the behavioral deficit, their involvement in a serial lesion greatly limits the amount of sparing on a spatial task such as DA. It appears that the anterior and posterior sectors may be capable of assuming the functions of the midprincipalis region (i.e., the focus for spatial-delay type tasks) when this focus is removed serially.

As a further examination of the role of the anterior-posterior sectors in the recovery process, one of the serial midprincipalis monkeys (No. 36A) was not sacrificed after completion of DA testing. This animal again relearned DA (Retention 3) and then received another lesion, a one-stage bilateral

ablation of the posterior third of sulcus
principalis. Two weeks following this last surgical
procedure, the monkey was tested again on DA
(Retention 4). Figure 10 shows the total DA
history of this monkey. The animal's preoperative
acquisition and retention (Retention 1) were

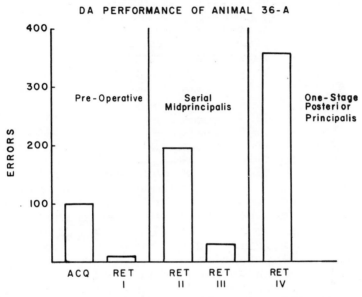

Figure 10. DA Performance of Monkey 36A: Errors
on acquisition and retention 1 (pre-operative
performance), on retentions 2 and 3 (after serial
midprincipalis lesions), on retention 4 (after
one-stage posterior principalis lesions).

normal. After receiving a serial midprincipalis
lesion, the monkey was impaired on DA (Retention
2) but did relearn the task within 1000 trials.
Performance on Retention 3 indicates that DA was
well retained by this midprincipalis monkey.
However, after the removal of the posterior sector
of sulcus principalis, the monkey was unable to
relearn DA within 1000 trials (Retention 4). For
this monkey, the posterior sector of sulcus
principalis was involved in the recovery of DA performance after the serial midprincipalis ablation.
     While the results of the third experiment
demonstrate that adjacent intact cortical tissue
is involved in the recovery process, the

possibility that more distant cortical regions may play some role still remains. To assess this question, we examined the role of three cortical association areas, the frontal periarcuate area, the inferior parietal lobule, and the posterior sector of the inferotemporal cortex, in recovery of function after serial lesions.

Fifteen monkeys participated in this experiment. All monkeys learned DA preoperatively and then were assigned to one of four groups. Four monkeys received one-stage bilateral ablations of the periarcuate sulcus in the frontal lobes (PA); three monkeys had one-stage bilateral removals of the inferior parietal lobule (IP); three monkeys received one-stage bilateral ablations of the posterior sector of the inferotemporal cortex (IT); and five monkeys remained unoperated at this time (SP).

Two weeks following surgery (or after two weeks of rest for the unoperated monkeys) all animals were retrained on DA (Retention 1). As shown in Table 2 all monkeys relearned DA with little difficulty and much positive savings. There were no significant differences among the groups on this first DA retention.

When the monkeys completed the first DA retention, they received serial ablations of the principal sulcus. In the first operation, the entire sulcus in the left hemisphere was removed; ten weeks later the principal sulcus in the right hemisphere was ablated. Two weeks following the second operation, all animals were tested again on DA (Retention 2), then on DR, and finally on PR. The same apparatus and procedures employed in previous studies were also used in this investigation. Following PR testing, all animals were sacrificed.

Figure 11 shows reconstructions of representative lesions from the four operated groups (PA, IP, IT, SP). The blackened regions represent the one-stage lesions (periarcuate, inferior parietal, infero-temporal). The stippled regions demarcate the dorsolateral extent of the serial ablations of sulcus principalis.

Table 2 shows the results for the total number of spatial errors (compiled by adding the errors on DA Retention 2, DR, and PR). All of the IP and

Table 2

Errors Compiled by PA, IP, IT, and SP Monkeys on
Spatial Tasks

	DA Acquisition	DA Retention 1	Total Spatial Errors
PA-74	82	22	715
PA-98	94	5	951
PA-32A	203	75	888
PA-50	231	11	1069
Mean	153	28	906
IP-2A	242	17	909
IP-3A	92	39	821
IP-4A	191	0	759
Mean	175	19	830
IT-60	176	28	801
IT-61	132	18	821
IT-59	382	43	923
Mean	230	30	848
SP-73	154	0	506
SP-14A	134	115	611
SP-29A	69	0	697
SP-45A	244	2	730
SP-42A	117	0	588
Mean	144	31	626

S P - 2 9 A

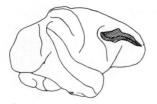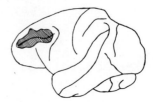

P A - 7 4

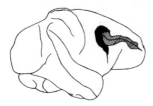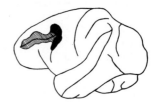

I P - 2 A

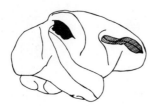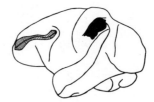

I T - 6 1 - 7 2

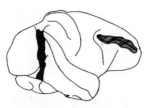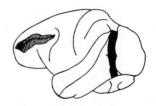

*Figure 11. Reconstructions of representative
lesions from the PA, IP, IT, and SP groups. The
blackened areas indicate one-stage lesions;
stippled areas indicate the serial removals of
sulcus principalis.*

IT monkeys and three of the four PA monkeys made more total errors than did the five monkeys receiving only serial sulcus principalis lesions (SP). All statistical analyses comparing the performance of the SP monkeys with the performance of any one of the other three groups were significant (p .05). No significant differences appeared in comparisons of the error scores of the PA, IP, and IT groups.

It is apparent from these results that a variety of diverse sectors of the intact cortex are involved in sparing of function after serial ablation of sulcus principalis. Tissue both proximal (i.e., posterior principalis) and distal (i.e., periarcuate, inferior parietal, and inferior temporal) to the principal sulcus appear to exert an influence on functional reorganization. It should be remembered that one-stage removals of either periarcuate, inferior parietal, inferotemporal or posterior principalis cortex produce no discernable DA impairment. Nonetheless serial ablation of sulcus principalis plus one-stage ablation of any of the aforementioned structures have been shown to preclude the sparing of DA. Thus, the integrity of each of these cortical areas appears to be necessary to preserve the sparing which would ordinarily accompany sequential sulcus principalis lesions. These findings stand in marked contrast to previous research involving restitution of sensory (Meyer 1958; Doty 1961; Pasik and Pasik 1971) and motor (Glees and Cole 1950) function in which rather precisely delimited areas have been implicated in the recovery processes. In our studies, the very diversity of the structures that have been shown to influence the serial lesion phenomenon suggests the possibility that the entire association cortex may be involved in functional reorganization following sequential removal of sulcus principalis in the mature primate.

The present findings also underline some pertinent differences between recovery after infant and serial lesions. Despite some parallels between the two phenomena (e.g., recovery after dorsolateral but not after orbital frontal lesions), the data available at this time can be interpreted to suggest that these two types of recovery may be mediated by different neural mechanisms. The evidence provided by Kling and Tucker (1968) points to subcortical mechanisms in recovery after early lesions. While destruction of the caudate nucleus prevented recovery after early frontal lesions, removal of a large area of posterior association cortex (including the inferior parietal lobule) did not affect such behavioral sparing. In contrast to these infant results, the present investigation emphasizes the role of cortical structures in recovery after serial lesions. One-stage bilateral removal of the inferior parietal region (as well as the peri-arcuate and inferotemporal areas) did interfere with recovery after serial frontal lesions. While future studies may indeed show that subcortical structures are also involved in the serial lesion phenomenon, such findings will not detract from the present evidence that intact cortical structures are more crucial for sparing after serial than after early frontal lesions.

In addition to the differential role of cortical and subcortical structures in the recovery process, the early and serial lesion phenomena may also be separated by the importance of temporal factors. Harlow and his collaborators (1964, 1970) have demonstrated that recovery after early lesions is dependent upon the age of the monkey at the time of surgery. Ablation of the frontal cortex must occur within the first 12 months of life if any appreciable sparing is to occur. While we have not systematically investi-gated the role of temporal factors (i.e., time between serial removals) in serial lesions, the sequential ablations of sulcus principalis in the first and in the fourth experiment did differ in time between operations and the rate of ablation. In the first experiment, the monkeys with serial lesions received four operations spaced three weeks apart, with one bank of the principal sulcus removed in each operation. In the last experiment, the monkeys receiving only serial sulcus principalis lesions (SP group) had two operations spaced 10 weeks apart, with the entire sulcus of one hemisphere removed in each operation. Since both groups of animals received the same behavioral tasks postoperatively (DA retention, DR, and PR) in the identical sequence, their behavioral performances may be compared. Table 3 shows the total errors compiled by both serial groups on the three spatial tasks. It is evident from this comparison that the monkeys receiving four operations three weeks apart made fewer errors (p < .05) than did the serial animals receiving two operations 10 weeks apart. Thus, despite the shorter temporal interval between lesions, the animals with the slower rate of lesion production (amount of tissue destroyed per operation) demonstrated greater recovery of function. While temporal factors (the earliness or lateness of the lesion) seem to be crucial for early lesions, rate of lesion development rather than time between operations may be a more important variable in determining the amount of recovery after serial lesions.

Finally, it is important to consider how recovery of function might be achieved. Rosner (1970) has differentiated between two possible mechanisms, reestablishment and reorganization. Reestablishment refers to the reappearance of the affected function. This could occur either through the dissipation of diaschisis or through the adoption of the function by intact neural structures. Reorganization, however, would involve the operations of the residual system of brain structures of which the ablated region was once a part.

These two mechanisms presumably can be further differentiated. On the one hand, reestablishment might be expected to foster a set of behavioral functions which are both qualitatively and quantitatively similar to the original behavior. The performance of the serial stage mid-principalis animals suggests the operation of such a mechanism. On the other hand, the concept of reorganization implies that the recovered function may be fundamentally different from the original behavior, i.e., that the animals may have acquired the ability to reachieve similar "ends" by virtue of a set of different "means". Morgan (1951) has alluded to such a possibility in his analysis of the effects of sequential removal of sensory cortex in dogs and primates. Morgan argued that

Table 3

Total Spatial Errors by Monkeys with Two- and Four-Stage Ablations of Sulcus Principalis

Two-Stage S̲s	Total Errors
73	506
14A	611
29A	697
45A	730
42A	588
Mean	626

Four-Stage S̲s	Total Errors
36	212
52	511
46	423
39	427
62	394
Mean	393

the serial ablation procedure enabled the subjects to assimilate new perceptual strategies (during the interoperative interval) into the residual of previously acquired sensory discriminations. Thus recovery could be viewed as a form of sensory substitution in which the remainder of a neural system continues to operate, but on the basis of different informational parameters. This view is partially supported by the reported deleterious effects of interoperative sensory deprivation on recovery of function (e.g. Meyer

1958).

        If one assumes, as have a number of
investigators (e.g., Konorski 1967; Gentile and
Stamm 1972; Goldman, Rosvold, Vest and Galkin
1971), that 1) the dorsolateral prefrontal cortex
serves as an integrator of spatio-proprioceptive
information, and 2) proprioceptive cues are the
sensory basis of DA performance, then the
sequential removal of sulcus principalis may
force the animal to utilize other, albeit less
salient, cues to perform this task. Interoceptive
stimuli, such as vestibular cues which have been
shown to play a role in certain spatial learning
tasks (e.g., Rosen and Stein 1969; Douglas 1966;
Beritoff 1965), may be involved as may some
exteroceptive stimuli. In the latter case, the
animal would no longer be performing traditional
DA, although his behavior would comply with the
reinforcement contigencies inherent in a win-shift
strategy. However, regardless of whether the
animal is employing interoceptive or exteroceptive
stimuli in place of proprioceptive cues, there is
no reason to believe that either of these
classes of stimulation are as salient in the
WGTA - DA situation as is proprioceptive information. Furthermore, in order to employ either class
of stimulation, the animal must engage in the
equivalent of an extradimensional shift, a
process which is more difficult than intradimensional reversal shifts even in normal subjects
(Eimas 1966; Stevenson 1972). Either or both of
these factors might account for the initial DA
retention impairments after sequential principalis
lesions.

                        Summary

        A series of experiments dealing with recovery
(sparing) of function after serial ablation of the
prefrontal association cortex of monkeys have been
reported. While recovery occurred following serial
removal of the dorsolateral frontal region, serial
ablation of the lateral orbital cortex did not
lead to an attenuation of the behavioral deficits
associated with one-stage lesions of this area.
        These findings parallel the results from early
lesion studies, but examination of the mechanisms

underlying recovery demonstrated some important distinctions between the two recovery phenomena. While recovery after early lesions seems to depend upon intact subcortical structures (i.e., the caudate nucleus), recovery after serial frontal lesions appears to involve cortical mechanisms. The present evidence implicates the cortex immediately adjacent to a serially ablated focus as well as more distant anterior and posterior association areas as mediators of recovery. Examination of temporal factors also demonstrates some differences between early and serial lesions. The age of the organism at the time of surgery is critical in early lesion studies. Recovery after serial lesions, however, appears to depend more on the amount of damage produced in each operation than on the amount of time between sequential operations.

ACKNOWLEDGMENTS: The research reported in this paper was supported in part by grants NS06209 to Boston University and NS08606 to Clark University from the National Institute of Neurological Diseases and Stroke, and by a Research Career Development Award to Donald G. Stein. The authors acknowledge the assistance of Miss Carol Soeldner and Mr. Jeffrey Patrissi in conducting the investigations.

REFERENCES

Ades, H. and Raab, D.H. (1949). Effects of pre-occipital and temporal decortication on learned visual discriminations in monkeys. *J. Neurophysiol.* 12, 101-108.

Beritoff, J.S. (1965). "Neural Mechanisms of Higher Vertebrate Behavior", Boston: Little, Brown and Co.

Butter, C.M. (1969). Perseveration in extinction and in discrimination reversal tasks following selective frontal ablations in *Macaca Mulatta*. *Physiol. and Behav.* 4, 163-171.

Butter, C.M. and Snyder, D.R. (1972). Alterations in aversive and aggressive behaviors following orbital frontal lesions in rhesus monkeys. *Acta Neurobiologiae Exp.* 32, 525-566.

Butters, N. and Pandya, D. (1969). Retention of delayed-alternation: effect of selective lesions of sulcus principalis. *Science* 165, 1271-1273.

Butters, N., Pandya, D., Sanders, K. and Dye, P. (1971). Behavioral deficits in monkeys after selective lesions within the middle third of sulcus principalis. *J. Comp. Physiol. Psych.* 76, 8-14.

Doty, R.W. (1961). Functional significance of the topographic aspects of the retino-cortical projection. *In* R. Jung and H. Kornhuber (Eds.) "Neurophysiologie and Psychophysic des Visuelen Systems", Berlin: Springer-Verlag. pp. 229-245.

Douglas, R.J. (1966). Cues for spontaneous alternation. *J. Comp. Physiol. Psych.* 62, 171-183.

Eimas, P.D. (1966). Effects of overtraining and age on intradimensional and extradimensional shifts in children. *J. Exp. Child Psych.* 3, 348-355.

Gentile, A.M. and Stamm, J.S. (1972). Supplementary cues and delayed-alternation performance of frontal monkeys. *J. Comp. Physiol. Psych.* 80, 230-237.

Glees, P. and Cole, J. (1950). Recovery of skilled motor functions after small repeated lesions in motor cortex in *macaque*. *J. Neurophysiol.* 13, 137-148.

Goldman, P.S. (1971). Functional development of the prefrontal cortex in early life and the problem of neuronal plasticity. *Exp. Neur.* 32, 366-387.

Goldman, P.S. (1972). Developmental determinants of cortical plasticity. *Acta Neurobiol. Exp.* 32, 495-512.

Goldman, P.S. and Rosvold, H.E. (1970). Localization of function within the dorsolateral prefrontal cortex of the rhesus monkey. *Exp. Neur.* 27, 291-304.

Goldman, P.S., Rosvold, H.E. and Mishkin, M. (1970). Evidence for behavioral impairment following prefrontal lobectomy in the infant monkey. *J. Comp. Physiol. Psych.* 70, 454-463.

Goldman, P.S., Rosvold, H.E., Vest, B. and Galkin, T.W. (1971). Analysis of the delayed-alternation deficit produced by dorsolateral prefrontal lesions in the rhesus monkey. *J. Comp. Physiol. Psych.* 77, 212-220.

Gross, C.G. (1963). A comparison of the effects of partial and total lateral frontal lesions on test performance by monkeys. *J. Comp. Physiol. Psych.* 56, 41-47.

Harlow, H.F., Akert, K. and Schiltz, K.A. (1964). The effects of bilateral prefrontal lesions on learned behavior of neonatal, infant and pre-adolescent monkeys. *In* J.M. Warren and K. Akert (Eds.) "The Frontal Granular Cortex and Behavior", New York: McGraw-Hill. pp. 126-148.

Harlow, H.F., Thompson, C., Blomquist, A. and Schiltz, K. (1970). Learning in rhesus monkeys after varying amounts of prefrontal lobe destruction during infancy and adolescence. *Brain Res.* 18, 343-353.

Johnson, T.N., Rosvold, H.E. and Mishkin, M. (1968). Projections of behaviorally-defined sectors of the prefrontal cortex to the basal ganglia, septum and diencephalon of the monkey. *Exp. Neur.* 21, 20-34.

Kling, A. and Tucker, R.J. (1968). Sparing of function following localized brain lesions in neonatal monkeys. *In* R. Isaacson (Ed.) "The Neuropsychology of Development", New York: Wiley. pp. 121-145.

Konorski, J. (1967). "Integrative Activity of the Brain", Chicago: University of Chicago Press.

Meyer, D.R. (1958). Some psychological determinants of sparing and loss following damage to the brain. *In* H.F. Harlow and C.N. Woolsey (Eds.) "Biological and Biochemical Bases of Behavior", Madison: Wisconsin Press. pp. 173-192.

Mishkin, M. (1957). Effects of small frontal lesions on delayed alternation in monkeys. *J. Neurophysiol.* 20, 615-622.

Mishkin, M. (1964). Perseveration of central sets after frontal lesions in monkeys. *In* J.M. Warren and K. Akert (Eds.) "The Frontal Granular Cortex and Behavior", New York: McGraw-Hill. pp. 219-237.

Morgan, C.T. (1951). Some structural factors in perception. *In* R.R. Blake and G.V. Ramsey (Eds.) "Perception - An Approach to Personality" New York: Ronald Press Co. pp. 3-36.

Nauta, W.J.H. (1964). Some efferent connections of the prefrontal cortex in the monkey. *In* J.M. Warren and K. Akert (Eds.) "The Frontal Granular Cortex and Behavior", New York: McGraw-Hill. pp. 397-409.

Pasik, T. and Pasik, P. (1971). The visual world of monkeys deprived of striate cortex: effective stimulus parameters and the importance of the accessory optic system. *Vision Res. Supp.* No. 3, 419-435.

Rosen, J.J. and Stein, D.G. (1969). Spontaneous alternation behavior in the rat. *J. Comp. Physiol. Psych.* 68, 420-426.

Rosner, B.S. (1970). Brain Functions. *Ann. Rev. Psych.* 21, 555-594.

Rosvold, H.E. (1972). The frontal lobe system: cortical-subcortical interrelationships. *Acta Neurobiol. Exp.* 32, 439-460.

Stamm, J.S. and Rosen, S.C. (1972). Cortical steady potential shifts and anodal polarization during delayed response performance. *Acta Neurobiol. Exp.* 32, 193-209.

Stein, D.G., Rosen, J.J., Graziadei, J., Mishkin, D. and Brink, J.J. (1969). Central nervous system: recovery of function. *Science* 166, 528-530.

Stevenson, H.W. (1970). Learning in children. *In* P.H. Mussen (Ed.) "Carmichael's Manual of Child Psychology", Vol. 1. New York: John Wiley and Sons. pp. 849-938.

Stewart, J.W. and Ades, H.W. (1952). The time factor in reintegration of a learned habit lost after temporal lobe lesions in the monkey. *J. Comp. Physiol. Psych.* 45, 119-126.

Tucker, T.J. and Kling, A. (1969). Preservation of delayed response following combined lesions of prefrontal and posterior association cortex in infant monkeys. *Exp. Neur.* 23, 491-502.

LATE CHANGES IN THE NERVOUS SYSTEM: AN OVERVIEW

Norman Geschwind
Harvard Medical School
Cambridge, Massachusetts

It will be the purpose of this closing discussion to present a general overview of the problem of late changes in the nervous system. I will devote much of my attention to topics which have not been discussed in the earlier papers. While I will mention some important experimental findings in animals, I will give particular attention to the very rich literature on late changes in the nervous system in humans.

Let me say first how pleased I am that the word "plasticity" has occurred very rarely in the discussions at this meeting. It may be recalled that even in the very recent past a belief in "plasticity" led, apparently paradoxically, to a remarkable lack of solid experimental study of mechanisms of recovery. If the nervous system was so plastic it seemed adequate simply to assert this as a matter of faith and it was regarded as unnecessary to detail the effects of localized lesions, or to search for the mechanisms which accounted for recovery in some instances but not others. This meeting reflected a genuine and healthy change in spirit. There seemed to be agreement that one can speak about the differential effects of localized lesions, and also study the anatomical, physiological, pharmacological, and developmental mechanisms of late improvement or deterioration without any sense that these activities conflict.

I would like to make a second general point. The title of the meeting, with its stress on recovery of nervous function distorts the basic important issue. There have been at this conference several interchanges as to whether a particular change was favorable or unfavorable with respect to recovery. This issue is, however, peripheral to a more general question, i.e., "What is the sequence of events which occurs after you place a lesion in the nervous system?" The sequence may involve alterations in anatomy and pharmacology in the vicinity of the lesion and its connections, or

may involve responses by other intact portions of
the nervous system. There may be changes in overall function which in some cases are beneficial,
(in which cases we will speak of recovery), but
which in other cases are distinctly disadvantag-
eous.

The critical question is thus to specify the
changes in the nervous system and their mechanisms.
While we have been accustomed in the past to
thinking about the effects of a "fixed lesion of
the nervous system" it may in fact be the rule
that a sequence of changes follows all lesions,
and that perhaps one never achieves an equilibrium.
There are immediate changes, and changes occurring
over seconds, hours, days, weeks, months, and
indeed years.

Early Changes After Lesions

Let me first consider two examples of very
rapid changes, occurring in systems in which lack
of immediate recovery would lead to death within
minutes. Despite the special character of these
systems, these phenomena deserve study because
they may well have the same essential mechanisms
as slower phenomena and yet be easier to study
because of their rapid onset.

The first of these changes does not even take
place in the nervous system, but rather in the
conducting system of the heart. It would not
surprise me, however, if similar phenomena took
place in the central nervous system, particularly
in tonically or rhythmically firing systems. As is
well known, when one destroys the sinus node of
the heart a new but slower rhythm appears. One can
produce a series of such lesions further down the
conducting system, with the appearance of progressively slower pacemakers until one gets the so-
called idio-ventricular rhythm. With destruction
of the ventricular pacemaker the heart stops
beating. The mechanism of this has been well
studied (Hoffman and Cranefield 1960). It seems
that potential pacemaker cells in the heart are
identified by the fact that after each action
potential the transmembrane potential, after
returning to the baseline, slowly begins to rise.
This rate of rise is most rapid at the sinus node

so that the cells here stimulate themselves first and in turn stimulate other potential pacemakers before they fire themselves. If the sinus node is destroyed then a set of cells further downstream in the conducting system can now fire themselves. The new pacemaker is slower since the rate of rise of the baseline is slower than at the sinus node. The importance of this mechanism is that it gives a simple model whereby a whole hierarchy of neuronal systems could be released in turn to "take over" when the ones above are destroyed. But the slowing of the system is the price exacted for plasticity. Any reader interested in change in the nervous system should study this system, because of its simplicity and potential importance, by reading the account in Hoffman and Cranefield (1960).

A classic form of early change is seen in the crossed-phrenic phenomenon, first described by Porter (1894-1895) but studied by many later authors. When the spinal cord is hemi-sectioned at the C4 level the diaphragm of the sectioned side stops contracting. Respiration may return spontaneously on the hemisected side but usually only after a delay. If, however, the opposite phrenic nerve is cut or blocked (with paralysis of the opposite diaphragm), the diaphragm on the side of the cord section immediately begins to contract again. Dolivo (1953) showed, by physiological recording, that an increase in the rate of discharge of the phrenic nerve on the hemisectioned side takes place in the first inspiration after electronic block of the opposite phrenic nerve. This increase disappears in the first inspiration after the block is removed. There must, therefore, be a second pathway to the neurons of the phrenic nerve descending on the opposite side of the cord and decussating below the level of the cord hemi-section; a pathway apparently normally inactive but which under appropriate circumstances comes into play.

The two phenomena just discussed represent examples of immediate change, one in the cardiac conduction system, the other in the pathways controlling phrenic motoneurons. The mechanism underlying immediate recovery in these two examples is clearly not neuronal sprouting. It seems unlikely that supersensitivity of denervation would account for such immediate recovery (and in the case of the cardiac conducting system seems to be clearly not the essential factor). The automatic tendency of many people is to assume that such immediate effects must represent withdrawal of inhibition. This is not, however, necessarily the case since, there is no true inhibition of pace-maker cells outside the sinus node. Rather there is a process of what I suppose more appropriately corresponds to occlusion, i.e., the subordinate pacemakers are fired by the sinus node before they fire themselves and are thus functionally inactive. Clearly such a process could also take place in the nervous system. I am, of course, not ruling out withdrawal of inhibition as one cause of immediate "release" of a previously inactive area, but only wish to point out that it is not the only possible mechanism.

Changes of Slower Time-course

Let us turn now to yet another phenomenon in which a change after a lesion takes place not in seconds or minutes but over, perhaps, 3 days. Recently, Wall and Egger (1971) mapped the distinct areas of thalamus or cortex in which stimulation of the arm or the foot led to an evoked response in normal cats. After destruction of the nucleus gracilis (receiving the input from the lower spinal cord) no responses appeared in VPL or cortex to stimulation of the foot, while stimulation of the hand produced the usual map in both locations. After 3 days, however, a striking change occurred; The area in which stimulation of the hand led to evoked responses expanded both in the thalamus and the cortex, so that eventually the arm area took over what was formerly the leg area. The latency of responses to stimulation of the hand was the same in the leg area as it was in the true arm area, so that one can exclude stimulation via another synapse. How do we explain this phenomenon?

Wall (personal communication) has pointed out that while in Raisman's (1969) work, sprouting was not seen until six weeks, the type of function-al changes described by Wall and Egger begin within

three days after surgery and are over by ten days.
He therefore tends to regard sprouting as unlikely,
although anatomical studies have not yet been
carried out. He suggests that the synapses in the
leg area which responded to stimuli in the hand
area three days after destruction of the nucleus
gracilis were present before the experiment but
for some reason ineffective. This phenomenon thus
has a time course longer than that of the crossed-
phrenic phenomenon but probably still too rapid
to be accounted for by axonal sprouting.

Kirk and Denny-Brown (1970) and Denny-Brown,
Kirk and Yanagisawa (1973) have reported some
striking changes over time that may be similar to
some of the phenomena described by Wall and Egger.
They first studied the strip of intact sensation
which remained in the monkey when one dorsal root
was left intact but the three roots above and
below were sectioned intradurally. They found that
the area of remaining sensation might increase in
size over a period of up to two weeks. In later
experiments they sectioned the dorsal roots (above
and below the test root) distal to the ganglion.
In these cases they found a larger dermatome than
after intradural section which would increase
further in size over a week. If they then sectioned
the same roots proximal to the ganglion the dermatome would shrink, but this reduction in size
might not take place for 3 or 4 days. After the
size of the dermatome had stabilized the injection
of strychnine caused a striking, although transient, widening of the zone of remaining sensitivity. Transection of the cord below the spared
root or hemisection above it both widened the size
of the spared dermatome. They carried their
analysis further to show that the lateral portion
of Lissauer's tract mediated an inhibitory effect
since a lesion of this pathway in a neighboring
segment caused widening of the isolated dermatome.
The medial portion of the tract was shown to exert
a facilitatory effect since a lesion of it led to
narrowing of the dermatome, although strychnine
would again widen it, Denny-Brown points out that
L-DOPA has the same effect. It is of importance
to notice that these effects after section of
Lissauer's tract were not immediate but took
several days to reach their peak.

471

Late Changes in Man After Lesions of the Nervous System

Let us now turn to some of the phenomena seen in man, particularly since they may illuminate some of the changes which take place after a lesion. Some of these effects are probably not really relevant to the concerns of this conference, although some are important to recognize as possible sources of error in the analysis of experimental results. Thus it is not uncommon for patients with occlusive vascular disease to improve within a few days. On the one hand, in many of these cases, it is clear that there was no destruction of tissue but only temporary loss of function. On the other hand, patients may worsen after certain lesions, particularly after surgery, because edema appears usually reaching its peak about the third day. Subsequent recovery may simply result from the disappearance of edema. It is usually thought that the temporary effects of anoxia or edema are completely gone by three weeks. There is, however, a general impression that recovery after surgical lesions or trauma may take place over a longer time than after vascular disease. This, if confirmed, would suggest that perhaps local tissue changes may persist for longer than we have thought in the past; a point of possibly special importance for the animal investigator. It also seems clear that there is a group of patients who show progressive neurological changes because of the persistence of virus in some altered form in the nervous system ("slow viruses") or because of immunological responses to certain types of disease. Yet true neurological changes after apparently fixed lesions, occur at every level of the nervous system in man and the time course of these late changes may extend in some cases over many years.

Even at the simplest level of the nervous system we may not be able to explain all the phenomena we observe. Thus it is generally thought that sprouting occurs at intact nerve terminals after poliomyelitis so that some denervated muscle fibers are reinnervated, often with excellent functional recovery. On the other hand some patients after recovery from a peripheral neuro-

pathic illness, show the curious phenomenon of
"acquired myotonia", i.e., prolonged contraction
of muscle, with inability to relax (Krabbe 1934).
The affected muscles may become hypertrophied and
extremely powerful, but the patient may be incon-
venienced by his failure to relax normally. The
mechanisms of this disorder are far from clear.

Let us consider an even simpler example, the
classical Bell's palsy. A patient develops, without
obvious cause, unilateral paralysis in the distribution of the seventh nerve. He may recover
completely or partially. Early recovery may simply
indicate that a conduction block was removed in
intact nerve fibers. In other cases recovery may
take months, presumably indicating regeneration
of fibers. However, what is most curious is the
stereotyped nature of this recovery. Recovery of
the muscles closing the eye is almost never worse
than recovery of muscles moving the mouth. A
patient may recover eye closure perfectly without
any capacity to move the mouth, but the reverse
phenomenon must be rare. Another phenomenon seen
in some patients is movement of the corner of the
mouth when the eye closes. This may occur even
when there is no voluntary movement of the mouth.
In some cases eye closure leads to a massive
spasm of the corner of the mouth.

The usual explanation for these events is
anomalous regeneration of fibers, i.e., fibers
intended for the eye go to the muscles of the
mouth. But why does the reverse never, or so
rarely, occur? Thus I have never seen a patient
in whom movement of the mouth led to closure of
the eye. We do not know the reasons for the occurrence of one pattern of abnormal regeneration but
not the other. Random regeneration would not - at
first glance - appear to explain the findings.

Late Changes After Spinal Lesions

Let us now consider briefly the events which
follow spinal transection since they constitute
one instance in which environmental effects appear
to be important. Earlier observers noted that
after spinal transection, paralyzed muscles were
flaccid, manifesting the classic phenomenon of
spinal shock. The patient would eventually develop

a posture of strong flexion of the lower extremities. As care of the skin and bladder improved, however, it was found the patient would tend to go into a position of extension. This might be converted into flexion if a bladder or skin infection developed. In one patient whom I observed, the leg with a bed sore had gone into flexion while the other remained extended. One could speculate as to the origins of this phenomenon by pointing out that in man, cutaneous reflexes are primarily flexor reflexes. Is it possible that the posture of paraplegia in flexion represents the facilitation of flexion postures by the presence of noxious lesions of skin and bladder, i.e., an evironmental effect which leaves a permanent imprint?

Let us consider another spinal lesion in which late changes occur. Since about 1912 neurosurgeons have been placing lesions in the lateral spinothalamic tract to relieve pain. The operation typically produced analgesia below the lesion and relief from pain, but within a year the effects wear off. As a result, the operation has frequently been abandoned except for patients with advanced carcinoma. The mechanism of this often undesired recovery has still not been elucidated.

Let me turn to still another example of recovery at the spinal level. Nathan and Smith (1973) have recently described a series of patients, taken from a very large series of anterolateral cordotomies in the thoracic region, who developed paralysis of the ipsilateral leg after the operation. Later post-mortem study showed that the surgeon had typically made a large cut which in some instances had effectively cut all descending systems on one side of the cord. Despite the extent of the first lesion the patient regained considerable function in the leg, usually being able to walk. Following a second cordotomy at a different level which transected descending pathways on the opposite side both legs became paralyzed. It thus seems clear that while each leg is normally activated by pathways descending on the same side of the cord it can, after destruction of these pathways, be innervated usefully by tracts running down the opposite side of the cord and decussating below the thoracic region. Would equally dramatic results occur in the arm after a high cervical transection? I am not sure of the answer. I would only point out now, as I will repeat later, that the leg recovers better than the arm in other circumstances.

Late Changes After Lesions of Cerebellum and Brain-stem

Let us now turn to a consideration of changes after lesions at higher levels of the central nervous system. Striking recovery is repeatedly said to be a feature of extensive cerebellar removals in children, while human adults tolerate this procedure poorly. It is worth stressing this recovery of children since it is sometimes claimed that removal of the cerebellum is followed by much greater recovery in the young human than in the young animal, in contradiction to what some take to be the rule that recovery is better in animals. It is interesting to speculate on why young humans might tolerate cerebellar removals better than other animals. I support the perhaps far-fetched view that there are systems in the frontal lobe involved with the upright posture which depend only partially on cerebellar connections and are most highly developed in man.

At the level of the brain stem there occurs one of the most dramatic examples of late change in the nervous system, the syndrome of palatal myoclonus and olivary hypertrophy. It is of particular interest since it combines a late functional change with one of the most striking forms of histological change seen in the nervous system. It was especially studied by French neurologists and much of this work is summarized by Trelles (1968) and Lapresle and Ben hamida (1970). It is remarkable that it has not attracted more attention among non-clinicians.

In the typical case the patient may suffer an acute lesion, e.g., a small hypertensive ball hemorrhage, in one dentate nucleus. About a year later the patient develops a striking movement at about 140/minute involving the soft palate, pharynx and larynx, and termed, not altogether appropriately, palatal myoclonus. It may also involve the eyelids, the diaphragm and sometimes

475

even limb muscles. If the patient should die, post-
mortem reveals hypertrophy of the olive on the
side opposite the lesion, readily visible to the
naked eye. Microscopically, the neurons in the
olive are grossly enlarged with tremendous
thickening and tortuosity of the dendrites.
Binucleate neurons may be seen. Eventually the
neurons die and are replaced by extensive gliosis.
The same sequence of events can occur with a lesion
not in the opposite dentate nucleus but in the
ipsilateral central tegmental tract.

The evidence can be taken to suggest that the
neuronal hypertrophy occurs within a short time
after the lesion, preceding therefore by many
months, the appearance of the palatal myoclonus.
The sequence of anatomical events takes several
years for its full evolution. Arguments as to the
pathogenesis are still not settled. Trelles
believes that one is observing an anterograde,
trans-synaptic change resulting from destruction
of afferents to the olive coming in via the
dentate-olivary pathway, which decussates in one
superior cerebellar peduncle and descends to the
olive via the central tegmental tract. Since
lesions of the olive-cerebellar fibers do not
produce the syndrome, it seems unlikely that
retrograde changes are important. Furthermore the
massive and almost unique neuronal hypertrophy
remains unexplained. This lesion and its effects
clearly deserve more study, since it combines a
functional change with a readily visible series of
anatomical alterations.

Late Changes in Spastic Hemiplegics

Let us now turn to perhaps the most common of
all neurological conditions, the chronic spastic
hemiplegia. Late change is a characteristic feature
of this disorder. Even in the earliest days of
neurology there was awareness of the fact that certain movements typically recovered while others did
not. In the acute hemiplegia the limbs are often
completely flaccid. In the chronic state, however,
one finds a reasonably stereotyped pattern. In the
arm, weakness is more pronounced at the abductors
of the shoulder, the extensors of the elbow, wrist
and fingers, and the abductors of the fingers.

Separate movements of the fingers are strikingly poor. On the other hand, adduction of the shoulder, flexion of the elbow, and the grip are almost always much better preserved and in some instances strength may be normal in these movements. In the leg, one finds weakness of flexion and abduction of the hip, flexion of the knee and dorsi-flexion of ankle and toes while movements in the opposite direction are often very powerful. The partial recovery of the leg is more useful than that in the arm since it usually permits the patient to walk again.

Some of the deficits of the hemiplegic show even more dramatic recovery than what I have just described. In my experience conjugate gaze weakness resulting from a unilateral hemisphere lesion always recovers (but can be permanent after a pontine lesion), the recovery taking up to two weeks, but rarely longer. The same is true for tongue weakness. Indeed the only permanent weakness in cranial musculature seen after a unilateral hemisphere lesion is that of the opposite lower face and even this is often extremely mild. A second lesion in the opposite hemisphere may lead now to a dramatic degree of bilateral cranial muscle weakness.

The pattern of the recovery of strength is independent, as far as I can tell, of the size of the lesion producing hemiplegia. I have seen it in patients with small capsular lesions but I observed the same pattern in the patient of Smith (1966) who had undergone a complete hemispherectomy in adult life because of glioma of recent onset. Since this patient had undergone a total left hemispherectomy down to, and including thalamus, it seems clear that his right hemisphere must have been capable of the residual movements of flexion and adduction of the right upper extremity, extension and adduction of the right lower extremity, and the almost totally preserved movements of the cranial musculature on the right side. The frequency of hemiplegia as a cause of chronic disability in man confers special importance on the elucidation of the mechanism of late changes after lesions in motor systems.

Recovery From Cortical Blindness

Let us now turn to a different system. It has sometimes been stated that cortical blindness recovers much better in the monkey than in man. Unfortunately we do not really have the basis for this comparison. It is perhaps possible to make lesions nearly confined to striate cortex in animals but in man the natural lesions usually extend well beyond the calcarine cortex. What is clear, however, is that, as Gloning *et al.* (1968) have shown, some degree of recovery occurs in nearly all cases of cortical blindness when they are followed over long periods of time. My own guess would be that some of this recovery is taking place at the collicular level.

Recovery From Aphasia

Let us now turn to the late effects of lesions which produce disorders of the higher functions. Although even today there is remarkable unawareness of the spontaneous recovery rate in aphasia the fact of recovery was observed by even the earliest workers in this field.

After some lesions the recovery rate is 100% or very close to this level. Thus, transient disorders of speech may occur with lesions of the supplementary motor area or the thalamus but within a few weeks or months the deficit becomes very mild or disappears. A distinct, severe memory disorder can occur after a left unilateral hippo-campal lesion as in the case of Geschwind and Fusillo (1966) but usually shows marked recovery in a few months, while bilateral lesions, of course, produce permanent severe effects.

There is a fair amount of data on recovery from aphasia. In children who become aphasic the recovery rate is nearly 100%. Byers and McLean (1962) described a group of children all of whom were left with permanent right hemiplegias but in all of whom the aphasias cleared completely over several months or years. There is the mistaken notion in the minds of some people that only very young children recover so well, but actually Byer's series ranged up to 10 years in age and my own limited experience confirms excellent recovery even this late. Byers, however, pointed out that the children paid a price for this recovery because, despite the disappearance of aphasia they all showed a drop in school performance in all areas. I will return later to this issue of the nearly 100% recovery in childhood aphasia since it raises some important theoretical issues.

While recovery from aphasia in children is often recognized, there is widespread unawareness of the rates of significant recovery in adult aphasia. A very simple observation confirms that adult aphasias frequently evolve over long periods of time. One need only compare the patient who is hemiplegic three weeks after a vascular occlusion with a patient who is still aphasic at the same period. The patient who is significantly hemiplegic at three weeks rarely shows a dramatically improved picture at a year. Yet many patients severely aphasic at three weeks are significantly better at three months or a year. One patient whom I followed closely had shown no change between three months and one year and I advised him that I doubted that he could ever get back to his old job. A year later - two years from onset - he turned up in my office. Over the intervening year with no specific treatment he had improved to the point of being able to return to work - as a salesman. I know of other cases in which significant recovery has gone on over as many as six years.

An excellent source of data as to the recovery rate is found in Luria's (1970) series of penetrating brain wounds. Let us consider only the cases in which there were penetrating missile wounds directly over Wernicke's or Broca's areas, i.e., cases in which there was almost certainly a gross destructive lesion of one of the speech areas. In the initial stages about 95% of these patients were significantly aphasic, but at a year 34% had either no aphasia or only mild aphasia. I have no doubt that if one had waited several years the recovery rate would have risen further.

One must remember that as a result of this recovery rate, one's accuracy in the clinical localization of an aphasia drops with the passage of time. It is highest at perhaps six weeks after onset, when accuracy of localization probably

exceeds 80%. On the other hand one has to be
foolhardy to offer a confident localization after
several years. Thus I once saw a brain of a
patient who had become aphasic 18 years before and
had been aphasic for several years, but who shortly
before death showed no significant aphasia despite
a persistent right hemiplegia. At post-mortem
there was total destruction of the left peri-
Sylvian regions, i.e., of the entire classical
speech area.

Although spontaneous useful recovery in aphasia
therefore occurs in many cases we should not
forget that poor recovery is still the fate of
probably the majority of aphasics. The patient who
is hemiplegic three weeks after a vascular
occlusion has of course a much poorer prognosis
for recovery. One should, however, keep in mind
the occasional human who recovers from a massive
lesion in the motor system. Thus I recall one
patient who had made an excellent recovery from a
hemiplegia despite an infarct which at post-mortem
extended the entire length of the prerolandic
region and extended down from the ventricle! Yet,
I have seen other patients with permanent hemiplegias who at post-mortem had much smaller
lesions that were sometimes difficult to find. My
own guess is that humans develop much more severe
hemiplegias than animals and that the differences
in severity of hemiplegia represent a major
species difference. In other words I do not agree
with the view that humans have more severe
hemiplegias only because their lesions are larger
or involve more systems. I suspect that it is
difficult if not impossible to give a monkey a
permanent severe spastic hemiplegia regardless of
the extent of lesions in one hemisphere, while in
man such a deficit is readily and frequently
produced.

We have some interesting although limited
information as to which patients manifest better
recovery from aphasias. The data of Gloning *et al.*
(1969) support the notion that left-handers are
likely to become aphasic regardless of which hemisphere is damaged, i.e., they have twice as great
a chance of becoming aphasic as do right-handers.
In striking contrast it is very rare for a right-
hander to become aphasic from a right hemisphere

lesion. Left-handers tend to recover better from the aphasias produced by right hemisphere than left hemisphere lesions. On the other hand they recover better on the average from left hemisphere lesions than do right-handers. Luria's (1970) and Subirana's (1969) data point in the same direction: left-handers recover better from aphasias than right-handers. Furthermore right-handers with a history of left-handedness among parents, siblings, or children, recover on the average better than right-handers without such a family history. Left-handers on the average appear to have a different kind of brain organization than right-handers.

Late Changes After Other Lesions of the Nervous System

Let me turn to two other examples of late changes after "fixed lesions". These examples are important for two reasons. They often take many years and they are both deteriorations rather than recoveries. One is the curious phenomenon that was of great interest to many of the French neurologists and was described in detail by Yakovlev (1954), i.e. "cerebral paraplegia in flexion". Patients with long-standing brain lesions may, after many years, start to assume increasingly, a posture of flexion similar to that seen in spinal lesions. The mechanisms may not be dissimilar to that which we mentioned speculatively for spinal paraplegia in flexion.

The long-term effects after frontal lobotomy are another example of late change. Control studies carried out years ago when these operations were still common, showed that in the first years after the operation, the lobotomized patients were performing as well as matched unoperated controls on a wide variety of tests. It was something of a surprise therefore, to discover that follow-up studies carried out several years later, showed a late decline among the operates in several areas (Hamlin 1970). This very late decline is dramatic. A clue as to the cause from some recent observations of Yakovlev (personal communication) who has been studying the brains of a large number of lobotomized patients, which he compares to controls of the same age. He finds that

481

the brain of the recently lobotomized patient is, except in the immediate vicinity of the lesion, essentially the same size as that of controls. If he compares, however, let us say, the brain of a 60 year old man, lobotomized 20 years earlier at age 40 with that of a normal 60 year old, he finds a marked diminution in size in the operated brain. The longer the time from lobotomy the greater the shrinkage. It seems likely that extensive trans-synaptic and transneuronal degeneration is taking place.

There is another set of late functional changes after nervous system lesions that, at least in the present state of technical advancement, have been observed only in man. These are the illusions or hallucinations that follow lesions in sensory systems. The best known of these is the phantom limb which is, as is well known, present almost invariably immediately after amputations. With the passage of time the phantom undergoes a character-istic shortening. In patients who are blind, striking illusory visual experiences may occur. Lhermitte (1951) and other French authors have particularly remarked on the occurrence of such illusory experiences in patients with chronic retinal disease. Hecaen and Ropert (1963) have discussed the occurrence of the similar appearance of auditory hallucinations in some patients with slowly progressive deafness. The stereotyped nature of the changes in the phantom limb, and of the late visual and auditory hallucinations we have just discussed makes it likely that we are dealing here with effects of chronic denervation, but we have no clear notion of the possible anatomical or physiological changes corresponding to these subjective changes.

Mechanisms of Change After "Fixed" Lesions

In this section I would like to review briefly some of the elementary mechanisms of late changes after "fixed" lesions of the nervous system. I will not discuss them in detail since some of them, although not all, have been discussed extensively at this meeting.

Some of the immediate changes must depend either on removal of inhibition, or on what I have

called above removal of <u>occlusion</u>, although this
may not quite be the right term. One problem in
any study of lesions in the nervous system is
that many immediate changes may take place of
which we may be unaware. Thus we know that conjugate gaze deficits after frontal lesions clear up
in at most, two weeks, but usually in a much
shorter time. Are there cases in which the deficit
lasts only for seconds or does not occur at all?
If this occurred frequently we might be failing
to take into account the major participation of
some areas in certain functions under normal
conditions.

When we turn to longer term changes, some other
mechanisms must be considered. Regeneration of
transected nerve fibers certainly occurs in the
peripheral nervous system, and may lead to some of
the phenomena of aberrant regeneration which are
rather difficult to explain. We continue to assume
that this type of regeneration of the main body of
the axon does not occur in the central nervous
system in higher animals. Theories as to this
phenomena have varied, some claiming that the CNS
neuron is incapable of regeneration, but more
generally it has been assumed that mechanical
factors prevent effective regeneration. The
presence of glial scarring is usually stressed.
It has also been suggested that collateral sprouting might, by taking up space on axons, leave no
space for longer regenerating fibers.

A recent paper by Ferlinga *et al*. (1973),
proceeding from the observation that animals who
accept skin homografts also show regeneration of
cord, tested the hypothesis that autoimmunity to
nervous system was the causal factor in animals
who did not show cord regeneration. They claimed
that in three of their adult rats who had received
immunosuppressant treatments they found evidence
of functional regeneration across a spinal transection. This work clearly deserves watching but
it would be premature to specify its ultimate
significance.

One can be fairly sure that collateral
sprouting occurs in denervated muscle in man,
e.g., in poliomyelitis. It, of course, seems
highly likely that collateral sprouting is
important in the recovery from spinal shock. It

seems reasonable indeed, to believe that it must occur in a wide variety of circumstances and must be a common cause of late effects, whether useful or not. Do the "environmental" effects on cases of spinal transection which lead to paraplegia in flexion operate by favoring the sprouting of particular collaterals, or by some other mechanism? We obviously cannot answer this on the basis of current knowledge.

Denervation supersensitivity clearly occurs in some obvious cases, such as in patients with a long-standing Horner's syndrome. It seems likely that denervation supersensitivity as discussed at this meeting plays a significant role in late changes after CNS lesions. Another phenomenon seen in man is increased activity of remaining portions of the sympathetic nervous system when some portions are destroyed. Thus patients who have lost sweating over the trunk and lower extremities after thoraco-lumbar sympathectomy often complain of grossly increased sweating over the face. I do not know whether the mechanisms of this increased production of transmitter in intact areas is known nor whether similar phenomena occur in the central nervous system.

I can only briefly mention a whole series of other possible pharmacological phenomena. The return of certain "lost functions" in response to drugs may well reflect an aspect of denervation supersensitivity. The nervous system of course responds not only to neurotransmitters in the strict sense but also to many hormones, releasing factors and even in special ways, to much simpler substances (e.g., the special effects of CO_2 in the respiratory centers). Long-term changes in the response to such substances have barely been studied.

I have already mentioned transsynaptic degeneration (i.e., death of the neuron distal to the one lesioned) and transneuronal degeneration (i.e., death of a neuron one synapse removed from the original one lesioned). This has been well known for years in certain systems, e.g., in the lateral geniculate after lesions of optic nerve and in the secondary trigeminal pathways after fifth nerve lesions. Another well-known example is the atrophy of the opposite cerebellum seen in

some patients with long-standing childhood hemiplegias, but rarely, if ever, after adult-onset
lesions. Recent studies suggest, however, that
such degenerations are much more common than was
previously realized. The extent of such degeneration probably increases with the years. Furthermore it is now clear that not only do anterograde
degenerations beyond synapses occur in the CNS,
but also retrograde transsynaptic and transneuronal degenerations. The full importance of these
phenomena has certainly not been explored.

Some Factors Influencing Late Changes

In this section I will shift to a somewhat
different level of analysis. Whatever the intimate
mechanisms of late change are they do not occur
uniformly in all circumstances and we will now
consider some of the factors which modify their
occurrence.

Species differences are of course of major
importance. As I have noted, it is usually said
that animals recover better than man. In one
important sense this is true, in that severe
losses of the higher functions after unilateral
lesions occur almost exclusively in man. Nottebohm
(1970) has shown that dominance effects occur in
birds, but the neural basis of this is not known.
Dominance has not so far been detected in any
mammal other than man, and it is not yet known
whether the mechanisms of unilateral preference
in man and the bird are related. In many cases the
lack of precisely similar lesions makes it difficult to compare man with other animals. It seems
likely that cats tolerate visual cortical lesions
better than monkeys, but comparison of monkey and
man is not easy for reasons discussed earlier.
There is as I have noted suggestive but not
conclusive evidence that in childhood, humans
tolerate cerebellar lesions better than animals.

I do not wish, however, to suggest that the
importance of species differences has been over-
estimated. I suspect that on the contrary, there
has been a tendency in some areas to neglect these
differences. Thus some authors who write on the
motor system are likely to mix together feline,
simian and human data. I believe that for many

485

reasons it will be important to separate carefully the effects of lesions of motor systems in
different species.

It is, of course, conventionally assumed that
early lesions are less damaging than later ones.
It is probably the case, however, that the differential effects of lesions at different ages cannot
be summarized by any simple formula. While it seems
to be true in man that early cerebellar lesions
are tolerated better than later ones, it is not at
all clear that early hemiplegias fare any better
than those occurring in adult life. Furthermore,
it seems possible that lesions of the caudate and
putamen have more serious effects in childhood.
Frontal lobotomy was said by some to have far more
severe unwanted effects in children than adults.

There are also several instances in which
superior childhood recovery is either clearly
documented or substantially supported by the data,
and yet is neglected in many discussions. Thus,
as I have already noted, there is very substantial
recovery from childhood lesions producing aphasia.
Despite this fact Penfield and Roberts (1959)
argued that certain regions of speech cortex
could be removed with little permanent disability,
but did not point out that this might be true only
in young patients or those with early lesions.
Yet nearly all their cases had lesions dating
from childhood and producing epilepsy for many
years. It would appear difficult to conclude that
the removal of a piece of cortex chronically
damaged since childhood would have the same effects
as those of destruction of a normal region of
cortex in the adult with no previous brain disorder.

It is my personal belief that failure to
separate childhood from adult lesions had led to
considerable confusion as to the effects of
callosal lesions. Thus, some authors describe the
syndrome produced in patients who have undergone
therapeutic callosal section as the syndrome of a
pure callosal lesion in a normal brain. These
normal syndromes are milder than the syndromes by
Liepmann (1908) or by Geschwind and Kaplan (1962).
The argument is made that the more severe syndromes
indicate that the callosal lesions were occurring
in brains that were otherwise not normal. A little

reflection, however, leads to some doubt as to this argument. It is obvious that therapeutic callosal surgery is not carried out in normal brains and that in all cases it has in fact been carried out for neurological disease, i.e., epilepsy, usually of long duration. Furthermore some of the operated cases have had clear evidence of gross brain disease, e.g., calcified brain lesions in X-ray.

It seems to me that a much more likely explanation is that milder syndromes occur when callosal surgery is carried out in patients with epilepsy of several years duration and dating back to childhood, while more severe syndromes are seen even with quite limited lesions when there is the sudden onset of a callosal lesion in a previously normal brain in the adult. Space does not permit me to go into a detailed discussion of the published cases. I doubt, however, that anyone at this conference would question the value of studies of early versus late callosal lesions in animals.

It could be advanced that the remarkable paucity of striking findings in patients with agenesis of the corpus callosum supports the argument I have just given that early callosal lesions have milder effects. Although this would support my argument I am reluctant to draw this conclusion on the basis of present evidence. Thus the diagnosis of agenesis has been made in the cases studied almost exclusively on the basis of X-ray findings. However post-mortem study of one such patient showed that while indeed there was total absence of the corpus callosum the anterior commissure was markedly enlarged, a situation similar to that normally seen in the kangaroo. It is conceivable that it is not the earliness of the lesion which accounts for the mildness of the syndrome but rather the fact that anterior commissure is larger.

There is a situation in which I suspect the childhood lesion might be more crippling than the same lesion in later life. I am referring to the lesions which in the adult lead to the classical Korsakow's syndrome, i.e., severe difficulty in the acquisition of new knowledge with a prolonged retrograde amnesia usually of several years' duration. Oddly enough this syndrome has not to my knowledge been described in childhood despite the fact that head injuries which often cause a transient Korsakow's syndrome in adult life are extremely common in the first decade. I suspect that Korsakow's syndromes do occur in this age group but are not recognized because the syndrome is much more severe than that seen in the adult. Thus, in the adult, aphasia is not part of the syndrome, perhaps because the retrograde amnesia does not extend back to the period of language acquisition. However, aphasia might be common in the childhood Korsakow's because the period of language acquisition would be affected. Similarly one could speculate that, if it existed, the congenital Korsakow's syndrome would give a picture of the grossest mental deficit, since the patient would fail to learn. The adult Korsakow's, despite the failure to learn, still retains enough old knowledge, which when combined with less affected capacities for abstraction, permits the attainment of very high scores on intelligence tests. If it should turn out that the child does not manifest a Korsakow's syndrome (either congenital or acquired), we would still be left with the question as to why adult lesions should cause the syndrome while childhood lesions do not. I might add that there may well also be a species difference, since it is not clear that a similar syndrome can be produced in animals.

This leads us naturally to the fact that, while most patients with certain congenital anomalies often show gross impairments, other patients with the same anomalies show little deficit. Thus many patients with agenesis of the callosum are mentally defective but others appear to be normal. Yakovlev has pointed out to me that while holotelencephaly, one of the grossest congenital anomalies, is usually associated with severe mental deficit, it has been found to be present in one case in an adult of superior intelligence. Work such as that presented by Altmann at this conference may help to elucidate these phenomena.

Serial Lesions in Man

This discussion leads us naturally to a consideration of serial lesions which have played so large a part in this conference. The nature of the data in man is such that it is very difficult to assess whether serial effects occur. There are in fact a very large member of situations in which one is in effect seeing a serial lesion. Most brain tumors produce their effects gradually. An example of the effects of gradual onset is shown by lesions of the frontal eye-field. Lesions of sudden onset, usually vascular occlusions, may produce conjugate deficit clearing in at most two weeks. But tumors in the same region almost never lead to eye-movement disorder. It appears that the compensation which takes place over two weeks after the acute lesion takes place imperceptibly during a lesion of slow onset. While the situation for the frontal eye-field is clear-cut, it is not certain whether gradual onset is always associated with milder disability. Part of the difficulty is that even enormous tumors are sometimes associated with very little disability. If they are externally compressive they may simply have moved brain structures slowly without damaging them. Infiltrative tumors may grow between normal structures without damaging them. In other words, although serial effects may - and I suspect - must, occur, it is too difficult to evaluate the clinical evidence.

Perhaps the most impressive example of possible serial effect I know of was a patient described to me who had undergone repeated operations to remove tumor from his left temporal lobe. After the final operation he had only a thin rim of temporal lobe remaining at the base and along the medial surface. After each operation he had become aphasic but had each time recovered essentially to normal, even after the last operation when there was no useful temporal speech cortex remaining. The reason why even in this case one cannot be sure of a serial lesion effect is that, as I have noted earlier, a certain number of patients even with acute permanent lesions recover very well from aphasia. One would require a larger series to be sure that the recovery rate was still higher in serial lesions.

Effects of Learning on Late Changes

Let us consider briefly the influence of
overlearning on subsequent recovery, a factor
which has received a fair degree of attention in
the animal literature. The question is whether a
previously overlearned performance will recover
better after a lesion. It would appear, at least
on superficial examination, that overlearning
cannot play a very large role in recovery in man.
Thus the very existence of large numbers of
permanent severe aphasias argues against the
importance of overlearning. Language must be, for
the majority of humans, the most overlearned
skill they possess, but they are nonetheless not
protected in most cases against the consequences
of unilateral lesions. On the other hand overlearning can be shown to exert some effects, but
of quite small magnitude. Thus, many aphasics will
be able to write their own names perfectly well
but nothing else. However, even this highly overlearned task may be as severely affected in some
patients as any other attempt at writing.

It has sometimes been argued that specific
training of one hemisphere can affect the process
of recovery either adversely or favorably. The
suggestion has been made that cerebral dominance
for language is a secondary effect of learning to
write. It is argued that use of the right hand for
language trains the left hemisphere, and that the
illiterate patient is therefore at an advantage
since he is more likely not to have educated only
one-half of the brain. There is not much strong,
positive evidence for this view, and there are
several arguments against it. In the first place,
the overwhelming predominance of left hemisphere
lesions in aphasia was observed at a period when
the majority of patients, at least in the
Continental European countries, were illiterate.
A further argument against this view is that in
left-handers the side of the lesion producing a
permanent severe aphasia has no fixed relationship
to the hand used for writing.

It has also been suggested that training of the
minor hemisphere might insure that language was

learned by both sides, thus protecting the patient against future unilateral lesions. While one cannot confidently conclude that such training is never beneficial there is evidence to suggest that at least in some cases it is apparently of little effect. This comes out dramatically in a case described by Nielsen (1962), of a left-hander who had always written with his right hand. He sustained in adult life what was probably a callosal infarction and lost the ability to write with the right hand, although it was intact from a motor point of view. He could, however, write correctly with his left hand. The mechanism seems to be clear. The patient's right hemisphere was dominant for language. His left hemisphere had always written passively under the control of the right hemisphere and could no longer write when it was cut off from the right hemisphere. Despite fifty years of practice the left hemisphere had never really learned to write but had always remained under control of the right hemisphere which was where the learning had primarily taken place.

There is one situation in which training seems to affect recovery. Sparks and Geschwind (1968) showed that a patient with a callosal lesion showed inability to report the words presented to the left ear in a dichotic listening task. With repeated trials the left ear performance rose in certain conditions to about 35% correct. The authors suggested that the ipsilateral auditory pathway was suppressed by the presence of competing inputs in the contralateral pathway, but that training could lead to increased capacity to handle the ipsilateral stimulus. The later study of Milner *et al.* (1968) confirmed these results in a larger series of patients.

Epilepsy as a Factor in Late Changes

Let me turn now to yet another possibly very important factor in late effects - epilepsy. Epilepsy has perhaps received less attention as a factor in late changes than it deserves from those working with animals. It may be argued by any experimenter that his animals have been closely observed and that no seizures were seen. While

this may give us some confidence as to the occurrence of major motor seizures it does not include
the many types of epilepsy that may have little or
no external motor effects, e.g., classical temporal lobe epilepsy in those cases where there is no
progression in the attacks to the obvious grand
mal convulsion. Even grand mal convulsions are
easier to miss in animals since neither they nor
their litter mates complain to the experimenter.

Epilepsy plays a double role in the scenario
of late changes both as an effect and a cause. On
the one hand epilepsy itself is often a late
change after a "fixed" lesion. Thus epilepsy comes
on with high frequency after many brain lesions,
particularly penetrating wounds. Epilepsy may
appear within days of a lesion or may not appear
until many years later - even 20 years. The late
onset of epilepsy after a lesion need not be too
surprising since the slow growth of glial scars
at a site of damage could account for it. What is
more surprising, and may be especially interesting
to study both anatomically and pharmacologically,
is the fact that in a very large percentage of
patients, post-traumatic epilepsy eventually
undergoes "spontaneous cure" and the patient is
seizure-free without medication.

While epilepsy can be a late effect of a lesion
it can also be a cause of late changes. Here again
it probably plays a multiple role, acting either
as a lesion itself, or as a factor in recovery.
At the level of overall behavior, studies such as
those of Slater, Beard and Glithero (1963),
Falconer (1973), and Blumer and Walker (1967)
illustrate the high incidence of behavioral
alterations in patients who suffer from temporal
lobe epilepsy. While it usually takes several
years for these behavioral alterations to become
obvious, they can come on even in 2 or 3 years
after the initiation of seizures. Some recent
studies in animals have shown that even a single
seizure in the amygdala can lead to effects on
behavior lasting for days (Belluzzi and Grossman
1969). What the mechanism is of such long-lasting
effects is not known, but certainly deserves
study.

The epileptic focus can apparently act in some
ways as a lesion. It therefore seems conceivable

that a long-standing seizure focus might, in some manner, act as a slowly progressive lesion, which might have analogies with the serial lesion paradigm. It is conceivable that repeated seizure activity, in, for example, one of the speech areas might, by repeatedly paralyzing it, set off the processes of recovery, so that when the focus is finally ablated there is little permanent focal deficit. This might suggest a useful experimental paradigm for studying serial lesion effects without actual destruction of one of the areas.

The epileptic focus may, however, also act in a quite different way, i.e., as a stimulus rather than as a paralyzing lesion. Thus there has been considerable study of the phenomenon of the mirror focus. If an epileptic lesion is established at one site in the brain, one will eventually see, in some instances, the development of a new independent focus in the homologous region of the opposite side, which will remain as a source of epilepsy even when the primary focus is removed. The mirror focus may be a very important model not only for late changes after injury but even for normal behavior. Morrell (1961a, b) has in fact suggested that the formation of a mirror focus essentially represents a model of the learning process.

Another example of the positive effects of seizures is seen in the experiments of T.C. Erickson (1940). He pointed out that a seizure starting in the hand area in the experimental animal would eventually spread to the leg area of the same side in a classical Jacksonian march. A cut between the arm and leg areas led at first to failure of the seizure to follow its accustomed course. The seizure would, however, follow a new route, going to the opposite hemisphere and then being relayed back, thus reaching the leg area of the original side by a circuitous route. Severing the corpus callosum would prevent the use of this roundabout route.

This experiment as well as the establishment of the mirror focus raises an important possibility. Is it conceivable that repeated seizures might in fact be a means of hastening recovery by "opening unused pathways"? If this were true then the detailed mechanisms would be well worth study.

Do seizures lead to sprouting, or do they alter pharmacological sensitivity, in distant regions? In any case epilepsy may be a common factor in late change and may well deserve much further investigation by the animal experimenter.

If one reviews rapidly the last few pages he may see that the determinants of recovery may be difficult to disentangle. Most patients who have had cortical excisions or surgical callosal sections have shown relatively milder syndromes than might have been expected on the basis of experience with vascular lesions in the adult. The surgical patients who had undergone these therapeutic procedures have nearly always had brain disease dating back from childhood. They have suffered from epilepsy dating back to child-hood and have had many severe seizures. The surgical procedures have nearly always been carried out in early adult life. They recover better than the older adult with an acute lesion and a previously normal brain. But why do they recover better? Is it the earliness of the origi-nal insult to the brain, the early onset of epilepsy, the repetitive seizures, or the surgery in early adult life, or some combination of these which account for this better recovery? Clearly we do not yet known the answer.

Mechanism of Recovery from Childhood Aphasia

It is commonly stated that the child recovers from aphasia by use of the other hemisphere. There are, however, two senses in which the patient might be "using" the other hemisphere. One could conceive that language was learned with the major hemisphere, and that after it was damaged, language was relearned by the minor hemisphere. This is, however, probably not the case, since the rate of recovery is much too rapid. For example, I saw a ten year old boy who was left with a permanent hemiplegia after an operation for removal of a massive glioma from the left hemisphere. He was severely aphasic immediately after the operation and one month later. By three months, however, his language was essentially normal, although he had been continuously hospitalized, with little or no specific language therapy.

494

It seems much more likely that the child learns language with <u>both</u> hemispheres, but that only the major hemisphere performs in both the production and comprehension of language. After destruction of the major hemisphere the minor hemisphere eventually comes to use its learning.

It seems clear that a similar mechanism must also play a part in those cases in which excellent recovery takes place in adults. Thus Dejerine and André-Thomas (1912) described a left-handed woman who developed a massive right hemisphere lesion which led to a permanent left hemiplegia. She was severely aphasic in all modalities for six months and then began to recover. By the time of her death two years later, her language functions were essentially normal, with the exception of writing which did not recover. (The failure of recovery of writing is a matter of special interest which I will not discuss. It is dealt with by Heilman *et al*. 1973). Post-mortem revealed destruction of the right hemisphere so extensive that recovery could have taken place only on the left. Such an excellent recovery over two years in middle life could not have been result of relearning by the minor (in this case, left) hemisphere. We must again assume that learning of language had taken place in both hemispheres, but that the minor hemisphere was somehow prevented from comprehending or producing language until the major hemisphere was destroyed.

If language is indeed learned with both hemispheres we are faced with several additional questions. Why is recovery not immediate in the child, and what takes place in the succeeding months to "release" the learning on the other side? Even more important are the implications for the adult. If language is present in both hemispheres at age 10, is it still there at age 50? Clearly it is in the 30% of aphasics who recover well. What of the 70% who show poor recoveries? Has the language that was present in the minor hemisphere in childhood somehow been lost? Or, is it still present, but suppressed in some manner? This is a matter of importance for the recovery of the aphasic. If those who do not recover still have language in the minor hemisphere, then some means should be available, conceivably surgical or pharmacological, to revive this suppressed activity. If on the other hand the language formerly present has been lost, my guess would be that there is little hope for significant recovery.

Consider briefly the mechanisms which prevent the right hemisphere from taking part in the language activities and which keep it suppressed in so many adult aphasics. One's first temptation is to assume that the inhibition is mediated via the corpus callosum. Indeed one often hears the suggestion that callosal section might benefit the adult aphasic. Although the inhibition in child-hood might be initially mediated callosally, it seems unlikely that this is the mechanism for the continued inhibition in the adult aphasic. The lesion producing the aphasia destroys the callosal fibers arising in the cortical region which have been destroyed. A very large left hemispheric destructive lesion may almost totally destroy the callosal fibers arising from that hemisphere, and yet recovery is typically very poor after such huge lesions. It seems likely that the locus of the suppression in the right hemisphere must lie in that hemisphere itself. I use the term "suppression" since the mechanism is not clear. Conceivably some structure in the right hemisphere inhibits the speech areas in the strict sense of the term. On the other hand, one might be dealing with atrophy of the cells or terminals as a result of long disuse - an atrophy reversible in the child and in many adults.

It is clear that if the right hemisphere mediates recovery from aphasia it must in some way respond to destruction of all or part of the left. The recovery may takes months or years. There is a tendency to presume that sprouting or denerva-tion sensitivity must account for such favorable late changes, while transsynaptic or transneuronal degeneration account for non-recovery or late deterioration. One can, however, readily conceive of the possibility that the degenerations might account for recovery, if the neurons which die are mediating inhibition of the speech area on the right. Conversely, it is easy to picture mechan-isms by which sprouting or denervation supersensi-tivity could interfere with recovery.

Shrinking Retrograde Amnesia

There is another instance in which the evidence is clear that recovery depends not on relearning, but on reactivation of learning which is already present. It is well known that bilateral medial temporal destruction leads to a permanent difficulty in the acquisition of new knowledge. Less well known is the fact that a left unilateral medial temporal lesion produces a memory disorder lasting several weeks (Geschwind and Fusillo 1966). While the difficulty in acquisition of new knowledge is present there is also a prolonged retrograde amnesia. As the memory disorder disappears the retrograde amnesia also vanishes with the return of the apparently lost memories. Clearly these memories were not lost. They obviously depended on the left medial temporal region for their activation. After destruction of the left medial temporal region they can eventually be reactivated by the right temporal region.

A similar phenomenon is seen in some patients after head injury who show difficulty in acquiring new knowledge and suffer from prolonged retrograde amnesia. The patient recovers and the retrograde amnesia shrinks, which again suggests that the memories were not lost, but simply incapable of activation (Russell and Nathan 1946; Benson and Geschwind 1967).

Recovery by Employment of Alternative Pathways

In some instances sparing of certain functions or their recovery occurs because an alternative pathway is available to replace the one destroyed. This particularly clear in the case of patients with apraxia, i.e., suffering from lesions which prevent a verbal command from reaching the appropriate motor region. Thus consider the patient with a callosal lesion. He may fail to carry out verbal commands with his left hand. On the other hand in some instances he apparently carries out a certain number of commands with his left hand. There is more than one mechanism which could account for this. Thus the right hemisphere might comprehend the commands and carry them out. On the other hand the commands might be understood only

by the left hemisphere and be carried out by means
of ipsilaterally descending motor systems. Careful
examination of many patients suggests that this
latter mechanism must account for many of the
cases. Thus consider the patient with a callosal
lesion who responds to the verbal command to show
the use of a hammer with his left hand. The normal
responds to this command by pretending to hold a
hammer in his left hand, but the patient responds
by using his closed left fist as a hammer. The
patient is, however, quite capable of making the
correct movement, since given an actual hammer he
handles it quite correctly.

Consider the mechanism of this performance.
When one gives the normal a verbal command to
carry out with his left hand, the command is
transmitted across the callosum and eventually the
pyramidal system is activated, producing a movement
containing its full complement of fine distal
movements. In the callosal patient the command is
transmitted ipsilaterally via non-pyramidal motor
systems, and as a result lacks the fine distal
components. In the same patient placing the hammer
in the left hand transmits somesthetic information
to the right hemisphere so that the pyramidal
system can again be activated.

There are other forms of evidence to support
this notion. In patients with lesions disconnect-
ing the speech region from the pyramidal system,
certain types of movement are typically preserved
to verbal command, e.g., eye movements, and
movements of the trunk. We know that eye movements
have no representation in the pyramidal system and
that trunk movements have little representation.
Thus, the class of movements which typically
travel via non-pyramidal pathways are preserved.
For a fuller account see the discussion of the
apraxias in Geschwind (1965).

Further support comes from the recent
demonstration by Brinkman and Kuypers (1973) that
one can make animals with appropriate lesions use
either pyramidal or non-pyramidal motor systems by
manipulation of the sensory input. These animals
show the same phenomenon seen in humans although
it takes more elaborate techniques to demonstrate
it. Axial movements may also be strikingly
preserved or show dramatic recovery after brain

lesions causing actual comprehension deficit. As I
have already pointed out, the speech areas of the
left hemisphere have access to non-pyramidal motor
systems. It is striking, however, that in patients
with left hemisphere lesions producing severe
comprehension deficits for all classes of language,
there is still often excellent comprehension of
eye-movement and trunk commands. I found this to
be the case in my examination of the patient of
Smith (1966) mentioned above who had undergone
total removal of the left hemisphere. In other
words it appears as if the right hemisphere can
understand this special class of commands, even
when it does not understand other aspects of
language.

Effects of Other Lesions on Recovery

There is one important mechanism of recovery
that has received some attention from animal
experimenters in the past although it has not been
discussed at this meeting. This is the effect of a
second lesion in improving performance. Perhaps
the most clear-cut example of this in man is the
improvement in Parkinsonism which may occur after
a surgical lesion in the VL nucleus of the thalamus. This is in fact one of the few non-trivial
applications of this approach. By trivial applications we mean such procedures as interrupting
the reflex arc to abolish spasticity be section of
either ventral or dorsal roots. The term "trivial"
signifies the lack of deep theoretical interest
regardless of therapeutic usefulness.

Over the years a large number of procedures of
this type have been attempted mostly for the
correction of abnormalities of motor function,
either Parkinsonism, athetosis, or hemiballismus.
Perhaps the most interesting are the ones in which
lesions were placed in the pyramidal system,
either in cord, peduncle, or even in area 4 for
the correction of movement disorder, e.g., Putnam
(1940), and Bucy et al. (1946). The striking point
of these procedures was not only the improvement
of the movement disorder but also the lack of
striking weakness in many cases after the surgery.
One might argue as many authors have that these
results simply indicate how unimportant pyramidal

lesions really are in producing paralysis. An
alternative interpretation is that the two lesions
are reciprocal, i.e., the pyramidal lesion diminishes the effect of the lesion in the basal
ganglia, but in turn the basal ganglia lesion
diminishes the effect of the pyramidal lesion.
Although this concept would fit in with the idea
of balanced systems it has not been studied
systematically. In some cases drugs might act as a
reversible lesion of a competing system. Thus one
common although not universal view is that Parkinsonism is benefited either by replacing the
dopamine lost as a result of the nigral lesion or
by blocking the antagonist cholinergic system.

Use of Alternative Strategies

In some cases apparent recovery can take place
when the patient learns to use a strategy which
circumvents the direct effects of the neural
lesion. I myself believe that the use of such
strategies must be regarded conceptually as being
of a different order from the types of mechanisms
we have been discussing until now. It is not
recovery based on redundant but latent learning
in an intact portion of the central nervous system.
It is not based on the use of alternative pathways.
At the level of cellular mechanisms it is not
based on sprouting, denervation supersensitivity
or any of the other mechanisms mentioned. I think
it is important to separate this group of
mechanisms since they can be treacherous in
misleading us.
A classic if simple and obvious animal
experiment is the one in which a rat with a right
hemiplegia still manages to turn right at a
choice point in a maze by turning left in a
complete circle. No one was misled by this. On the
other hand it is possible that reports of
"spontaneous" emptying from totally denervated
bladders were incorrect. The patients had perhaps
learned to empty the bladder by repeated Valsalva
maneuvers. Such "tricks" would be of little
interest in deeper understanding of bladder
physiology, while true spontaneous voiding from a
denervated bladder would be of major interest.
The use of such strategies is quite evident in

some apraxic patients. For example, consider a patient with a callosal lesion who apparently carried out verbal commands correctly with both the right and left hands. The fact that the left hand performed correctly might tempt one to assume that either the right hemisphere understood the commands or that the left hemisphere was carrying them out by means of ipsilateral pathways. Careful examination of the patient, as we shall see, ruled out both these explanations and made it clear that the patient was using a "trick."

The clue to these findings was the way in which the patient carried out verbal commands. He would respond rapidly to commands to use his right hand. When given a command to use his left upper limb, e.g., "Show me how you salute with your left hand" the patient would first carry out the command with his right hand and would only then carry out the movement with the left arm. If the examiner prevented the patient from carrying out the movement with the right hand the patient was unable to carry it out with his left; he would, in fact, struggle to release the right hand. Once the right hand was freed he would carry out the movement with it and subsequently make the same movement with the left. The explanation seems clear. The patient, or rather the left hemisphere of the patient, had learned that by signalling non-verbally it could get the right hand to imitate the movement. Clearly no language comprehension by the right hemisphere was necessary for this performance, but one could be easily fooled. This patient illustrates a phenomenon that is commonly seen in the clinic.

Individual Variation

One extremely important factor is often overlooked in man, and is rarely considered in animal work. I am referring, of course, to individual variation, i.e., differences in the effects of lesions which are attributable to what one might describe as host variation. Despite the tremendous interest in individual differences dating back for nearly a century there has been comparatively little attention paid to variations in the nervous system that might account for different responses to lesions. Indeed such variations from case to case have sometimes been taken as evidence against the "doctrine of localization" although even the classic localizers realized that the same lesion did not always lead to the same permanent effects.

Individual variations in height, weight, eye color are readily perceived and cannot be overlooked. Variations in intellectual function have been studied very extensively. Within the past few years there has begun to appear a considerable literature on individual differences in drug responses. The lack of interest in individual differences in the nervous system is probably the result of two factors. First, experimental study of this problem in man is difficult. One can measure eye-color or the ability to taste phenylthiocarbamide in a large kinship but one can rarely observe more than one brain lesion in a large family. The second reason is that individual variations in structure in the brain have until now been much more difficult to delineate than variations in, let us say, height or eye-color.

To my knowledge little attention has been paid to this factor in animals. Differences in strains of rats in learning ability, drug responses, or susceptibility to disease have been studied, as well as strains with congenital disorders of nervous development. I know of no study of either strain or individual differences in effects of lesions, nor has there been study of differences in anatomy, e.g., are there strains of rats in which the caudate is very large relative to the remainder of the brain and do these rats show different susceptibility to lesions? Furthermore I don't know if anyone has made the attempt to breed strains of animals which are particularly susceptible or particularly resistant to certain lesions. This might represent a very fruitful approach to the problem of late changes.

It seems clear that individual variation is of major importance in man. We know that some patients recover extremely well from certain lesions which are permanently crippling to other patients. We know a little about the source of some of these individual differences, e.g., left-handers respond

to certain brain lesions differently from right-
handers and tend to show better recovery. But we
know little more than this. Although it has sometimes been suggested that sex may affect recovery
from certain lesions in man there has been little
systematic study of this problem.

It is my guess that among the major sources of
individual variation are differences in size of
anatomical structures between individuals. We know
in fact that certain differences of this type are
very large. Thus it was generally assumed (see,
for example, Bonin 1962) that the two cerebral
hemispheres of man differed at most slightly from
each other. Geschwind and Levitsky (1968) demonstrated, however, that there are anatomical
differences between the hemispheres which are
readily visible to the naked eye. The area which
is larger on the left is the planum temporale, a
portion of Wernicke's area lying on the upper
surface of the temporal lobe. Other investigators
have not only confirmed our work but have also
shown that these differences are present at birth
(Wada 1969; Teszner 1972; Witelson and Pallie
1973), which certainly rules out post-partum
environmental effects and makes it likely that
these differences are genetic. One important
aspect of the findings is the fact not merely of
left-right differences, but also the remarkable
degree of variation from brain to brain. We found
that in 65% of the cases the planum was bigger on
the left, equal on the two sides in 24%, while in
11% it was bigger on the right. It seems likely
that those people with a larger planum on the left
are different from those with equal plana or a
larger planum on the right. There are, however,
large variations even within each group. Thus in
some people the planum on the left is 5 times as
large as it is on the right, while in others it
is only slightly larger. In cases with equal plana,
one sometimes finds a small planum on each side,
while in others this region is large on both
sides. It seems likely that each of these patterns
corresponds to a difference in function. Furthermore it is probably not unreasonable to guess that
cases with different types of pattern of the plana
on the two sides will show different patterns of
late change after aphasia-producing lesions. It

also seems likely that such right-left and individual differences will be found in many sites in
the human brain. It is also conceivable that the
distribution of patterns is different in the two
sexes which may explain the much lower frequency
in females of disorders of language development.

ACKNOWLEDGMENTS: Some of the work reported here
was supported by Grant NS 06209 from the National
Institutes of Health.

REFERENCES

Belluzi, J.D. and Grossman, S.P. (1969). Avoidance learning: long-lasting deficits after temporal lobe seizures. *Science* 166, 1435-1437.

Benson, D.F. and Geschwind, N. (1967). Shrinking retrograde amnesia. *J. Neurol. Neurosurg. Psychiat.* 30, 539-544.

Blumer, D. and Walker, S.E. (1967). Sexual behavior in temporal lobe epilepsy. *Arch. Neurol.* 25, 260-264.

Bonin, G.V. (1962). *In* V.B. Mountcastle (Ed.) "Interhemispheric Relations and Cerebral Dominance", Baltimore: Johns Hopkins Press, pp. 1-6.

Brinkman, J. and Kuypers, H.G.J.M. (1973). Cerebral control of contralateral and ipsilateral arm, hand, and finger movements in the split-brain rhesus monkey. *Brain* 96, 653-674.

Bucy, P.C., Keplinger, J.E., and Siqueira, E.B. (1964). Destruction of the "pyramidal tract" in man. *J. Neurosurg.* 21, 385-398.

Byers, R.K. and McLean, W.T. (1962). Etiology and course of certain hemiplegias with aphasia in childhood. *Pediatrics* 29, 376-383.

Dejerine, J. and André-Thomas (1912). Contribution à l'étude de l'aphasie chez les gauchers. *Revue Neurologique* 24, 213-266.

Denny-Brown, D., Kirk, E.J. and Yanagisawa, N. (1973). The tract of Lissauer in relation to sensory transmission in the dorsal horn of spinal cord in the macaque monkey. *J. Comp. Neurol.* 151, 175-200.

Dolivo, M. (1953). "Crossed phrenic phenomenon" et phénomène phrénique bilatéral. *Helvet. Physiol. Pharmacol. Acta* 11, 251-269.

Erickson, T.C. (1940). Spread of the epileptic discharge. *Arch. Neurol. Psychiat.* 43, 429-452.

Falconer, M.A. (1973). Temporal-lobe resection for epilepsy and behavioral abnormalities. *New England J. Med.* 289, 451-455.

Feringa, E.R., Gurden, G.G., Strode, L.W., Chandler, W. and Knake, J. (1973). Descending spinal motor tract regeneration after spinal cord transection. *Neurology* 23, 599-608.

Geschwind, N. (1965). Disconnection syndromes in animals and man. *Brain* 88, 237-294 and 585-644.

Geschwind, N. and Fusillo, M. (1966). Color-naming defects in association with alexia. *Arch. Neurol. Psychiat.* 15, 137-146.

Geschwind, N. and Kaplan, E. (1962). A human cerebral deconnection syndrome. *Neurology* 12, 675-685.

Geschwind, N. and Levitsky, W. (1968). Human brain: left-right asymmetries in temporal speech region. *Science* 161, 186-187.

Gloning, I., Gloning, K., Haub, G. and Quatember, R. (1969). Comparison of verbal behavior in right-handed and non right-handed patients with anatomically verified lesion of one hemisphere. *Cortex* 5, 43-52.

Gloning, I.K., Gloning, K. and Hoff, H. (1968). "Neuropsychological Symptoms and Syndromes in Lesions of the Occipital Lobe", Paris: Gauthier-Villars.

Hamlin, R.M. (1970). Intellectual functions 14 years after frontal lobe surgery. *Cortex* 6, 299-307.

Hécaen, H. and Ropert, (1963). Les hallucinations auditives des otopathes. *J. de Psychologie Normale et Pathologique* 60, 293-324.

Heilman, K.M., Coyle, J.M., Gonyea, E.F. and Geschwind, N. (1973). Apraxia and agraphia in a left-hander. *Brain* 96, 21-28.

Hoffman, B.F. and Cranefield, P.F. (1960). "Electrophysiology of the Heart", New York: Blakiston.

Kirk, E.J. and Denny-Brown, D. (1970). Functional variation of the dermatomes in the macaque monkey following dorsal root lesions. *J. Comp. Neurol.* 139, 307-320.

Krabbe, K.H. (1934). The myotonia acquisita in relation to the postneuritic muscular hypertrophies. *Brain* 57, 184-194.

Lapresle, J. and Ben Hamida, M. (1970). The dentato-olivary pathway. *Arch. Neurol.* 22, 135-143.

Lhermitte, J. (1951). "Les Hallucinations", Paris: Doin.

Liepmann, H. (1908). "Drei Aufsätze aus dem Apraxiegebiet", Berlin: Karger.

Luria, A.R. (1970). "Traumatic Aphasia", The Hague: Mouton, pp. 27-76.

Milner, B., Taylor, L. and Sperry, R.W. (1968). Lateralized suppression of dichotically presented digits after commissural section in man. *Science* 161, 184-185.

Morrell, F. (1961a). Electrophysiological contributions to the neural basis of learning. *Physiol. Revs.* 41, 443-494.

Morrell, F. (1961b). Lasting changes in synaptic organization produced by continuous neural bombardment. *In* J.F. Delafresnaye, A. Fessard and J. Konorski (Eds.) "CIOMS Symposium on Brain Mechanisms and Learning", Oxford: Blackwell.

Nathan, P. and Smith, M. (1973). Effects of two unilateral cordotomies on the motility of the lower limbs. *Brain* 96, 471-494.

Nielsen, J.M. (1962). "Agnosia, Apraxia, Aphasia", New York: Hafner. pp. 186-187.

Nottebohm, F. (1970). Ontogeny of bird song. *Science* 167, 950-956.

Penfield, W. and Roberts, L. (1959). "Speech and Brain-Mechanisms", Princeton: Princeton University Press.

Porter, W.T. (1894-1895). The path of the respiratory impulse from the bulb to the phrenic nuclei. *J. Physiol.* 17, 455-459.

Putnam, T.J. (1940). Treatment of unilateral paralysis agitans by section of the lateral pyramidal tract. *Arch. Neurol. Psychiat.* 44, 950-976.

Raisman, G. (1969). Neuronal plasticity in the septal nuclei of the adult rat. *Brain Res.* 14, 25-48.

Russell, W.R. and Nathan, P.W. (1946). Traumatic amnesia. *Brain* 69, 280-300.

Slater, E., Beard, A.W. and Glithero, E. (1963). Schizophrenic-like psychoses of epilepsy. *Brit. J. Psychiat.* 109, 95-150.

Smith, A. (1966). Speech and other functions after left (dominant) hemispherectomy. *J. Neurol. Neurosurg. Psychiat.* 29, 467-471.

Sparks, R. and Geschwind, N. (1968). Dichotic listening in man after section of the neocortical commissures. *Cortex* 4, 3-16.

Subirana, A. (1969). Handedness and cerebral
dominance. *In* P.J. Vinken and G.W. Bruyn
(Eds.) "Handbook of Clinical Neurology",
Vol. 4. Amsterdam: North Holland. pp. 248-272.

Teszner, D. (1972). Etude anatomique de l'asymétrie
droite-gauche du planum temporale sur 100
cerveaux d'adultes. Thèse pour le Doctorat en
Médecine, Université de Paris.

Trelles, J.O. (1968). Les myoclonies vélo-
palatines. *Rev. Neurol.* 119, 165-171.

Wada, J. (1969). Presentation at Ninth International Congress of Neurology, New York.

Wall, P.D. and Egger, M.D. (1971). Formation of
new connexions in adult rat brains after
partial deafferentation. *Nature* 232, 542-545.

Witelson, S.F. and Pallie, W. (1973). Left hemisphere speculization for language in the
newborn: Neuroanatomical evidence of asymmetry,
Brain 96, 641-646.

Yakovlev, P.I. (1954). Paraplegia in flexion of
cerebral origin. *J. Neuropath. Exp. Neurol.*
13, 267-295.

Subject Index

A

Acetylcholine, 346
Activity
  exploratory, 397-404, 413-417
  frontal lesions and, 348-354
  hippocampal lesions and, 129-144
Acute drug action, 341-342
Adipsia, 206
Adrenergic neurons, regeneration in,
  111-123
Aging, recovery of function and, 413-417
α-methyl-p-tyrosine, 238, 353-354,
  356-360
Amphetamine, 218, 221, 226, 227, 276,
  287, 343-352, 356, 360, 363-365
  effects on hyperphagia, 343-345
Amygdala, 448
  regeneration in, 120
  serial lesions in, 380-391, 397-404
Amygdalectomy, 120, 153, 157, 226-229
  social behavior and, 228-229
Anorexia, 343
Anterior neocortex, 221-222
Aphagia, 343, 355-360, 404-413
Aphasia, 1-2, 13, 176
  childhood, 478-481, 486-488, 494-497
  recovery from, 1-2, 204, 208-210, 245,
    478-481, 486, 489-490, 494-497
Apraxia, 293-294, 311, 501
Aspiration lesions, 237-238, 376-378
Ataxia, 275, 294-302, 314, 317
Atropine, 204
Avoidance behavior, 153, 217-219, 227,
  350-354, 363-365, 380-391, 397-404
Axonal growth, see also Collateral sprout-
  ing, Sprouting, Regeneration, 203, 205
anomalous, 65, 71, 73, 78-80, 82-91,
  94, 98-100, 113-115, 144, 149, 152,
  483, 496

B

Behavioral compensation, see Compensa-
  tion, behavioral
Behavioral plasticity, see Recovery
Bell's palsy, 473
Bilateral symmetry, recovery of function
  and, see Contralateral homologue
Brainstem, 14, 288, 397
Broca's area, 479

C

Canaries, 204
Castration, behavioral effects of, 204
Catecholamines, 344, 346, 352-354, 356,
  358, 363
Cats
  hyperphagia in, 343
  recovery in, 222-226, 243-244, 255,
    269
  serial lesions in, 245, 253, 397
  visual system of, 152
Caudate nucleus, 449
  afferent connections of, 154, 165-166,
    361
  aphagia and, 358
  delayed reward and, 429, 449
  development of, 166-167, 169
  lesions of, 166, 309, 358, 363-365,
    381-391
  serial lesions of, 381-391

Cerebellar lesions, behavioral effects of,
    129-144, 288, 294-304, 311-317,
    475-476
Cerebellar tremor, 275, 294-304, 314, 317
Cerebellum, 5, 10, 484-485
    basket cells of, 130
    behavioral plasticity of, 129-144, 475,
        484-486
    dentate nucleus of, 279, 311, 475-476
    development of, 129-144
    granule cells of, 130, 294-304
    interpositus nucleus, 279, 294-304, 311
    stellate cells of, 130
Cerebral dominance, 207-210, 480-481,
    485, 494-497, 503
Cerebrum, 7, 13
Chlorpromazine, 346
Cholinergic receptors, 363
Chronic drug action, 342-343
Cingulate cortex, 448
Circling behavior, 360-362
Clarke's nucleus, 307, 309, 312
Clinical study of recovery, 1-2, 204,
    207-219, 468-470, 472-504
Cognitive skills
    in aphasia, 208-211
    development in humans, 175-199
Collateral sprouting, 20-21, 111-123,
    152-153, 169, 175, 269-270, 284,
    308-310, 312, 318, 320, 365, 392-397,
    483
Compensation, behavioral, 149-150,
    152-153, 162, 164, 166, 169, 206-207,
    254-255, 278, 292, 316, 319, 459-461
Conditioned avoidance, 217-219, 227
Conditioning, 67-68, 279-280, 288, 289,
    290-292, 308, 313, 319-320
Contralateral homologue, recovery
    mediated by, 395-396, 412, 480-481,
    485, 494-497
Contralateral paralysis, see also
    Hemiplegia, 10
Corpus Callosum, 10, 486-488, 490-491,
    496, 497-498
Corpus striatum, 10
Cortex, see also separate areas, 470
Cortex, localization of faculties in, 11-15

Corticospinal tract, 271-277, 281, 287,
    300-301
Cytoarchitectonic maps, 289, 470

D

Deafferentation, 282, 304-310, 314
Degeneration
    axonal, 74-75, 80, 86, 152, 166
    transneuronal and transsynaptic, 482,
        484-485, 496
Delayed response deficits, 150-151, 154,
    157-169, 345-346, 381-392, 411-415,
    417-418, 429-461
Denervation supersensitivity, 20, 268-270,
    284, 315, 318-319, 339-367, 416,
    470, 494
Development, neural
    of cats, 157, 243, 252, 255
    of cerebellum, 129-148
    cortical lesions and, 237, 243-244,
        413-421, 478-479, 486-488
    deafferentation and, 307-308
    dyslexia and, 175-199
    of hamsters, 66-101
    of hippocampus, 129-148
    of humans, 175-199, 478-481, 486-488,
        494-497
    language disorders and, 175-199,
        478-486, 486-488
    of monkeys, 150-169, 237
    of rats, 129-144, 157, 271, 413-421
    recovery and, see Recovery, development
        and,
    regeneration and, see Regeneration,
        developmental studies of
    of visual system, 65-101, 152
    X-radiation and, 129-148
Diaschisis, 16, 21-22, 219, 284, 308, 391,
    421, 459
Disease model of developmental dyslexia,
    176-177, 199
Dishabituation, 317
Disuse atrophy, 276
Disuse supersensitivity, see also
    Denervation supersensitivity, 340
Dogs, serial lesions in, 153

Dopamine, 344, 352-353, 358, 366, 500
Dorsal roots, 269, 270, 303, 304, 307,
    310, 313, 318, 471
Dorsolateral cortex, *see* Frontal cortex,
    dorsolateral
Drug sensitivity after brain damage,
    339-367, 404-413, 470
Drugs, effect on recovery, 20, 204,
    217-218, 220, 226, 276, 287, 339-367
Dyskinesia, 151
Dyslexia, 175-199

E

Electrophysiological regeneration evidence,
    31-41, 53-59, 318
Emotionality changes, 226-229
Enactive representation, 195
Enucleation, 239
Environmental effects on recovery, 203,
    238, 473-475, 484
Environmental enrichment, 238
Epilepsy
    mirror focus of, 493
    recovery and, 486-487, 491-494
Equipotentiality, 16, 265-268, 278, 314
Exploratory behavior, 397-404
Extrapyramidal system, 287

F

Falck-Hillarp method, *see* Regeneration,
    histofluorescence evidence for
Fastigial nucleus, 295, 303
Feedback mechanisms, 304, 307-309, 314
Fink-Heimer stain, 69, 72, 82-91
Flower spray endings, 303
Flux discrimination, recovery of, 217-222
Frog visual system, 51-53, 98
Frontal cortex, 13, 149-169, 242, 280,
    345-354, 356, 360-361, 429-462,
    481-483, 486
    activity and, 348-354
    aphagia and, 356
    circling behavior and, 360-362
    dorsolateral, 150-151, 154, 157-169,
        345-346, 431-439
    orbital, 150-151, 159-169, 439-448

serial lesions of, 381-398, 411-421
Frontal lobotomy, 481-482, 486
Functional reorganization, 268, 278, 315,
    318-320, 395, 457, 459

G

Gliosis, 120, 394, 476, 483
Glucoreceptors, 411-412
Goldfish visual system, 34-38, 45, 48-49,
    51, 53-59, 97-98
Go-no go tasks, 162, 439-448

H

Hamsters
    adulthood lesions in, 66-67, 69, 73-75
    development of, 65-103
    heart, sinus node of, 468-470
    instrumental conditioning of, 67-68
    neonatal surgery in, 66-67, 69, 73-75,
        78-80, 83, 98
    pattern discrimination by, 66-71
    visual system of, 65-103
Hemiplegia, *see also* Contralateral
    paralysis, 4, 476-478, 480, 486, 495
Hemispherectomy, 152, 477
Hierarchical rerepresentation, 15-16,
    20-21, 175, 320-321
Hippocampal lesions, 129-144, 153,
    362-365, 380-391, 395-396, 478
Hippocampus
    behavioral plasticity of, 129-144,
        363-364, 381-391, 395-396
    connections in rat, 117-119
    dentate gyrus of, 130
    development of, 129-144, 153
    granule cells of, 130
    memory deficits and, 478
    neuroplasticity of, 99, 129-144
    serial lesions in, 380-391, 395-396
Humans
    language disorders in, 175-199
    recovery of function in, 468-470,
        472-504
Hypermetria, 294, 295
Hyperphagia, 343

Hypothalamic satiety, 343-345
Hypothalamus, *see also* separate nuclei,
  366, 448

I

Iconic representation, 195, 198
Individual differences, recovery and,
  501-504
Inferior colliculus, 79, 83
Inferotemporal cortex, 454-461
Inferotemporal lobe syndrome, 206-207
Inhibition, 15-16, 287-288, 292, 305-306,
  317, 320, 470-471, 482, 496
Insulin induced hypoglycemia, 404-413
Intelligence quotient of dyslexic children,
  178-181, 199

J

Joint receptors, 303

K

Korsakow's syndrome, 487-488

L

Language
  acquisition, 175-199
  disorders, *see also* Aphasia, dyslexia,
    175-199, 208-210
Latent learning in recovery, 375-376, 500
Lateral geniculate body, 69, 72, 86, 96,
  119-121, 308, 484
Lateral hypothalamus
  drug-induced recovery in, 355-360
  lesions in, 21, 206-207, 229, 343-345,
    355-360
  recovery in, 21, 206-207, 343-345,
    355-360, 404-413
  regeneration in, 21
Learning aids recovery, *see also* Latent
  learning, Pretraining, Retraining,
  490-491, 495
Lesion technique and recovery, 237-238
Lesions aid recovery, 225-230, 499-500
Limbic system lesions, *see* Separate
  structures

Localization of function, 1-29, 315
  cardiovascular theory of, 2-10
  encephalic theory of, 2-29
  motor control, 11, 14
  phrenological theory of, 11-14
  recovery and, 203, 373-375, 429-430,
    450, 502
  ventricular theory of, 2-9
Longitudinal study of recovery, 129-144,
  175-199

M

Mapping, *see* Cytoarchitectural maps,
  Electrophysiological regeneration
  evidence, Spatial maps
Mass action, 16, 278, 315
Maturational retardation, 176-199
Medial forebrain bundle, regeneration in,
  113-114, 117, 119
Medial geniculate body, 79-80
Mice
  drug studies in, 362-365
  frontal lesions in, 350-354
  serial lesions in, 245-246
Mind
  localized in brain, 2-29
  localized in cardiovascular system, 2-10
  localized in ventricles, 2-10
  theories of history, 1-29
Monkeys
  developmental studies of, 150-169
  recovery of function in, 150-169,
    206-207, 243, 271-321, 345-346,
    429-462, 471, 480, 485
Motivation aids recovery, 206, 208-211,
  276, 416
Motor cortex, 11, 14, 151-152, 156, 237,
  272-273, 279-280, 289-294, 300-303,
  312, 313, 315, 319, 449
Motor system, recovery in, 129-144,
  265-321

N

Neostigmine, 204
Nerve growth factor, 20, 115, 238
Neurospecificity, 203

Neurotransmitters, *see also* separate
   substances, 341, 346, 484
Norepinephrine, 118, 344, 352-353, 358,
   366

O

Object discrimination reversal, 162-163,
   168
Occipital cortex, *see also* Striate cortex,
   69-71, 96, 152, 217-226, 242
Occlusion, recovery and, 470, 483
Occlusive vascular disease, *see* Stroke
Olfactory bulb
   developmental studies of, 99
   regeneration in, 99, 121
Open field activity, 413-417
Optic nerve, 34-37, 45-47, 50, 53, 75-78,
   484
Optic tectum, *see* Tectum, optic
Orbital cortex, 150-151, 159-169,
   439-448

P

Paraplegia, 474
Paresis, 285
Parietal cortex, 28, 454-461
Parkinson's disease, 499-500
Passive avoidance deficits, 153, 350-354,
   363-365, 380-391, 397-404
   time course of, 363-365
Pattern discrimination, 66-71, 152,
   154-155, 219-220, 382-383
Perception, 3, 175, 195
Periarcuate area, 293, 454-461
Perceptual discrimination and reading, 195
Perseveration, 435-436
Phantom limb phenomenon, 482
Phrenic nerve, 469
Physostigmine, 346
Poliomyelitis, 472
Postcentral cortex, 19, 301
Posterior neocortex, 217-226
Premotor cortex, 279, 289-294, 311, 316
Pretraining aids recovery, 220-221,
   249-252, 277, 301, 313-314, 375
Principal sulcus, *see Sulcus principalis*

Prospective potency, 18-19, 22
Pyramidal lesions, 282, 310, 312, 319
Pyramidal system, 498, 499
Pyramidal tract, 274, 279-289, 316, 320
Pyramidectomy, 151, 157
Pyramidotomy, 271, 275, 277, 281, 283,
   285-292, 310, 315
Pyramids, decussation of, 10, 12

R

Radio-frequency lesions, 237-238, 378
Rats
   aphagia in, 355-360
   brain development in, 129-144
   circling behavior in, 360-362
   frontal lesions in, 346-350, 360-362
   hippocampal connections in, 117-119
   septal lesions in, 225-229
   serial lesions in, 217-222, 245-256,
      376-421
   visual system of, 71, 152, 217-222
Reading skills, measurement of, 175-199
Recovery of function, *see also* individual
      areas of the nervous system and
      mechanisms
   clinical, 1-2, 204, 207, 210, 468-470,
      472-504
   developmental studies of, 18-19, 21-22,
      65-101, 129-144, 149-169, 237,
      243-244, 270-271, 307-310, 312,
      373, 413-421, 430, 475-476,
      485-488
   failure to find, 248-250, 278, 307,
      417-419, 439-448, 461-462
   history of, 1-29
   mechanisms of, *see also* individual
      mechanisms, 20, 149, 162, 217-218,
      268-270, 339-367, 391-392,
      395-396, 449-461, 470, 480-481,
      494-497
   serial lesion studies of, 19, 217-219,
      245-256, 373-421, 431-462,
      489-490
   theories of, *see also* individual theories,
      15-22, 149-153, 162-166, 175-176,
      204-205, 219, 254-255, 265-268,
      284, 315-321, 391, 394-395, 449-491

time course of, 150-169, 243-245,
   248-249, 340-341, 360-365,
   391-398, 404, 419-420, 448,
   458-459, 468-504
variables influencing, *see also* individual
   variables, 206, 208-211, 219-221,
   225-230, 270-280, 312-314, 375,
   416-419, 485-504
Redundancy, 253, 268, 278, 394
Reflex movements, 279, 284, 287, 307,
   319, 474-475
Regeneration, *see also* Axonal growth,
   Collateral sprouting, Sprouting, 20-22,
   37, 46-59, 78, 89, 91, 94-95, 267,
   392-397, 483, 494
   Bodian stain for, 46
   chemical affinity and, 47-51, 96-97
   developmental studies of, 49-52, 54,
      65-101, 129, 270
   electrophysiological evidence of, 32,
      53-59, 318
   Fink-Heimer stain evidence of, 69, 72,
      82-91
   histofluorescent evidence of, 20,
      113-123, 394
   mechanical factors in, 20, 49, 89-91, 94,
      100, 152
   nerve growth factor and, 20, 115
   of peripheral nerve fibers, 111
   in visual system, 31-41, 45-59, 65-103
Reticulospinal system, 272
Retina, 32, 46, 50-59, 86
Retino-tectal system, *see also* Visual
   system, 31-41, 45-59
   action potentials in, 32
   holographic analysis of, 39-41
   locus specificities in, 32-41
   neuroplasticity in, 31-41, 45-59, 65-103
   postsynaptic recording in, 37
   scotoma and, 36, 51-59
   spatial mapping in, 31-41, 46-49, 75-80,
      82-91, 94-99
Retraining aids recovery, 17, 21-22, 176,
   204-206, 208, 210, 219
Retrograde amnesia, 487-488, 497
Reversal learning, 162-163, 168, 381-391,
   433-448

S

Scopolamine, 345, 352, 363-364
Scotoma, 36, 51-59
Sensory neglect, 226, 294
Sensory relay nuclei, 280, 313
Septal lesions, 117, 118, 153, 226-229
   developmental studies of, 153
   emotionality following, 226-229
   recovery following, 226-229, 362-365
   social behavior and, 226-229
Septum, 117-120, 448
   regeneration in, 117-120
Sequential lesions, *see also* Lesions aid
   recovery, 217-219, 225-230
Serial lesion recovery
   and infant recovery, 438-440, 447-448,
      457-458, 462
   and intact cortical structures, 449-461
Serial lesions, 245-250, 373-419, 429-461
   acquisition after, 245-250, 375-418
   of association cortex, 245
   in cats, 245, 253, 397
   developmental studies of, 413-421
   in dogs, 253
   of frontal cortex, 376, 381-391,
      411-419, 429-461
   in humans, 489-490
   interoperative interval of, 248-249,
      391-398, 412, 419-420, 448
   interoperative treatments, 217-219, 375
   of limbic system, 245, 380-391,
      395-396, 397-404
   in mice, 245
   in monkeys, 245, 429-461
   of occipital cortex, 217-219, 430
   of postcentral cortex, 19
   of precentral cortex, 19
   in rats, 217-222, 245-256, 376-421
   retention after, 250-252, 375, 431-461
   of reticular formation, 245
   in senescent animals, 411-421
   of sensory neocortex, 245
   of somatosensory cortex, 245-256
   of *Sulcus principalis*, 431-439
   survival rates following, 250
Serotonin, 346-358

SUBJECT INDEX

Sex differences
  language disorders and, 504
  recovery and, 417-419, 503-504
Short term memory, 208-211
Social behavior, 226-229
Somatosensory cortex, 237-256, 303
  primary projection zone, 240-241, 273
  second somatic projection area, 240-241
Spatial behavior deficits, 346, 381-392,
    411-415, 417-418, 429-461
Spatial maps, 31-41, 46-49, 75-80, 82-91,
    94-99
Species differences in recovery, 485-488
Spinal cord, 14, 269, 271-272, 279-289,
    308, 312, 470, 473-475
  Clarke's nucleus of, 307, 309, 317
  corticospinal tract of, 271
  lateral spinothalamic tract of, 474
  nucleus gracilis of, 470-471, 499
Spinal shock, 284, 473-475, 483
Spontaneous movement, 279
Sprouting, 81, 416, 469-473, 494, 496
  collateral, see Collateral sprouting
Stress, recovery and, 415, 419
Striate cortex, see also Occipital cortex,
    243, 478
  regeneration in, 69-71, 96
Striatum, see also separate nuclei, 366
Stroke, 1-2, 204-205, 207-210, 472-473,
    480, 489, 491
Substantia nigra lesions
  aphagia induced by, 358
  circling behavior induced by, 360-362
Substitution, 149-150, 175, 205, 219, 221,
    254, 268, 278, 292
Sulcus principalis, 150, 431-439, 449-461
Superior colliculus, see Tectum, optic
Strychnine, 471
Symbolic representation, 195
Syrian hamster, see Hamster

T

Tactile behavior, lesion effects on, 154,
    238-256, 272, 276, 277, 281, 290-292,
    311, 319, 396

Tectum, optic, 32, 34-41, 46-49, 52-59,
    65-103, 225-226
  connections of, 71-75, 81
  electrophysiological experiments on, 32,
    37-38, 58, 96
  lesions of, 68-69, 72-75, 78-80, 83,
    86-88, 95-96, 98, 101, 225-226
  mediates recovery, 449, 478
  recovery in, 68-69, 74, 96, 225-226
  synaptogenesis of, 81
Temporal lobe lesions, 497
Testosterone, see Castration
Thalamus, 71, 166-167, 169, 239,
    248-250, 275, 303, 470, 478, 499
  recovery in, 248-250
Triggered responses, 281, 288-289, 310,
    320
Turning response to visual stimuli, 68,
    73-79

U

Unlearned behaviors recover, 397-413

V

Ventricles, 2-10
Ventromedial hypothalamus, 153, 229,
    343-345
Vermis lesions, 295, 303
Vestibular cues, 461
Vestibular system, 303, 305
Vicarious function, 219-222, 255,
    265-268, 278, 287, 315, 316, 319,
    449-461
Visual cortex, see Striate cortex,
    Occipital cortex
Visual system, see also Retino-tectal
    system
  developmental studies of, 65-101, 203
  early experience and, 203
  of hamsters, 65-103
  neuroplasticity of, 65-103, 203, 217-226
  of rats, 71, 152, 217-222
Visual tasks, see also Pattern
    discrimination, 68, 73-79, 206-207,
    217-226, 381-391, 440-448

515

W

Water consumption, 406-413
Weight regulation, 404-413
Wernicke's area, 479

X

X-radiation, behavioral development and, 129-144

A 4
B 5
C 6
D 7
E 8
F 9
G 0
H 1
I 2
J 3